PROGRESS IN LIVER TRANSPLANTATION

DEVELOPMENTS IN GASTROENTEROLOGY

Pena, A.S., Weterman, I.T., Booth, C.C., Strober W., eds: Recent advances in Crohn's disease
ISBN 90 247 2475 9

Motta, P.M., Didio, L.J.A., eds: Basic and clinical hepatology
ISBN 90 247 2404 X

Rachmilewitz, D., ed.: Inflammatory bowel diseases
ISBN 90 247 2612 3

Fleischer, D., Jensen, D., Bright-Asare, P. eds: Therapeutic laser endoscopy in gastrointestinal disease
ISBN 0 89838 577 6

Borriello, S.P., ed: Antibiotic associated diarrhoea and colitis
ISBN 0 89838 623 3

Gips, Ch.H., Krom, R.A.F., eds: Progress in liver transplantation
ISBN 0 89838 726 4

PROGRESS IN LIVER TRANSPLANTATION

edited by

CHRIS H. GIPS
Division of Hepatology
University Hospital Groningen
Groningen
The Netherlands

RUUD A.F. KROM
Liver Transplantation Unit
Mayo Clinic
Rochester, Minnesota 55905
U.S.A.

1985 SPRINGER-SCIENCE+BUSINESS MEDIA, B.V.

Library of Congress Cataloging in Publication Data

Main entry under title:

Progress in liver transplantation.

   (Developments in gastroenterology)
   Includes index.
   1. Liver--Transplatnation. I. Gips, Christiaan
Hendrik. II. Krom, Ruud A. F. III. Series.
[DNLM: 1. Liver--transplantation.
W1 DE997VYB / W1 770 P964]
RD546.P72 1985   617'.556   85-5101

ISBN 978-94-010-8722-3   ISBN 978-94-009-5018-4 (eBook)
DOI 10.1007/978-94-009-5018-4

Copyright

Table of contents

Preface

This book – the first multicenter book on orthotopic liver transplantation – reflects the progress in this field. The first 'experience in hepatic transplantation' was documented in 1969 by Starzl and his group in Denver in the classic of the same name. It was followed in 1983 by 'Liver transplantation', edited by Calne, in which the experience of the Cambridge-King's College Hospital team was laid down. Apart from these the book of Lie and Gütgemann appeared in 1974. These books are fundamental for all who want to become involved with experimental and clinical liver transplantation.

Developments in liver transplantation are fast (faster than the production of this book) and new knowledge now not only is coming from the pioneer centers but also from their off-spring, scattered over the world. In only a few years there has been an enormous increase in the number of liver transplantations and certainly there have been performed at least as many transplants since 1980 as between 1963 – the start of clinical liver transplantation – and 1980. Even if our understanding is better, many problems are the same as twenty years ago and for some there may be a long way to go before they are solved.

Experimental liver transplantation constitutes a basis for the clinical work and attention is given to several aspects. Alterations in Disse's space and their relation to rejection seem important as is the role of the veiled cells which may be related to Kupffer cells. Blood transfusions prior to grafting may find its rationale in the experiments in rhesus monkey, where they seem to mitigate the hepatocellular type of rejection. Rejection has its own characteristics in electron microscopy and in fine needle aspiration cytology. Orthotopic transplantation of liver segments is of relevance in paediatric liver grafting.

During transplantation, metabolic and circulatory responses and their handling are of paramount importance, as is coagulation. Blood bank logistics are crucial in any liver transplant program.

Bacterial, fungal and viral infections exert their influence on the immune status of the recipient of the liver graft and thereby interact with the immunosuppressive regimen. Progress has been made in the prevention of infections, both bacterial and viral. Because of the clinical impact of cytomegalovirus (CMV) infections and of their immunological interactions, these are dealt with in more detail. CMV-negative recipients presumably are best helped by receiving liver and blood products from CMV-negative donors. Genetically determined donor-recipient interactions also exert their influence on the recipient and the role of the Kupffer cells in the handling of viral infections merits special attention. The immunosuppressive regimen has seen a change in most but not all centers from azathioprine-steroids to cyclosporine-low dose steroids. It can still be argued whether the improved survival seen in the last few years has been due to the new immunosuppressive regimen, but certainly the spectrum of side-effects has changed. In the monitoring of the recipient the liver biopsy has proven to be of importance and monoclonal antibodies have found their way to the immuno-histopathologist. Fine needle aspiration cytology, less invasive, is promising. Relative measurements of hepatic arterial and portal flow using radionuclides help in differentiating rejection from other conditions.

Liver transplantations have been performed for many types of disease and in all stages of liver disease. Some diseases have proved not to be suitable for liver transplantation and sometimes not so much the disease itself but the stage of disease proved to be a contra-indication. For this book, the adult series of Cambridge-King's College Hospital, the tumor patients of Hannover and the paediatric patients of Pittsburgh-Denver have been analyzed in separate chapters and multi-center surveys are found in the overview and in the four-center analysis. Prediction in the individual patient of excessive blood loss during transplantation proved difficult with the Child-Turcotte classification. Reliable parameters are those of impaired renal sodium and water handling. In paediatric liver transplantation it may be difficult to obtain a suitable sized donor liver and a reduced sized adult orthotopic liver graft can solve the problem.

The organisation of liver transplantations is complex because several disciplines are involved. Complex too, in part for the same reason, is multiple organ procurement. Compilation of the liver transplantations done in Europe shows a change from few to many, often smaller, centers, indicates the need for donor organs and also that a registry is timely.

The progress in liver transplantation is reflected in the improved survival of the last few years. From the four-center analysis can be learned that patients still living after 1 year spent a very small proportion of their time in hospital and that more than 80% has resumed their former activities. Liver transplantation has advanced to a treatment modality but many efforts, multicenter and multidisciplinary, have to be made before it can be regarded as a moderate-risk procedure. One of these efforts is this book.

Groningen – Rochester, Minnesota

C.H. Gips
R.A.F. Krom

Acknowledgements

We wish to thank Mrs. Martha Messchendorp and Mrs. Joke G. van Bree-Riksman for excellent secretarial assistance and Mr. Boudewijn F. Commandeur, Martinus Nijhoff, for his compliance.

Note to the reader

In this book 'cyclosporine' denotes cyclosporine A (Sandimmune[R], Sandimmun[R]) also written Cy-A or CyA. Ciclosporin, the word proposed by the WHO has not been used as it had not gained the 'recommended' state when the proofs were read.

List of contributors

L. Achterhof, Donor Centre, Red Cross Blood Bank Groningen-Drenthe, Oostersingel 59, 9713 EZ Groningen, The Netherlands

J. Ahonen, Fourth Department of Surgery, Helsinki University Central Hospital, Helsinki, Finland

H. Balner, TNO Primate Centre, Rijswijk, The Netherlands

J.M. Beelen, Bloodgrouping Laboratory, Groningen University Hospital, Oostersingel 59, 9713 EZ Groningen, The Netherlands

H. Bismuth, Unité de Chirurgie Hépato-Biliaire, Inserm U17, Hôpital Paul Brousse, Villejuif, France

J.C.C. Borleffs, Department of Internal Medicine, Utrecht University Hospital, Catharijnesingel 101, 3511 GV Utrecht, The Netherlands; formerly: TNO Primate Centre, Rijswijk, The Netherlands

C.E. Brölsch, Department of Surgery, University of Chicago, 5841 South Maryland Avenue, Chicago, IL 60637, USA; formerly: Klinik für Abdominal- und Transplantationschirurgie, Medizinische Hochschule Hannover, Postfach 610180, D-3000 Hannover 61, FRG

C.M.A. Bijleveld, Department of Pediatrics, Groningen University Hospital, Oostersingel 59, 9713 EZ Groningen, The Netherlands

R.Y. Calne, Department of Surgery, University of Cambridge Clinical School, Addenbrooke's Hospital, Hills Road, Cambridge CB2 2QQ, UK

F.J. Carmichael, Department of Anaesthesia, Addenbrooke's Hospital, Cambridge CB2 2QQ, UK

H. Creutzig, Department of Radiology, Medizinische Hochschule, D-3000 Hannover 61, FRG

P.C. Das, Red Cross Blood Bank Groningen Drenthe, Oostersingel 59, 9713 EZ Groningen, The Netherlands

H.F. Eggink, Laboratorium voor de Volksgezondheid in Friesland, Jelsumerstraat 6, 8917 EN Leeuwarden, The Netherlands

B. Eklund, Fourth Department of Surgery, Helsinki University Central Hospital, Helsinki, Finland

J.V. Farman, Department of Anaesthesia, Addenbrooke's Hospital, Cambridge CB2 2QQ, UK

J.C. Gartner, University Health Center of Pittsburgh, University of Pittsburgh, Pittsburgh, PA, USA

C.H. Gips, Division of Hepatology, Groningen University Hospital, Oostersingel 59, 9713 EZ Groningen, The Netherlands

H. van Goor, Department of Surgery, Groningen University Hospital, Oostersingel 59, 9713 EZ Groningen, The Netherlands

E.B. Haagsma, Division of Hepatology, Groningen University Hospital, Oostersingel 59, 9713 EZ Groningen, The Netherlands

M.R. Harrison, Peterborough District Hospital, Peterborough, UK

P. Häyry, Transplantation Laboratory, University of Helsinki, Helsinki, Finland

K. Höckerstedt, Fourth Department of Surgery, Helsinki University Central Hospital, Helsinki, Finland

H.F.W. Hoitsma, Department of Surgery, Free University Hospital, De Boelelaan 1117, 1007 MB Amsterdam, The Netherlands

D. Houssin, Unité de Chirurgie Hépato-Biliaire, Inserm U17, Hôpital Paul Brousse, Villejuif, France

H.J. Houthoff, Department of Pathology, University of Amsterdam. Formerly: University Hospital and University of Groningen, Oostersingel 63, 9713 EZ Groningen, The Netherlands

G.W. van Imhoff, Division of Hematology, Groningen University Hospital, Oostersingel 59, 9713 EZ Groningen, The Netherlands

S. Iwatsuki, Department of Surgery, University Health Center of Pittsburgh, University of Pittsburgh, Pittsburgh, PA, USA

G.M.Th. de Jong, Division of Hepatology, Groningen University Hospital, Oostersingel 59, 9713 EZ Groningen, The Netherlands

A. Kauste, Fourth Department of Surgery, Helsinki University Central Hospital, Helsinki, Finland

C. Korsbäck, Fourth Department of Surgery, Helsinki University Central Hospital, Helsinki, Finland

R.A.F. Krom, Liver Transplantation Surgery, Mayo Clinic, Rochester, MN 55905, USA; formerly: Department of Surgery, Groningen University Hospital, Oostersingel 59, 9713 EZ Groningen, The Netherlands

W. Lauchart, Klinik für Abdominal- und Transplantationschirurgie, Medizinische Hochschule Hannover, Karl-Wiechert-Allee 9, D-3000 Hannover, FRG

I. Lautenschlager, Transplantation Laboratory, University of Helsinki, Helsinki, Finland

M.J. Lindop, Department of Anaesthesia, Addenbrooke's Hospital, Cambridge CB2 2QQ, UK

J.J. Malatack, University of Pittsburgh, University Health Center of Pittsburgh, Pittsburgh, PA, USA

J.M. Middeldorp, Department of Clinical Immunology, Groningen University Hospital, Oostersingel 59, 9713 EZ Groningen, The Netherlands

J. Neuberger, Liver Unit, King's College Hospital and School of Medicine and Dentistry, Denmark Hill, London SE5, UK

P. Neuhaus, Klinik für Abdominal- und Transplantationschirurgie, Medizinische Hochschule Hannover,Postfach 610180, D-3000 Hannover 61, FRG

R. Neuhaus, Klinik für Abdominal- und Transplantationschirurgie, Medizinische Hochschule Hannover, Karl-Wiechert-Allee 9, D-3000 Hannover, FRG

R. Orko, Fourth Department of Surgery, Helsinki University Central Hospital, Helsinki, Finland

R. Pichlmayr, Klinik für Abdominal- und Transplantationschirurgie, Medizinische Hochschule Hannover, Postfach 610180, D-3000 Hannover 61, FRG

B. Portmann, Liver Unit, King's College Hospital and School of Medicine and Dentistry, Denmark Hill, London SE5, UK

B. Ringe, Klinik für Abdominal- und Transplantationschirurgie, Medizinische Hochschule Hannover, Postfach 610180, D-3000 Hannover 61, FRG

H.W. Roenhorst, Delfzicht Hospital, Jachtlaan 50, 9934 JD Delfzijl, The Netherlands; formerly: Department of Clinical Immunology, Groningen University Hospital, Oostersingel 59, 9713 EZ Groningen, The Netherlands

K. Salmela, Fourth Department of Surgery, Helsinki University Central Hospital, Helsinki, Finland

B.F. Scharschmidt, Department of Medicine and Liver Center, University of California, San Fransisco, CA 94143, USA

B. Scheinin, Fourth Department of Surgery, Helsinki University, Central Hospital, Helsinki, Finland

T.M. Scheinin, Fourth Department of Surgery, Helsinki University Central Hospital, Helsinki, Finland

G.P. Schröter, Department of Pediatrics and Surgery, University of Colorado Health Sciences Center, 4200 East Ninth Avenue, Denver, CO 80262, USA

B.W. Shaw Jr., University Health Center of Pittsburgh, University of Pittsburgh, Pittsburgh, PA, USA

M.J.H. Slooff, Department of Surgery, Groningen University Hospital, Oostersingel 59, 9713 EZ Groningen, The Netherlands

C.Th. Smit Sibinga, Red Cross Blood Bank Groningen-Drenthe, Oostersingel 59, 9713 EZ Groningen, The Netherlands

T.E. Starzl, Department of Surgery, University Health Center of Pittsburgh, University of Pittsburgh, Pittsburgh, PA, USA

J. Swieringa, Red Cross Blood Bank Groningen-Drenthe, Oostersingel 59, 9713 EZ Groningen, The Netherlands

E. Taskinen, Transplantation Laboratory, University of Helsinki, Helsinki, Finland

T.H. The, Department of Clinical Immunology, Groningen University Hospital, Oostersingel 59, 9713 EZ Groningen, The Netherlands

F.-J. Vonnahme, Universität des Saarlandes, Pathologisches Institut, D-6650 Hamburg, FRG

D. van der Waaij, Laboratory for Medical Microbiology, Groningen University Hospital, Oostersingel 59, 9713 EZ Groningen, The Netherlands

J. Waltje, Red Cross Blood Bank Groningen-Drenthe, Oostersingel 59, 9713 EZ Groningen, The Netherlands

H. Wesenhagen, Department of Anaesthesiology, Groningen University Hospital, Oostersingel 59, 9713 EZ Groningen, The Netherlands

E. von Willebrand, Transplantation Laboratory, Helsinki University Central Hospital, University of Helsinki, Helsinki, Finland

R. Williams, Liver Unit, King's College Hospital and School of Medicine and Dentistry, Denmark Hill, London SE5, UK

K. Wonigeit, Transplantation and Immunology Laboratory, Klinik für Abdominal- und Transplantationschirurgie, Medizinische Hochschule Hannover, Karl-Wiechert-Allee 9, D-3000 Hannover, FRG

B.E. Zitelli, University Health Center of Pittsburgh, University of Pittsburgh, Pittsburgh, PA, USA

Section 1

LIVER TRANSPLANTATION: AN OVERVIEW

1. Liver transplantation (1963–1983): A review of results of the centers Pittsburgh, Cambridge, Hannover, Groningen, Innsbruck and Paris

R.A.F. KROM

History of liver transplantation

Transplantation research started in 1950, mainly focussed on renal transplantation and immunobiology. In 1953 research in liver transplantation was begun by Starzl and became a clinical reality in 1963 [1] when three patients with biliary atresia received transplants. However, the results of liver transplantation remained poor until the early 1970s, when long-term survival became more frequent. In 1968 Calne started his program at Cambridge in close cooperation with Williams in London. The main topics of research in those days were immunosuppressive agents and regimes, the biliary anastomosis and biliary sludge, and hepatotrophic factors.

In 1975 Pichlmayr in Hannover and in 1978 Bismuth in Paris and Margreiter in Innsbruck started their liver transplantation program, followed by Krom and Gips in Groningen in 1979, Wolf in East Berlin in 1980 and Häyry in Helsinki in 1982. At the moment a number of new centers are developing in the USA and Europe.

This interest in clinical liver transplantation was renewed as a result of Starzl's move from Denver to Pittsburgh and the successful expansion of his program to more than 100 liver transplantations in 1983.

Overall results until 1983 (Table 1)

From 1963 to 1983 555 liver transplantations have been performed (Table 1). Of these transplants, a total of 155 patients were alive in 1983; 81 patients survived more than one year; 23 more than 5 years and 5 even beyond 10 years (Table 2). The actuarial one-year survival was 35%. The results of more recent years are further improving to 60 and 70% [1].

Primary diagnosis (Table 3)

The three most common diagnoses, for which liver transplantation has been performed, are tumor, cirrhosis and biliary atresia. Other frequent diagnoses are antitrypsin deficiency and Budd-Chiari syndrome.

Table 1. Overall results (1963–1983) of the six participating centres (results of questionnaire).

Results until 1983	Start of program	Number of liver transplantations	Alive
Denver	1963	184	
Pittsburgh	1980	109	293	89
Cambridge/KCH	1968	138	24
Hannover	1975	78	20
Paris	1978	11	1
Innsbruck	1978	9	4
Groningen	1979	26	16
1963–1983		555	155

Table 2. Survival data (1963–1983) of the six participating centers (results of questionnaire).

Alive 1983	Total	1 year	5 years	10 years
Pittsburgh/Denver	89	45	18	5
Cambridge/KCH	24	16	4	–
Hannover	20	10	1	–
Paris	1	1	–	–
Innsbruck	4	2	–	–
Groningen	16	7	–	–
Total	155	81	23	5

Table 3. Total number liver transplantations that have been performed for the three most frequent indications (1963–1983) (results of questionnaire).

	Primary liver tumor	Cirrhosis	Biliary atresia
Pittsburgh[a]	27	125	62
Cambridge/KCH	49	61	2
Hannover	38	20	8
Innsbruck	6	3	–
Groningen	1	20	–
Total until 1983	121	229	72

[a] Until May 1982.

Liver tumor

Until 1983, 121 patients with a primary liver tumor have been treated with liver transplantation. Only 4 of all patients who had been transplanted in Denver/ Pittsburgh before 1982 for liver tumor survived one year. The majority of the 11 patients that survived the operative procedure died with tumor recurrence [4].

Also in Cambridge only 10 out of 25 patients survived one year, but 6 of these patients died later with tumor recurrence [3]. In Hannover ± 50% of the patients has been transplanted for primary liver tumor. The results are disappointing as ± 80% of the patients died due to recurrent disease within the first and second year after liver transplantation. However, all centers have individual long-term survivors, emphasizing the need for meticulous preoperative screening for extra-hepatic metastases, and perhaps on the histological type of the liver tumor.

Cirrhosis

A total of 229 patients had been transplanted for end-stage liver cirrhosis prior to 1983, and the majority suffered from chronic active cirrhosis (CAC). Out of 61 patients with a variety of other cirrhotic liver diseases, 19 were known to have alcoholic liver cirrhosis. Before 1980 the results were moderate, with one-year survival at ± 30%. Since then, however, the results have improved to reported one-year survival rates of 60–70%.

Principally patients with end-stage liver cirrhosis are ideal candidates for liver transplantation, because they lack the risk of rapid recurrence of primary disease as in patients with liver tumor. However, the often poor physical condition makes liver transplantation a risky surgical procedure with substantial operative mortality. An important problem is the coagulation abnormalities, intrinsic to the deterioration of liver function, with subsequent massive peroperative bloodloss. Many of these patients died postoperatively due to multi-organ failure.

Obviously, there are two ways to approach these problems. Firstly it may be necessary to exclude patients whose liver function has deteriorated too far. Groningen evaluated the preoperative data of the patients in relation to blood-loss. This relation was significantly positive regarding parameters belonging to the hepatorenal syndrome and to synthetic liver function, as coagulation factors and anti-thrombin III and albumen [5] (Chapter 21).

According to these data it is possible to detect these poor-risk patients and to improve patient selection. Secondly one can search for better surgical techniques and ways to normalize the peroperative coagulation status or to reduce the peroperative bloodloss. Pittsburgh recently introduced the porto-caval axillary venous bypass [4] in order to decrease the portal hypertension and to restore the systemic circulation during the anhepatic period. Bloodloss and hemodynamics improved markedly by this procedure.

Previously Cambridge used an arteriovenous bypass to diminish the venous trapping of the blood and to improve the arterial blood pressure. Although success has been reported this procedure has not been routinely used. Most centers started to use an autotransfusion system. Coagulation prevention by both heparin and citrate was used.

Biliary atresia

Only Denver/Pittsburgh has major experience with pediatric liver transplantation. More than 50% of the children suffered from biliary atresia, but also patients with congenital metabolic diseases, such as α-1-antitrypsin deficiency, Wilson's disease and glycogen storage disease, received transplants. The results of pediatric liver transplantation from 1963 through 1979 were somewhat better than for adults but have improved markedly since then [2]. Very likely cyclosporine-A contributed to this improvement of the one-year survival from 38% to 70%, although within the new organisation at Pittsburgh cooperation with the pediatricians has also played an important role. At the other centers children have received transplants only occasionally. Lack of suitable donors and feelings about the moral justification of liver transplantation in children have limited the total number. It can be expected that with the increased life expectancy and the diminished need for the use of prednisone with cyclosporine-A the pediatricians will consider liver transplantation more frequently in the future.

Immunosuppression

Until the introduction of Cyclosporine-A in 1978 immunosuppression had been achieved by various regimes of corticosteroids and azathioprine optionally in combination with antilymphocyte globulin or thoracic duct drainage. During that era complications in liver transplantation consisted mainly of biliary complications (25%), sepsis (± 20%) and rejection (± 10%). Especially the bacterial sepsis, sometimes related to biliary problems, was believed to hamper the prognosis of liver transplantation. Corticosteroids enhance the incidence and seriousness of bacterial infections.

Gram-negative sepsis carries a high mortality. With the use of Cyclosporine-A these complications seem to have become less frequent. The effect on the incidence of viral infections however remains questionable. The beneficial effect of bacterial infections is counterbalanced by the adverse effect on renal function, and the uncertainty of metabolic and toxic properties. This is characterized by the uncertainty about the way of administration, oral or intravenous, and relationship between plasma levels and toxicity. The incidence of rejection seems to increase, as apparently the number of retransplantations for rejections in Pittsburgh has increased to ± 20%. An easy availability of donors contributed to a policy of early retransplantation. Therefore the figure of 20% retransplantation cannot be compared to the generally accepted 10% incidence of rejection leading to graft loss. The overall survival in Pittsburgh has substantially increased to 60–70% since the introduction of Cyclosporine-A. However, Groningen has achieved 60% one- and two-year survival while using the old-fashioned regimen with corticosteroids and azathioprine. Improved results of liver transplantations are therefore multifactiorial and are not only caused by a change in immunosuppressive regimes.

Matching, typing and rejection

For prospective crossmatching and HLA-typing, the necessary time is usually not available. In order to keep the preservation time as short as possible and certainly not exceeding the maximum storage duration of 8–10 h.

As it is considered to be important not to violate the ABO blood type barrier, suitable liver donors are selected on blood type only. This is based on the experiences in other organ and tissue transplantation, where hyperacute rejection will occur when the ABO-barrier is violated. However, in liver transplantation at least 11 cases are known in which the ABO-match was incompatible. In only one case fatal rejection could be diagnosed (Table 4), and long-term survivals have been observed.

A cytotoxic crossmatch can only seldomly be performed prospectively, but will often be done retrospectively. Twenty-two patients are known to have undergone transplantations despite a positive retrospective crossmatch. Acute rejections have been reported in only 2 patients and the long-term survivors are also noted. The occurrence of fatal acute rejection in these cases does not differ from the 10% fatal rejection in liver transplantation in general as reported in the literature. The conclusion may be that the liver is acting differently and is immunologically more favourable than other organs. However, only hypotheses exist to explain this phenomenon.

It will not be surprising that HLA- and DR-matching have also no noticeable influence on patient survival. In 90% of the transplantations in Groningen, the

*Table 4.*Incompatibilities: Number of incompatibilities between donor and recipient in ABO blood group system, and retrospective positive crossmatches.

	No. of patients	Acute rejection	Survival
Blood group	11	1	1–500 days
Crossmatch	22	2	2 years

donor was compatible with only 2 antigens or less. No difference existed between the group of living and deceased patients.

The immunobiology of the liver has to be an important area of research in the coming years.

Size of the donor liver

In selecting the donor the equality of size to the recipient is important. A donor liver that grossly exceeds that of the recipient's will create serious spatial and hemodynamic problems during closure of the abdomen. Also, a donor liver that is too small provides technical difficulties, due to the discrepancies in the size of the vessels and bileducts, that can create hemodynamic complications.

European centers have reported eight patients in whom incompatibility of size had created a fatal course. It is generally accepted that the difference in size or weight of the donor and the recipient should not exceed 25%.

Biliary drainage

Biliary drainage has been considered as the Achilles heel of liver transplantation, as illustrated by the changing preference for various biliary anastomoses. Septic cholangitis or biliary leakage were the most frequent and often lethal complications. Presently three types of biliary anastomoses are commonly used: choledocho-choledochostomy, choledocho-jejunostomy with Roux-Y loop and gallbladder conduit as described by Calne. The complication rate is ± 20% while mortality related to the biliary anastomosis is ± 10%. As the arterial blood supply of the donor bileducts is totally dependent on the patency of the arterial anastomosis, the surgical technique has to be meticulous. If arterial thrombosis occurs the extrahepatic bileduct will become necrotic with subsequent disruption of the biliary anastomosis and development of liver abcesses. The mortality related to this complication is ± 100%.

Long-term surviving patients

At the beginning of 1983, 155 patients were reported to be alive; of them, 109 have survived for more than one year and 28 longer than 5 years. Five patients have already lived more than 10 years beyond their liver transplantations. Most of the long-term survivors are rehabilitated and participate in daily life by having a full-time job or taking care of home and family.

A number of problems remains: The delayed growth of transplanted children, especially of those treated with corticosteroids, can lead to emotional problems, while osteoporosis in the elderly PBC patients may lead to a significant shortening of statue. The use of Cyclosporine-A might improve these complications while introducing others like chronic nephrotoxicity. The effect of long-term immunosuppression on tumor development de novo is not really known, although the incidence has been increasing. Presently, the life expectancy with a transplanted liver is totally unknown, but the increasing number of long-term survivors and the good quality of life makes liver transplantation worthwhile.

Future of liver transplantation

The improved results of liver transplantation have created hope for many otherwise doomed liver-diseased patients. In many medical centers around the world renewed interest has arisen and new liver transplantation programs are being considered. In order to determine the present status of liver transplantation in relation to clinical application and research the National Institutes of Health organised a consensus development conference in June of 1983 [6]. The members of the panel came to the following conclusion (Chapter 27):

> After extensive review and consideration of all available data, this panel concludes that liver transplantation is a therapeutic modality for end-stage liver disease that deserves broader application. However, in order for liver transplantation to gain its full therapeutic potential, the indications for and results of the procedure must be the object of comprehensive, coordinated, and ongoing evaluation in the years ahead. This can best be achieved by expansion of this technology to a limited number of centers where performance of liver transplantation can be carried out under optimal conditions.

This conclusion might be the best guide for the next generation of liver transplantation.

Acknowledgements

The author thanks the participating centers for their cooperation in collecting the necessary data by completing the various questionnaires.

References

1. Starzl TE, Machioro TL, Von Kaulla KN: Homotransplantation of the liver in humans. Surg Gynaecol Obstet 117: 659–696, 1963.
2. Starzl TE, Iwatsuki S, Thiel DH van, Gartner JC, Zitelli BJ, Malatack JJ, Schade RR, Shaw BW Jr, Hakala TR, Rosenthal JT, Porter KA: Evolution in liver transplantation. Hepatology 2 (5): 614–636, 1982.
3. Calne RY: Liver transplantation for liver cancer. World J Surg 6: 76–80, 1982.

4. Iwatsuki S, Klintmalm GBG, Starzl TE: Total hepatectomy and liver replacement (Orthotopic liver transplantation) for primary hepatic malignancy. World J Surg 6: 81–85, 1982.
5. Krom RAF, Gips CH, Houthoff HJ, Newton D, Waay D van der, Beelen JM, Haagsma EB, Slooff MJH: Orthotopic liver transplantation in Groningen (The Netherlands, 1979–1983). Hepatology 4: 61S–65S, 1984.
6. National Institutes of Health: Summary of the Consensus Development Conference in Liver Transplantation (June, 1983). Volume 4, no. 7.

Section 2

EXPERIMENTAL LIVER TRANSPLANTATION

2. Experimental liver transplantation

P. NEUHAUS, C.E. BRÖLSCH, B. RINGE and R. PICHLMAYR

Experimental liver transplantation

The first transplantation of the whole canine liver was described by Welch in 1955 [1]. Eight years later T.E. Starzl performed his first human liver transplantation and for a long time he alone carried the burden of frequent clinical failure and overall disheartening results in this field [2].

Many other centers had an experimental transplant program but never really started a clinical program. Problems studied were organ preservation, the immunological reaction against the transplanted organ and the prevention and treatment of rejection. Technical problems, high costs and the difficult interpretation of sometimes very disappointing results dampened enthusiasm so that up till now clinical liver transplantation has been established at only a very few centers.

Failures in liver transplantation almost always result in the patient dying from liver insufficiency, multiorgan failure and sepsis. The underlying cause may be the recipient's preoperative condition, problems with the donor and organ preservation, technical problems, problems of patient management, during and after surgery problems with rejection and the side effects of immunosuppression and rejection therapy. Experimental findings have in most instances deepened understanding of these complex processes but in some cases have also influenced clinical transplantation in a negative fashion, especially with regard to the importance and severity of rejection phenomena.

For a long time the transplanted liver was regarded as an immunologically-privileged organ since it was known from experimental data in pigs that liver transplantation in Swine Leucocyte Antigen (SLA) incompatible donor recipient combinations was possible without immunosuppression. Moreover Calne, Bockhorn and Flye demonstrated a specific, protective effect of the transplanted liver on subsequent kidney and skin allografts [3–5].

The general validity of this immunological privilege should at least have been questioned since Starzl had already shown in 1969 that lethal rejection is the regular outcome after allogeneic orthotopic liver transplantation in dogs not receiving immunosuppression [6]. With some exceptions Calne, Myburgh and recently our own group found that monkeys also underwent severe rejection and death without immunological modification or immunosuppression [7–9]. Interestingly Flye reported in 1983 that the incidence of rejection in SLA identical inbred miniature pigs was similar to that of outbred domestic pigs with a mean survival time of more than 150 days. In contrast recipients of SLA mismatched grafts died rapidly from fulminant hepatic rejection with a mean survival time of only 14.6 ± 3.6 days [5].

One way of obtaining more information on immunological questions determining the fate of transplanted organs seemed to be the use of genetically well-defined, identical animals in large experimental groups. At the moment this is only possible with inbred and congenic rats. In an outstanding study Zimmermann examined the survival of orthotopic liver allografts in 22 different rat strain combinations. He found extreme differences in survival times ranging from prompt rejection in six, delayed rejection in five, to prolonged and indefinite survival in seven combinations [10]. Moreover Engemann was able to show that the surgical technique used in liver transplantation in rats not only influenced early postoperative failure or success but also immunological behaviour. In a fully Major Histocompatibility Complex (MHC) different strain combination he found long-term acceptance of liver grafts without any immunosuppression. This could only be observed however if the hepatic artery had been anastomosed. In such cases 65% of recipients survived indefinitely whereas all recipients in the non-arterialised group died by day 22 [11].

It has been claimed that acute rejection in clinical liver transplantation occurs less often and is not as severe as in kidney transplantation. It is also clear that technical problems such as the loss of arterial blood supply inevitably result in graft failure. The human situation differs considerably from that of other animals but is most closely approximated in subhuman primates as wide experience with kidney transplantation in rhesus monkeys has shown [12]. Therefore clinically relevant immunological questions can only be answered with confidence in this animal model whereas basic investigations on immunological mechanisms can be carried out in the rat model.

Questions to be answered by these experimental studies are what is the reason for the apparently different, lower immunological reactivity after liver transplantation compared with transplantation of other organs? Is there perhaps no real immunological difference but only a difference in the functional damage after rejection?

As possible explanations for the so-called lower immunological reactivity after liver transplantation, several experimental observations have been put forward. In 1976 Davies found differences in the expression of MHC antigens on liver and kidney cells [13]. In our group, Wonigeit used in vitro techniques such as Mixed Lymphocyte Culture (MLC) and Cell Mediated Lympholysis (CML) to demonstrate a donor specific loss of cytotoxic T-lymphocytes (CTL) production in several of our human liver recipients after transplantation [14].

Whereas both MLC and CML are positive before transplantation, the CML response against donor cells is lost after transplantation. This could be demonstrated in our longest survivor who was transplanted in 1975. A recent reexamination of these findings in the same patient has revealed that this phenomenon is stable over a period of 7 years. The same phenomenon has also been demonstrated in rats by Kamado, Davies and Roser who have presented clear evidence that clonal deletion is the underlying mechanism [15].

Paralysis of the immune system through antigen overload may also be a factor and the loss and replacement of Kuppfer cells, thought to be closely related to the dendritic cells in the kidney, by recipient type cells after liver transplantation has been brought into the discussion. This replacement of Kuppfer cells by recipient type cells has recently been observed clinically in a 7-year-old child with sea blue histiocyte syndrome where the obviously extrahepatic storage disease recurred in the Kuppfer cells of the transplanted liver [16].

Not to be underestimated are extra-immunological factors related to the surgical procedure. Liver graft recipients are highly compromised hosts before, during and after transplantation. They are not only subjected to maximal stress and periods of prolonged shock during cross-clamping of vessels and the anhepatic phase, but blood flow to the most important immunological organs, namely the spleen and the entire intestine with its lymphatic organs, is considerably disturbed. Although these factors have not yet been investigated clinically or experimentally, blood loss and its replacement have certainly been documented by Myburgh and others as being of importance for the immunological answer [17]. In 1974 Myburgh showed a significant difference in the survival times of liver transplanted baboons which had either been transfused with donor blood during surgery or were given only human or baboon plasma for volume replacement. Both groups were treated postoperatively with polyspecific baboon alloantiserum and donor bone marrow cells. The mean survival time for the group receiving donor blood was 51 days, for the other groups 13 and 17 days respectively.

An attempt has also been made to explain the difference in immunological reactivity with a lower susceptibility of the liver to effector mechanisms. The large liver cell mass with its ample functional reserve and extraordinary regenerative capacity was suggested as the reason why severe rejection, in kidney transplantation leading to complete loss of organ function, can be overcome by the liver graft recipient. We think this phenomenon occurred in our liver grafted rhesus monkeys where all animals underwent severe rejection one week after transplantation. Some animals died immediately while others survived this first episode, showed partial liver regeneration and then died from a subsequent rejection episode or chronic liver failure due to chronic or repeated rejection episodes 4 weeks to 4 months later [9].

Interestingly the question also rises here of the blood supply and normal physiological conditions for the transplanted liver, the importance of which has been elegantly shown by Engemann [11]. The sinusoidal circulation within the space of Disse between liver cells and endothelial lining of the blood vessels has been subjected to investigation. Observations by Vonnahme from our own group reveal changes in this area after transplantation in man and monkeys that may very well be of importance for the expression and development of clinical rejection.

Understanding of the immunological factors influencing liver transplantation is poor and other influences like the recipients' preexisting disease are of equally great importance. Here only the clinical experiment can and has given an answer to the problem. Thus Starzl has clearly shown that liver cell based inborn errors of metabolism can be corrected by liver transplantation and that, on the other hand, extrahepatic diseases affecting the liver can certainly recur [16]. Apart from that it would be very helpful to have an animal model which closely resembled the pathophysiological and anatomical sequelae of chronic active hepatitis and cirrhosis so that surgical, anaesthetic and postoperative management under these circumstances in relation to the human situation could be studied. But with the exception of general rules for fluid and volume replacement, the value of antibiotics and the need for glucose and antacid therapy, not much can be learned from animal experiments for postoperative patient management.

Nevertheless attention should be drawn to antibiotic therapy. Since dog experiments on liver ischemia some 60 years ago, it is known that an ischemically damaged liver looses its natural capability of clearing portal blood from endotoxins and bacteria. It is also known that, after transplantation, the liver almost completely looses its Kupffer cells. Thus the liver recipient is very much compromised in his ability to handle bacteria which come from the intestines and cause severe infectious complications, even under immunosuppression. The work of the Groningen group of Van der Waaij on selective decontamination of the bowel of animals such as rhesus monkey has therefore been transferred to clinical liver transplantation and apparently has been very successful [18].

Another aspect of postoperative care where animal studies can at least underline clinical observations is the deleterious effect of prolonged artificial ventilation. As Calne stated some time ago, a patient who does not get off the respirator soon after transplantation will almost certainly die. This has also been our experience. From studies on extracorporeal auxiliary liver perfusion we learned that homogeneous portal blood flow is mainly dependent on extrahepatic intraabdominal and intravascular pressure changes which lead to a kind of passive 'pump circulation' through the liver like a sponge that is soaked with fluid and squeezed out again [19]. The conclusion is that the liver, like the lung, is also hemodynamically damaged during prolonged respirator treatment and develops gross functional impairment. This in turn promotes infection, sepsis and liver insufficiency. There are good reasons for believing that the underlying cause is the hemodynamic alteration during artificial ventilation.

Let me now move to the more familiar, at least for most of us the more familiar, field of surgical technique. Without any doubt the ground here was prepared in experimental studies by Welch, Moore, Starzl, Mikaeloff, Fonkalsrud, Mieny, Terblanche, Calne and others [1, 2, 20–24].

Apart from auxiliary liver transplantation there were two problems most extensively studied in a number of experimental protocols (1) organ preservation and assessment of graft viability after harvesting and (2) technique of biliary anastomosis. As Starzl wrote in 1975 'about one third of all deaths after liver transplantation are due in one way or another to trouble with bile duct reconstruction'.

Liver preservation for clinical transplantation is now performed in all centers by simple gravity flushing and cooling of the organ and subsequent storage either with an intracellular type of electrolyte such as is used in kidney transplantation or else with a plasma protein fraction as recommended by Calne. Early experiments by Abouna, Eisemann, Elmslie and others on normothermic perfusion of the liver were complicated by rapid deterioration of the organ with shunts, inhomogeneous perfusion, partial thrombosis and microembolisms causing severe cell damage [25–27]. So interest turned to the inhibiton of metabolic processes by hypothermia. The use of various drugs such as chlorpromazine, prednisolone, isoproterenol and allopurinol and the composition of the perfusion solution, especially the electrolyte concentrations, were the subjects of many investigations, most of which were carried out in parallel to studies on kidney preservation. In 1960 Starzl was able to perform successful orthotopic liver transplantations in dogs after preserving the organs with Ringer's lactate [28]. Schalm [29] and Calne [30] in 1969 and 1972 could extend the hypothermic ischemia time to 3 and 5–7 h respectively by using dextran, plasma and glucose. Slapak in 1970 and Spilg in 1972 showed that moderate elevations in the potassium concentration of the perfusion fluid was beneficial for primate and pig livers [31, 32]. Abouna in 1971 reported the use of high potassium and magnesium concentrations in dextran-electrolyte solutions [33]. Longer preservation times up to 20 h were achieved by Mieny and Myburgh in 1971 with a dextran-electrolyte-sorbitose solution [34]. Calne in 1972 and Otte in 1973 were able to achieve similar preservation times with isoproterenol in Sack's and Collin's solutions respectively [30, 35]. But attempts to preserve the liver with hypothermic storage for 24 h have been consistently unsuccessful.

In 1979 Toledo-Pereyra reported the use of a modified hyperosmolar silica gel fraction for cold storage of the canine liver for 24 h. Five of six animals subsequently transplanted with the preserved organs survived for more than 5 days. If Sack's solution was used instead, only three of six animals survived. With Ringer's lactate all animals died. From these results it seemed evident that this modified silica gel fraction allows preservation times only previously achieved with continuous perfusion [36].

Another approach to preservation was continuous hypothermic perfusion with diluted blood, cryoprecipitated plasma, dextran, albumin or silica gel fractions. In kidney preservation, machine perfusion had been shown to give considerably longer preservation times and better functional quality. Brettschneider and other groups used diluted blood and after 11–15 h of preservation all animals survived whereas after 24 h only three of five animals survived [37]. Belzer, Petrie, Sung and Woods used cryoprecipitated plasma with other substances. Belzer's pigs all survived after 10 h cold perfusion [38]. Petrie and Woods reported that 12 of 19 dogs survived longer than 4 days after 24 h hypothermic pulsatile perfusion with cryoprecipitated plasma using the same techniques as in kidney preservation. The same group even reported successful liver transplantation after 48 h perfusion [39, 40]. Slapak [31] reported satisfactory hypothermic perfusion for up to 11 h with dextran, electrolytes and albumin and Toledo-Pereyra [41] in 1975 reported consistently successful liver transplantation after preservation for 24 h using hypothermic pulsatile perfusion with the silica gel fraction and high concentrations of potassium, glucose and albumin. However, as in his experiments with cold storage, he performed auxiliary transplantation. This may have been advantageous for animal survival in the early postoperative period. Although these and other investigations showed the beneficial effect of continuous perfusion, no consistent survival could be achieved with orthotopic transplantation after hypothermic preservation for 24 h. Moreover the perfusion machines were very complicated and not safe enough for use in human liver transplantation.

Another approach to preservation was hyperbaric oxygenation during cold storage or perfusion of the liver in high pressure Organ containers. Brettschneider [37] and Spilg [42] from Kapstadt reported favourable results with this method while other groups like that of Hinchcliff [43] in Bristol found no improvement.

Intermittent perfusion and hypothermic storage was introduced by Calne in order to combine the advantages of continuous perfusion with the lesser degree of vascular damage occurring during cold storage [44]. In this way the cooled liver could be provided with the necessary substrates and oxygen, the concentration of metabolites could be kept low and the danger of thrombosis and endothelial damage diminished. Lie reported consistent survival of all transplanted animals after 12 h preservation [45]. Idezuki also reported consistent survival after 8–9 h preservation using a dextran and electrolyte solution like Lie and three of his ten animals survived after 24 h preservation [46]. The use of plasma protein fractions and Sack's or Collin's solution by Calne and Kestens respectively resulted in better results for both groups than those obtained without intermittent perfusion. To summarise, attempts to achieve consistently good results in experimental liver transplantation after 24 h preservation have not yet been successful. The safest preservation method at the moment seems to be flush perfusion with an intracellular type electrolyte solution and possibly storage in a plasma protein solution.

During ischemia energy consuming processes stop functioning so a shift in extracellular and intracellular ions can be expected. Therefore in 1969 Collins introduced his intracellular type electrolyte solution with high potassium and magnesium and low sodium concentrations [47]. The osmolarity with 375 mosmol/l was kept well above physiological values in order to prevent edema. A physiological pH seemed of minor importance with pH values of 7 being regarded as optimal. However recent studies by Carter indicate that a pH of 7.4 is the borderline below which rapid deterioration of function can be expected. Lie even reported good results with liver preservation at a pH of 9 [48], but the buffer capacity of his solution was very small so that the pH of the venous effluent had already fallen to 7. The now widely used Euro-Collins solution has a pH of 7 so that a change here could possibly prove beneficial.

The discussion of experimental liver preservation would be incomplete without mentioning recent work on the use of prostacycline and Coenzyme Q by Monden and Marubayashi respectively [49, 50]. Monden has been able to preserve canine livers for 24 and even 48 h successfully by simple hypothermia in a modified Sack's solution containing prostacycline. When Marubayashi administered Co Q to the donor 1 h before perfusion, the hepatic energy charge after ischemia, as determined by ATP, ADP and AMP concentrations in the mitochondria, was significantly higher. The hepatic energy charge is closely connected to liver function after transplantation. This is one possible way to assess organ viability without transplantation. We have developed a perfusion apparatus in order to assess liver damage, function and morphological integrity after isolated normothermic perfusion. In this perfusion apparatus the liver can be kept in good macroscopic condition for 24 h and functional parameters remain basically normal as sequential BSP retention tests show. This could also be a new approach to preservation by continuous perfusion.

Generally liver preservation is the most interesting clinical problem for experimental investigation at the moment. The great advance in immunosuppression with Cyclosporine A has made evident shortcomings in the functional quality of the transplanted organs.

Another important field is the experimental and clinical problem with biliary drainage and the achievements made so far. The simple and crude method of cholecystoduodenostomy and cholecysto-jejunostomy has been abandoned for many reasons, not the least the numerous complications in man and experimental animals. The physiological end to end anastomosis of the common duct of donor and recipient resulted in many bile leakages and subsequent stenosis at the site of anastomosis. Moreover it seemed technically impossible in small animals or in children. However Krom [51] has shown that microsurgery can be used to perform a relatively safe end to end bile duct anastomosis and it has the advantage of preserving the natural sphincter which prevents ascending biliary infection. Choledocho-jejunostomy with a Roux-en-Y-loop has given good clinical results and is used in many cases where direct bile duct anastomosis is not possible. Calne [52] developed the gall bladder interposition between the recipient's and donor's common duct which also preserves the natural sphincter and gives a safe anastomosis. All these methods cannot be used in small experimental animals however. In rhesus monkeys Calne performed a cholecystoduodenostomy [7], Myburgh inserted a tube into the bile duct over which he performed an anastomosis [8]. We have developed a side-to-side anastomosis between the donor's and recipient's common duct which is easy to carry out even in the small bile ducts of rhesus monkeys and no stenosis can develop [53]. This method was first tried in the pig and then in 40 liver transplant experiments in monkeys without any failure. We have now started using it in clinical transplantation when possible, with good results so far.

Another example for experimental techniques which have been adopted in the clinic is the sequence in which the anastomoses are performed. In early monkey experiments we anastomosed the superior vena cava and portal vein and then released blood flow in these vessels. This resulted in considerable warm ischemia during subsequent cross-clamping of the aorta for the arterial anastomosis. When both the arterial and portal anastomosis were performed before reperfusion the liver, its initial appearance and enzyme loss improved greatly, showing the advantages of this approach. The same was seen in human transplantation where now usually all anastomoses are completed before restoring blood flow. This shows that problems and questions for experimental studies come from clinical situations but experimental problems can also influence clinical work.

References

1. Welch CS: A note on transplantation of the whole liver in dogs. Transpl Bull 2: 54–58, 1955.
2. Starzl TE: Experience in hepatic transplantation. WB Saunders, Philadelphia, 1969.
3. Calne RY, Sells RA, Pena JR et al.: Induction of immunological tolerance by porcine liver allografts. Nature 223: 472–476, 1969.
4. Bockhorn H: Die allogene Lebertransplantation. Res Exp Med 178: 177–199, 1981.
5. Flye MW, Rodgers G, Kacy S et al.: Prevention of fatal rejection of SLA-mismatched orthotopic liver allografts in inbred miniature swine by Cyclosporin-A. Transpl Proc 15: 1269–1271, 1983.
6. Starzl TE, Kaupp HA, Brock DR et al.: Studies on the rejection of the transplanted homologous dog liver. Surg Gynecol Obstet 112: 135, 1961.
7. Calne RY, Davies DR, Pena JR et al.: Hepatic allografts and xenografts in primates. Lancet I: 103–106, 1970.
8. Myburgh JA, Abrahams C, Mendelsohn D et al.: Cholestatic phenomenon in hepatic allograft rejection in the primate. Transpl Proc 3: 501–504, 1971.
9. Neuhaus P, Brölsch CE, Neuhaus R et al.: Der Einfluss von Bluttransfusionen auf die Überlebenszeit lebertransplantierter Rhesusaffen. In: Zelder O, Röhrer HD, Fischer M (eds.): Experimentelle und klinische Hepatologie. F.K. Schattauer Verlag, Stuttgart, New York, 1984, pp. 245–250.
10. Zimmermann FA, Knoll PP, Davies HS et al.: The fate of orthotopic liver allografts in different rat strain combinations. Transpl Proc 15: 1272–1275, 1983.
11. Engemann R, Ulrichs K, Thiede H et al.: Value of physiological liver transplant model in rats. Transplantation 33: 566–568, 1982.
12. Balner H: The DR system of rhesus monkeys: A brief review of serology, genetics and relevance to transplantation. Transplant Proc 12: 502–508, 1980.

13. Davies HFS, Taylor JE, Daniel MR *et al.*: Differences between pig tissues in the expression of major transplantation antigens: Possible relevance for organ allografts. J Exp Med 143: 987–992, 1976.
14. Wonigeit K, Bockhorn H, Pichlmayr R: Posttransplant changes in specific presursor T-cell reactivity: Comparison between liver and kidney allograft recipients. Transpl Proc 11: 1250–1255, 1979.
15. Kamada N, Davies HFS, Roser BJ: Fully allogeneic liver grafting and the induction of donor-specific unreactivity. Transplant Proc 13: 837–841, 1981.
16. Zitelli BJ, Malatack JJ, Gartner JC *et al.*: Orthotopic liver transplantation in children with hepatic-based metabolic disease. Transpl Proc 15: 1284–1287, 1983.
17. Myburgh JA, Smit JA: Acute normovolaemic haemodilution in orthotopic liver transplantation in the baboon. S Afr J Surg 12: 205–211, 1974.
18. Waaij D van der, Vries JM de, Lekkerkerk JEC: Eliminating bacteria from monkeys with antibiotics. In: Balner H, Beveridge WIB (eds.). Infections and immunosuppression in subhuman primates. Munksgaard, Copenhagen, 1970, p. 21.
19. Neuhaus P, Neuhaus R, Vonnahme F *et al.*: Verbesserte Möglichkeiten des temporären Leberersatzes durch ein neues Konzept der extracorporalen Leberperfusion. In: Schreiber HW (ed.) Chirurgie Foraum 83 für experimentelle und klinische Forschung. Springer, Berlin, Heidelberg, 1983, pp. 223–228.
20. Moore FD, Smith LL, Burnap TK *et al.*: One-stage homotransplantation of the liver following total hepatectomy in dogs. Transpl Bull 6: 103, 1959.
21. Mikaeloff P, Dureau G, Rassat JP *et al.*: Notre expérience de la transplantation orthotopique et heterotopique du foie chez le chien. Rev Mediochir Mal Foie 41: 51, 1966.
22. Fonkalsrud EW, Ono H, Shafey OA *et al.*: Orthotopic canine liver homotransplantation without vena caval interruption. Surg Gynecol Obstet 125: 319, 1967.
23. Mieny CJ, Moore AR, Homatas J *et al.*: Homotransplantation of the liver in pigs. S Afr J Surg 5: 109, 1967.
24. Terblanche J, Peacock JH, Hobbs KEF *et al.*: Orthotopic liver homotransplantation: An experimental study in the unmodified pig. S Afr Med J 42: 486, 1968.
25. Abouna GM: Pig liver perfusion with human blood. Brit J Surg 55: 761–768, 1968.
26. Elmslie RG, Mohan Rao M, Alp M *et al.*: Functional deficits in the isolated perfused pig liver. Surg Gynecol Obstet 7: 89–92, 1971.
27. Eiseman B, Soyer T: Prosthetics in hepatic assistance. Transpl Proc 3: 1519–1524, 1971.
28. Starzl TE, Kaup HA jun, Brock DR *et al.*: Reconstructive problems in canine liver homotransplantation with special reference to the postoperative role of hepatic venous flow. Surg Gynecol Obstet 111: 733–743, 1960.
29. Schalm SW, Terpstra JL, Drayer B *et al.*: A simple method for short term preservation of a liver homograft. Transplantation 8: 77–881, 1969.
30. Calne RY, Dunn DC, Gajo-Reyero R *et al.*: Trickle perfusion for organ preservation. Nature 235: 171–173, 1972.
31. Slapak M, Beaudoin JG, Lee HM *et al.*: Auxiliary liver homotransplantation: A new technique and an evaluation of current techniques. Arch Surg 100: 31–41, 1970.
32. Spilg H, Hickman R, Uys CJ *et al.*: Liver storage: 12-hour preservation of the pig liver. Brit J Surg 59: 307, 1972.
33. Abouna GM, Aldrete JA, Starzl TE: Changes in serum potassium and pH during clinical and experimental liver transplantation. Surgery 69: 419–426, 1971.
34. Mieny CJ, Myburgh JA: Succesful 20-hour preservation of the primate liver by simple cooling. Transplantation 11: 495–497, 1971.
35. Otte JB, Lambotte L, Squifflet JP *et al.*: Succesful orthotopic transplantation of the canine liver after prolonged preservation by initial perfusion and cold storage. Eur Surg Res 5: 273–281, 1973.
36. Toledo-Pereyra L: Successful orthotopic liver transplantation after preservation by simple hypo-

thermia. Transplantation 27: 291–293, 1979.

37. Brettschneider L, Daloze PM, Huguet D *et al.*: The use of combined preservation techniques for extended storage of orthotopic liver homografts. Surg Gynecol Obstet 126: 263–273, 1968.

38. Belzer FO, May R, Berry MN *et al.*: Short term preservation of porcine livers. J Surg Res 10: 55–61, 1970.

39. Petrie R, Woods JE: Successful 24-hour preservation of the canine liver. Arch Surg 107: 461–464, 1973.

40. Sung DTW, Woods JE: Forty-eight-hour preservation of the canine liver. Ann Surg 179: 422–426, 1974.

41. Toledo-Pereyra LH, Simmons RL, Najarian JS: Factors determining successful liver preservation for transplantation. Ann Surg 181: 289–298, 1975.

42. Spilg H, Hickman R, Uys CJ *et al.*: Twelve-hour liver preservation in the pig using hypothermia and hyperbaric oxygen. Brit J Surg 59: 273–276, 1972.

43. Hinchliffe A, Dent DM, Bowes JB *et al.*: Preservation of the pig liver using hyperbaric oxygen. In: Pegg DE (ed.) Organ Preservation. Churchill, Livingstone, Edinburgh, London, 1973.

44. Calne RY, Dunn DC, Gajo-Reyero R *et al.*: Trickle perfusion for organ preservation. Nature 235: 171–173, 1972.

45. Lie TS, Totovic V, Lagacé R *et al.*: Einfache Methoden zur Konservierung der Schweineleber. I. Dreistündlich intermittierende Perfusion in Hypothermie. Res Exp Med 160: 122–135, 1973.

46. Idezuki Y, Maki T, Kasahara K *et al.*: Twenty-four-hour preservation of the canine liver by squirt perfusion using a non-plasma-containing perfusate. Transpl Proc 3: 305–309, 1974.

47. Collins GM, Bravo-Shugaman M, Terasaki PI: Kidney preservation for transportation. Initial perfusion and 30 hours ice storage. Lancet 6: 1219–1222, 1969.

48. Lie TS, Ukikusa M: Significance of alkaline preservation solutions in liver transplantation Transpl Proc 16: 134–137, 1984.

49. Monden M, Fortner JG: Twenty-four- and 48-hour canine liver preservation by simple hypothermia with prostacyclin. Ann Surg 196: 38–42, 1982.

50. Marubayashi S, Dohi K, Ezaki H *et al.*: Preservation of ischemic rat liver mitchondrial functions and liver viability with CoQ. Surgery 91: 631–637, 1982.

51. Krom RAF, Gips CH, Newton D *et al.*: A successful start of a liver transplantation program. Transpl Proc 15: 1276–1278, 1983.

52. Calne RY: A new technique for biliary drainage in orthotopic liver transplantation utilizing the gall bladder as a pedicle graft conduit between the donor and recipient common bile ducts. Ann Surg 184: 605–609, 1976.

53. Neuhaus P, Neuhaus R, Pichlmayr R *et al.*: An alternative technique of biliary reconstruction after liver transplantation. Res Exp Med 180: 239–245, 1982.

3. Donor–recipient interactions in orthotopic liver transplantation in pigs

H.F.W. HOITSMA

Introduction

Since 1978 surgical experience in porcine orthotopic and auxiliary liver transplantation has been built up in our laboratory. After more than 180 transplantations, it has become a standard procedure with a success rate of more than 90%, and long-survival times are recorded. To achieve this high success rate we have intensively investigated and refined our anaesthetic management [1].

Although the skill of both anaesthesists and surgeons improved, we were still confronted with severe bleeding problems in several cases even when heparinisation was avoided. These problems were caused by administrations of A-O incompatible blood transfusions. Originally blood from the donor was given at random to the recipient. Fatal reactions after such transfusions were characterized by an acute rise of the pulmonary artery pressure which expresses an anaphylactic catastrophe in the pulmonary vascular system. Simultaneously, a marked fibrinogen decrease and invariable positive FDPs in the A-O incompatible series lead to intravascular coagulation. It is our opinion that the combination of an incompatible transfusion and a major surgical procedure favours the induction of intravascular coagulation followed by lethal hemorrhages. Our study indicates that if blood transfusions are required in major experimental surgery, blood should be typed preoperatively for A-O incompatibility and selected blood should be given instead of arbitrarily collected blood from random donors or abattoirs. It will definitely improve the transplantation results [2].

Based on our experience in experimental orthotopic liver grafting in pigs we came across various donor – recipient interactions which will be discussed in detail in the following chapters.

Liver allograft rejection in pigs; histology of the graft and the role of Swine Leucocyte Antigen-D

The porcine liver is often considered an immunologically-privileged organ as liver allografts in unrelated pigs can survive without any form of immunosuppression [3–6].

Although signs of rejection are noted, at least in pigs, liver allografts are immunologically privileged as compared to skin, heart and kidney grafts [4, 6, 7]. To gain a better understanding for this phenomenon on the rejection rate of orthotopic liver allografts in pigs from different herds was investigated. To define the role of histocompatibility between donor and recipient we have used the Mixed Lymphocyte Culture (MLC). Graft rejection was studied with respect to survival time and also by histology and biochemical monitoring of the function of the graft.

Materials and methods

Yorkshire pigs with an average weight of 20 kg from two separate herds were obtained from two different farms. Orthotopic liver transplantations were performed according to the technique described by Calne *et al.* [8]. Neither immunosuppressive nor antibiotic drugs were used. Donor and recipient were matched or mismatched for Swine Leucocyte Antigen-D (SLA-D) by testing the degree of MLC-stimulation of the recipient by donor lymphocytes.

Postoperatively needle biopsies of the graft and simultaneously blood biochemical tests were done at day 1, 4, 6, 8, 11, 15, 20 and 27 after transplantation and thereafter at weekly intervals until 8 weeks and at monthly intervals up to 4 months. After 4 months the animals were sacrificed and a final liver biopsy was taken during autopsy. In blood samples serum total bile acids, bilirubine, alkaline phosphatase and glutamate-oxalacetate transaminase were determined.

Results

Most of the SLA-D matched donors and recipients were littermates whereas all outbred pigs showed a positive reaction in the mixed lymphocyte culture. In the SLA-D matched couples almost all the recipient animals survived for 4 months, while the recipients of a SLA-D mismatched graft only survived 6–25 days.

The difference in survival time between SLA-D matched and mismatched recipients was statistically significant. Based on survival times and histological studies on liver biopsies taken at regular time intervals after transplantation, we could determine four types of transplantation reactions looking at the cellular infiltrate in the portal tracts:

- type I,   early rejection
- type II,   late rejection
- type III, transient rejection
- type IV,   no rejection.

Type I: A dense mononuclear infiltration of the portal tracts was observed at day 4 after transplantation. On day 6 an infiltrate of mainly lymphocytes and lymphoblasts was invading both the portal tracts and the parenchyma. Destruction of liver cells was noted and at autopsy the architecture of the liver was completely destructed. Early rejection was seen in animals with a survival time ranging from 6 to 10 days.

Type II: Infiltration of the liver was milder and restricted to the portal tracts and interlobular septa. Besides lymphocytes, mainly plasmacells were seen from the 8th day on. All the animals died from rejection of the graft. The survival time in type II varied from 10 to 25 days. Almost all the recipient animals with an early and late type of rejection received a graft from a SLA-D mismatched donor.

Type III: This type is characterized by a mild, transient infiltration of the portal tracts by mononuclear cells with minimal plasmacell involvement. The infiltration was found between day 4 and day 30 postoperatively and subsequently disappeared thereafter. All the animals survived. At autopsy macroscopically and microscopically normal livers were seen. This mild intransient type of rejection is observed only in recipients with an allograft from an SLA-D matched donor.

Type IV: No noteworthy histologic signs of rejection during the first four months after transplantation were seen. Almost all these recipients were matched for SLA-D antigens.

The biochemical parameters were tested simultaneously when liver biopsies were taken. The results revealed that only serum total bile acids were a very sensitive parameter in predicting liver rejection when compared with bilirubine, alkaline phosphatase and glutamate oxalacetate transaminase [9].

Conclusions

The results of this study clearly indicate that the fate of liver allografts in pigs largely depends on the degree of SLA-D histocompatibility between donor and recipient. Recipient animals that received a graft from an MLC (SLA-D) matched donor had significantly longer survival times than recipient animals that received a graft from MLC (SLA-D) mismatched donors [10].

SLA-D histocompatibility as measured in MLC is often accompanied by genetic relationship between donor and recipient. Lymphocytes of outbred couples always showed a positive rejection in the MLC (mismatched for SLA-D antigen) and liver transplantation was followed by histologically proven rejection in all such combinations. The finding that pigs from one herd are so closely related might explain the varying results from different groups concerning the privileged status of the liver for transplantation. That liver grafts still are privileged is based on the fact that skin transplants are invariably rejected within two weeks even in MLC littermate couples. The difference however, in take rate between liver and skin might be explained by the fact that more and other antigens play a part in grafting of the latter.

Cyclosporine A in orthotopic porcine liver transplantation: Long-term survival after short-term treatment

As demonstrated above, in MLC mismatched couples orthotopic porcine liver transplantation results in rejection of the graft. We have demonstrated an early type I and a late type II. In order to prevent rejection the effect of Cyclosporine A (CyA) was investigated. CyA exerts its immunosuppressive effect by eliminating only that part of the immune system, which relies on T-cell proliferation. It interferes with the T-cell dependent production of monokines (Il-1) by accessory cells and it blocks the receptor expression for these monokines on T-cells, resulting in the abrogation of lymfokine (Il-2) production. The expression of Ia-like antigens is diminished on alloactivated peripheral lymphocytes after treatment with CyA. We have chosen for a short-term and low dose treatment.

Materials and methods

Yorkshire pigs of two separate herds were obtained from two different farms. The animals were grafted when they were 20 to 30 kg in weight and 2 to 3 months of age. Antibiotic therapy was not applied.

Donor and recipient animals were mismatched for SLA-D, and SLA-D incompatibility was tested in the MLC.

CyA treatment was started at the day before operation and stopped at the 21th postoperative day. A solution of 0.1 g CyA per ml neutral oil (Miglyol, Dynamit Nobel AG, Troisdorf-Oberlar) was given intramuscularly. Four recipients received a dose of 10 mg/kg per day and ten recipients received a dose of 20 mg/kg per day. The control group consisted of 14 MLC mismatched host/recipient combinations receiving no Cya treatment.

Needle biopsies of the liver were taken at day 1, 4, 6, 8, 11, 15, 20 and 27 after transplantation, thereafter at weekly intervals until 8 weeks and at monthly intervals up to 4 months. After 4 months the animals were sacrificed and an open biopsy of the liver was taken. At the same time as the liver biopsies blood was taken by venapuncture for estimation of total bilirubin, alkaline phosphatase and glutamate oxalacetate transaminase and creatinine.

Results

Four liver allograft recipients received CyA in a dose of 10 mg/kg. One of these animals rejected the graft. The liver biopsies showed an infiltration of virtually pure plasmacells. This animal died at the 12th postoperative day. Liver function tests were elevated. Liver biopsies taken from two other recipients treated with 10 mg/kg revealed a transient infiltration of plasmacells. One of these accepted the graft and survived, the other animal died on the 31th postoperative day from a pneumonia. The fourth animal accepted the graft and had a long-term survival. The animal was sacrificed after 4 months because of lodging problems. Histology of the liver revealed no abnormalities as well as at autopsy as well as at the liver biopsies taken at regular times after transplantation. The biochemical profile did not show disturbances as well.

By doubling the dose of CyA, nine out of ten animals accepted their graft. Long-term survival was noted in six of these nine animals, while the other three died after 17, 22 and 46 days from infective complications. Liver biopsies of these nine animals revealed no signs of rejection and all liver function tests were normal. One out of the ten recipients treated with 20 mg/kg CyA rejected its graft in 14 days.

Histology showed that the portal tract of the liver of this animal was infiltrated mainly by plasmacells. An increase in serum bile acids reflected the rejection process with a prompt and marked increase in serum bile acids at the 5th postoperative day. Other liver function tests were elevated as well.

Recipients assigned to the control group received a liver allograft from a donor who was mismatched for SLA-D antigens as tested in the MLC. No CyA treatment was applied. The liver allografts were rejected in all but one of the 14 cases studied. Ten receptor animals died within 2 weeks after transplantation. The difference in survival time between CyA treated and untreated liver allograft recipients was significant ($p<0.01$, Wilcoxon test). Rejection of the graft in the control group was confirmed by the histology of the liver biopsies and the disturbed biochemical profile. The survival time of the recipients of a MLC mismatched liver allograft who were treated with CyA in a dose of 20 mg/kg during 3 weeks was comparable to the survival time of untreated recipients that got a MLC matched graft.

Regarding the nephrotoxicity of CyA, no kidney damage was observed. The serum creatinine level remained normal during CyA treatment until death.

No abnormalities in white blood cell counts and differentiation were noted.

Conclusions

In the first series a low dose of 10 mg/kg per day was given intramuscularly. In almost all the cases a pure plasma cellular infiltrate was seen in liver biopsies taken at regular times postoperatively. Although some were transient in most of the cases, this infiltrate led to destruction of the graft and subsequently to the death of the recipient. By doubling the dose to 20 mg/kg/per day, long survival times were obtained. Practically no infiltrating cells were noted in liver biopsies. These observations led to the conclusion that the survival time of recipients of a MLC mismatched liver allograft, who were treated with CyA in a dose of 20 mg/kg during 3 weeks, was equal to the survival time of untreated recipients transplanted with a MLC matched graft. CyA induces a state of graft acceptance in pigs. After 21 days of CyA treatment the immunosuppressive regimen can be discontinued. Long-term graft survival with no further signs of rejection is observed [11].

In the CyA immunosuppressed animals, five died from infections, mainly of the respiratory tract. This might be caused by CyA and can probably be overcome by the use of antibiotics. The most serious side-effect encountered so far by CyA is its nephrotoxicity [12]. This can be diminished by reducing the dose or by using conventional immunosuppression until renal function is satisfactory and then change to CyA. In our model CyA did not cause kidney damage. The low dose applied and the route of administration possibly circumvents nephrotoxicity.

Regarding the biochemical parameters, we have concluded that serum total bile acid estimation is a simple, sensitive and useful test for the follow-up of liver allograft rejection [9]. In the CyA treated MLC mismatched group the total serum bile acid estimations were normal and comparable to the profiles found in the untreated MLC matched group [11]. Other liver function tests were normal indicating that the dose of CyA used was not hepatotoxic. This was confirmed by the fact that these livers showed no histological abnormalities. When rejection occurred despite CyA treatment an increase in serum bile acids was noted as in untreated MLC mismatched couples.

Veiled cells in liver lymph: Their role in orthotopic porcine liver transplantation

It is well known that Ia, HLA-D and DR antigens play an important role in transplantation [13–16].

In pigs SLA-D antigens as determined in mixed lymphocyte culture are important for the outcome of graft survival [10].

The question is: Which cells start an immunological reaction and initiate rejection?

In which way is antigen presentation regulated?

In skin, the antigen presenting system consists of Langerhans cells, lymph born veiled cells and interdigitating cells from the lymphnodes [17–20]. Langerhans cells pick up antigens in the skin and migrate via efferent lymphatics as 'veiled cells' to the lymphnode. Veiled cells are strongly positive for immune response associated antigens and are characterized by actively moving cytoplasmatic veils

[17, 20]. When these cells enter the lymphnode they become 'interdigitating cells' presenting their antigens to the T-dependent area of the node and as such the T-lymphocytes. An immunological reaction is born. It is well known that not only veiled cells but also Langerhans cells and interdigitating cells are strongly Ia positive. In liver Kupffer cells are strongly Ia positive. Based on this knowledge we 'transplanted' this 'skin concept' to the liver. We have studied in our porcine experiments the cellular composition from the efferent pig liver lymph vessel in the hepatoduodenal ligament [21].

Materials and methods

Lymph from the efferent lymph vessels in the hepatoduodenal ligament was obtained during orthotopic liver transplantation experiments or during a laparotomy when pigs were under neurolept anaesthesia [1]. These lymphatics can be clearly seen, they stain within 60 s after injection of trypan blue in the liver. They come right from the hilar region of the liver and from the gallbladder wall. They enter small lymphnodes in this ligament. The first lymphnodes are mostly found in halfway down between the hilar region of the liver and the duodenum.

Lymph was collected from the vessel before entering the lymph gland by aspiration within a fine needle and a syringe containing a drop of heparin or by canulation of a suitable large lymphatic by inserting a Portex canula (pp 10, Portex Ltd, Hyth, Kent, England). Artificial breathing of the animal was stopped during a few seconds in order to prevent respiratory induced movements of the liver.

Results

Isolation of veiled cells from the liver lymph is performed according to a special technique [21]. Further determination of these veiled cells is possible by histochemical studies and moreover these veiled cells show a positive staining with anti Ia-serum indicating that they belong to Ia-bearing cells. Finally characterization of the typical movements of the cytoplasmatic veils is done using a time lapse cinematography. An important finding is that veiled cells can only be demonstrated in efferent liver lymph before entering a lymphgland. Lymph coming from a gland, from the cysterna chyli or from the thoracic duct does not contain veiled cells. Apparently these cells remain in the lymphnode. In a few cases we were able to collect liver lymph a couple of weeks after orthotopic liver transplantation. Again veiled cells were identified but their amount was considerably lower compared to the amount of veiled cells found in pig liver lymph before transplantation.

Conclusions

The finding of veiled cells in efferent liver lymphatics might be of great importance on the outcome of orthotopic liver transplantation. This is supported by the fact that these cells are Ia positive and by the great influence of SLA-D histo-(in)compatibility on the outcome of orthotopic liver transplantation in pigs.

The question is: Which cells are precursors of veiled cells? Our hypothesis is that monocytes from the bloodstream enter the liver and become Kupffer cells. A part of the Kupffer cells are residents, while others might leave the liver and become veiled cells in the liver lymph, enter a lymphnode in the hepatoduodenal ligament and act as interdigitating cells by presenting their antigens to the T-lymphocytes. A difference in SLA-D antigens itself might provoke an immunological reaction after transplantation. Accepting this hypothesis one may find new ways for immunosuppression.

Pretreatment of the graft in order to eliminate the veiled cells and their precursors with anti Ia serum or even better anti-veiled cell serum or a monoclonal antiserum might favour the outcome of graft acceptance. Irradiation of the graft in combination with cytostatic treatment will probably have the same effect [21]. All these speculations hopefully will give birth to further research programmes.

Orthotopic transplantation of liver segments

Since the success rate of liver grafting is rising, an increase of liver transplantation activities may be expected. There will be a greater need for donor livers of all sizes. It is obvious that a large liver cannot orthotopically be grafted into a small individual or even into children. In addition to this small donors are seldom available.

Transplantation of liver segments will therefore probably be a solution. We have studied this option in our animal laboratory, based on earlier experiences in porcine orthotopic liver transplantation. A 'hypothermic workbench' technique of extended left donor hepatectomy was developed to overcome size incompatibility in orthotopic liver grafting.

Materials and methods

Yorkshire pigs of either sex with a mean weight of 25 kg are used. In order to prevent rejection of the graft the transplanted couples are SLA-D matched. The donor operation is almost identical to the technique described by Calne [8]. Before hepatectomy is done the left hepatic artery, the cystic artery, the left branch of the portal vein and the left hepatic bile duct are resected. As a consequence of this a sharp demarcation line can be seen on the liver surface between the non-perfused left liver lobe and the perfused right liver lobe, indicating the anatomical border between the two liver halves. The liver is taken out in the usual way with a long segment of caval vein. In a 'hypothermic workbench' procedure the two liver lobes are separated following the demarcation line, starting left from the suprahepatic caval vein downwards to the right side of the gallbladder fossa, using a diathermic knife. In this way an extended left hemi-hepatectomy is achieved. Visible veins and bile ducts on the raw surface of the right liver segments are sutured with 6 × 0 prolene, followed by covering of the surface with isobutyl-2-cyanoacrylate or collagen fleece (Novacol®).

A graft thus prepared is orthotopically transplanted according to the technique described by Calne. It differs in a way that before recirculation of the graft all the vascular anastomoses are completed. At the same time the portal venous bloodflow and the arterial bloodflow through the graft is restored. Finally the bile duct is end-to-side anastomosed to the duodenum.

Results

Five animals who received a reduced size livergraft (one third of the original weight of the donor liver) had an uneventful recovery from the operation. Survival times up to 8 months were recorded. All the animals were SLA-D matched and no noteworthy signs of rejection were seen in liver biopsies taken at regular times postoperatively. The blood biochemical parameters were the same as seen after orthotopic transplantation of the whole liver.

Conclusions

Our technique of an extended left hepatectomy in a 'hypothermic workbench procedure' offers an adequate opportunity to overcome size incompatibility. It is clear that less than one third of the whole liver is enough to give vital support to a hepatectomized animal without giving rise to portal hypertension. Liver regeneration takes place in the usual way as is demonstrated after partial liver resection. No blood transfusions were needed during the transplantation procedure, because the use of isobutyl-2-cyanoacrylate or collagen Fleece (Novacol®) was most effective in sealing off the raw liver surface of the graft. Our experiments show that transplantation of liver segments is a realistic procedure [22].

It is clear that these experimental studies are necessary as a prerequisite for successful grafting of liver segments both in adults and children. Successful clinical application in children is reported from Paris (Chapter 22 and [23]) and from Hannover [24].

Acknowledgements

I wish to thank my medical colleagues Dr. S. Meijer, Dr. J.J. de Lange, drs. B.J. Dwars, drs. M.A.J.M. Hunfeld and Dr. J.J. Visser (biochemist), Dr. Ir. Adri A. Bom-van Noorloos and Dr. H.A. Drexhage (immunologists) and laboratory personnel for their contribution to make this experimental liver transplantation programme possible.

References

1. De Lange JJ, Hoitsma HFW, Meijer S: Anaesthetic management in experimental orthotopic liver transplantation in the pig. Eur Surg Res 16:360–365, 1984.
2. Hunfeld MAJM, Hoitsma HFW, Meijer S, Van Haeringen H, Rietveld FW: The role of A-O incompatible bloodtransfusions in porcine orthotopic liver transplantation. Eur Surg Res 16:354–359, 1984.
3. Bockhorn H, Lauchart W, Ringe B, Nedden H, Pichlmayr T: SLA-Testing und MLC-Reaktion beim Schwein und ihre Beziehung zur Abstossung von Haut- und Lebertransplantaten. Langenbecks Arch Chir Suppl Chir For 141, 1975.
4. Calne RY, White HJO, Yoffa DR, Binns RM, Maginn RR, Herbertson RM, Millard PR, Molina VP, Davis DR: Prolonged survival of the liver transplants in the pig. Br Med J 4:645, 1967.
5. Garnier H, Clot JP, Chomette G: Orthotopic transplantation of the porcine liver. Surg Gynaecol Obstet 130:105, 1979.
6. Starzl TE: Experience in hepatic transplantation. WB Saunders, Philadelphia, 1969.
7. Calne RY: Allografting in the pig. In: Calne RY (ed.) Immunological aspects of transplantation surgery. 1973, p. 296.
8. Calne RY, Yoffa DE, White HJO, Maginn RR: A technique of orthotopic liver transplantation in the pig. Brit J Surg 55:203, 1968.
9. Visser JJ, Bom-van Noorloos AA, Meijer S, Hoitsma HFW: Serum total bile acids monitoring after experimental orthotopic liver transplantation. J Surg Res 36:147–153, 1984.
10. Bom-van Noorloos AA, Visser JJ, Drexhage HA, Meijer S, Hoitsma HFW: Liver allograft rejection in pigs: Histology of the graft and role of swine leucocyte antigen-D. J Surg Res 37:269–276, 1984.
11. Bom-van Noorloos AA, Visser JJ, Drexhage HA, Meijer S, Hoitsma HFW: Cyclosporine A in orthotopic porcine liver transplantation. Long term survival after short term treatment. Eur Surg Res 16:329–335, 1984.
12. White DJG, Calne RY: The use of cyclosporine A immunosuppression in organ grafting. Immunol Rev 65:115, 1982.
13. Faustman D, Kraus P, Lacy PE, Finke EH, Davie JM: Survival of heart allografts in nonimmunosuppressed murine recipients by pretreatment of the donor tissue with anti Ia antibodies. Transplantation 34:302–305, 1982.
14. Lechler RI, Batchelor JR: Restoration of immunogenicity to passenger cell-depleted kidney allografts by the addition of donor strain dendritic cells. J Exp Med 155:31–41, 1982.
15. Persijn GG, Van Leeuwen A, Parlevliet J, Cohen B, Lansbergen Q, D'Amaro J, Van Rood JJ: Two major factors influencing kidney graft survival in Eurotransplant: HLA-Dr matching and blood transfusion(s). Transpl Proc XIII:150–154, 1981.
16. Schulak JA, Goeken NE, Ngkiem DD, Corey R: Effect of DR matching on rejection in first cadaver kidney transplantation. Transplantation 34:382–384, 1982.
17. Drexhage HA, Mullink H, De Groot J, Clarke J, Balfour BM: A study of cells present in peripheral lymph of pigs with special reference to a type of cell resembling the Langerhans cell.

Cell Tiss Res 202:407–430, 1979.
18. Kamperdijk EAW, Hoefsmit ECM: Birbeck granules in lymph node macrophages. Ultramicroscopy 3:137, 1978.
19. Silberberg-Sinakin I, Thorbecke GJ, Baer RL, Rosenthal SA, Beresowsky V: Antigen bearing Langerhans cells in skin dermal lymphatics and in lymphnodes. Cell Immunol 25:137, 1976.
20. Søeberg G, Binns RM, Balfour BM: Contact sensitivity in the pig. II Induction by intralymphatic infusion of DNP-conjugated cells. Int Arch All Appl Immunol 57:114, 1978.
21. Bom-van Noorloos AA, Drexhage HA, Kegel A, Meijer S, Hoitsma HFW: Veiled cells in liver lymph: Their role in orthotopic porcine liver transplantation. Transplantation (accepted for publication).
22. Hoitsma HFW, Meijer S, Dwars BJ, Hunfeld MAJM, Visser JJ: Orthotopic- and heterotopic auxiliary transplantation of liver segments. An experimental study in pigs. Eur Surg Res (submitted for publication).
23. Bismuth H, Houssin D: Reduced-sized orthotopic liver graft in hepatic transplantation in children. Surgery 367–370, 1984.
24. Brölsch CE, Neuhaus P, Burdelski M, Bernsau U, Pichlmayr R: Orthotope Transplantation von Lebersegmenten bei Kleinkindern mit Gallengangatresien. Chir For Exp Klin For: 105–109, 1984.

4. Blood transfusion and graft survival after liver transplantation in rhesus monkeys

P. NEUHAUS, C.E. BRÖLSCH, R. NEUHAUS, W. LAUCHART,
F. VONNAHME, K. WONIGEIT, J. BORLEFFS, H. BALNER
and R. PICHLMAYR

Introduction

The positive effect of blood transfusions on the results of kidney transplantation has been well established experimentally and clinically [1–5]. In addition it has been known for some time that survival after liver transplantation in pigs and rats is possible without any immunosuppression whereas kidney transplants are rejected in a regular fashion. Thus the transplanted liver was regarded as an 'immunologically privileged' organ [6–8]. It remained unclear, however, whether immunological modification, in particular preoperative blood transfusions, would have the same positive influence on transplant survival in liver transplantation as in kidney transplantation.

The aim of our study was to examine this question in a preclinical animal model. Rhesus monkeys are genetically closely related to man and thus are an ideal preclinical model for human organ transplantation. Moreover, in contrast to dogs, families or large populations of outbred animals are available. The major histocompatibility complex of rhesus monkeys has been subjected to detailed study and is similar to that of man as is the role of histocompatibility antigens and the effects of blood transfusions in graft survival after kidney transplantation.

Materials and methods

Unrelated adult male and female rhesus monkeys weighing between 4 and 10 kg were used. They were either imported directly from India or else had been bred at the Rijswijk Primate Center. Kinship among the imported animals could not be excluded but is unlikely. The animals were not preimmunised and all donor/recipient combinations were serological defined (SD) and lymphocyte defined (LD) incompatible. Orthotopic liver transplantation was performed in ten untreated donor/recipient combinations and in ten combinations receiving blood transfusions before surgery. Three transfusions of 20 ml fresh, unpooled whole citrated blood were given at biweekly intervals before transplantation, the last 2–3 weeks prior to operation. The blood donors were so selected that immunisation against SD antigens and the A- and B-locus antigens of the major histocompatibility complex Rh-LA, where donor and recipient differed, was avoided in order to minimise the chance of a positive crossmatch at the time of transplantation. No postoperative immunosuppression was carried out. The technique of liver preservation and orthotopic transplantation was similar to that used in man. However early experiments showed that the anastomosis of the hepatic artery and the portal vein before restoring blood flow to the liver gave better results. Initial blood flow through the liver with this technique was much more homogeneous than with portal perfusion alone.

A newly-developed, side-to-side choledocho-choledochostomy was used for the biliary anastomosis. So far no leakages or stenosis at the site of anastomosis have been observed [9].

During surgery the animals received glucose and electrolyte solutions as well as a donor blood transfusion. Two to three hours after transplantation all animals regained consciousness after all catheters had been removed.

Serum enzyme levels were measured on days 1, 3, 7, 14, 21 and 49. Liver needle biopsies were carried out on days 7, 21 and 49. Death of the animal was regarded as the end point of the experiment. The cause of death was determined through autopsy and histological examination of all organs. Animals dying from other causes apart from rejection such as technical failure were excluded from the study.

Results

In the control group which did not receive blood transfusions, six of ten animals died between 6 and 9 days after transplantation from fulminant rejection. Four animals survived for more than 22 days and were therefore regarded as long term survivors. In the second group which received pretransplant blood transfusions, eight of ten animals were long term survivors. The average survival time in both groups differed significantly with 7 and 32 days respectively (Figure 1).

There was a good correlation between serum levels of GOT and GPT (ASAT and ALAT) and the occurrence of rejection. After an initial rise due to preservation damage, both groups of animals had SGOT-values between 100 and 500 U/l. In the untreated group GOT-values underwent a second increase between days 5 and 10. This was observed in all animals, including the long term survivors (Figure 2). Long-term survivors in the blood transfusion group did not show this second increase however. This was also observed with SGPT-levels. Alkaline phosphatase, gamma-GT and bilirubin levels revealed significant cholestasis in both experimental groups (Figure 3).

Liver biopsies from both groups revealed heavy infiltration by round cells on day 7 with cholestasis as a sign of classic rejection (Figure 4). In the transfused group cellular infiltration of the sinusoids and the degree of necrosis was less

SURVIVAL TIME OF RHESUS MONKEYS AFTER LIVER TRANSPLANTATION
WITHOUT IMMUNOSUPPRESSION

GROUP	TRANSF.	SURVIVAL TIME (DAYS)	MST (DAYS)	% LONG TERM SURVI- VORS (22 DAYS)
I	Ø	6,6,6,6,7,9, 22,33,44,116	7	40% (4/10)
II	+	6,8, 26,27,32,33, 40,45,79,95	32	80% (8/10)

Figure 1. Survival times of rhesus monkeys after liver transplantation with and without preoperative blood transfusions.

marked however. Histological signs of recurrent or continuous rejection became more pronounced after 14, 21 and 49 days. The architecture of the liver lobule was destroyed, round cell infiltration and massive fibrosis with regenerative nodules developed (Figure 5). Recurrent rejection also caused massive vascular changes with fibrinoid necrosis, intimal hyperplasia and alterations in the media. All animals died from liver failure due to repeated rejection.

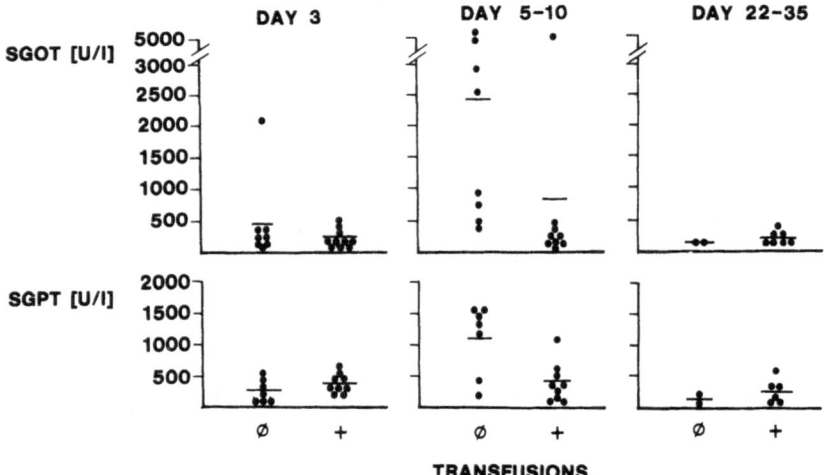

Figure 2. Serum transaminases after liver transplantation in rhesus monkeys with and without preoperative blood transfusions.

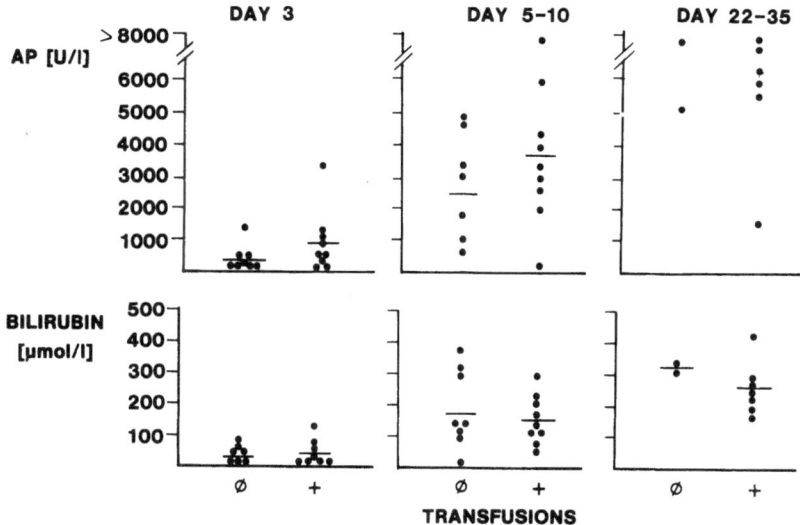

Figure 3. Alkaline phosphatase and bilirubin after liver transplantation in rhesus monkeys with and without preoperative blood transfusions.

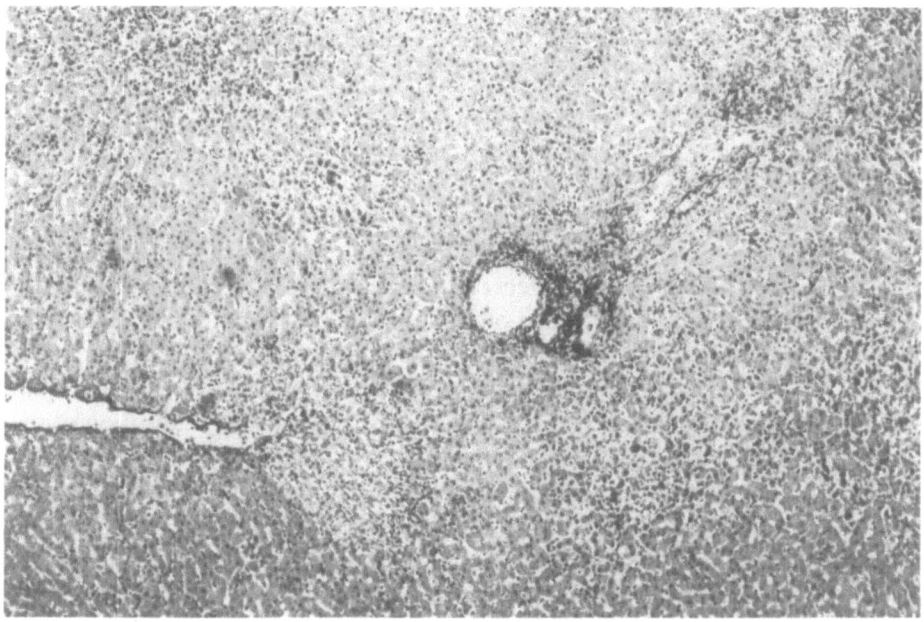

Figure 4. Acute rejection on day 7 after liver transplantation. The portal triad is completely infiltrated by round cells. So-called bridging necroses can be seen from periportal field to right upper corner. Zonal necrosis is evident around central and sublobular veins (left lower corner). Round cells are also present between hepatocytes and in sinusoids (×55).

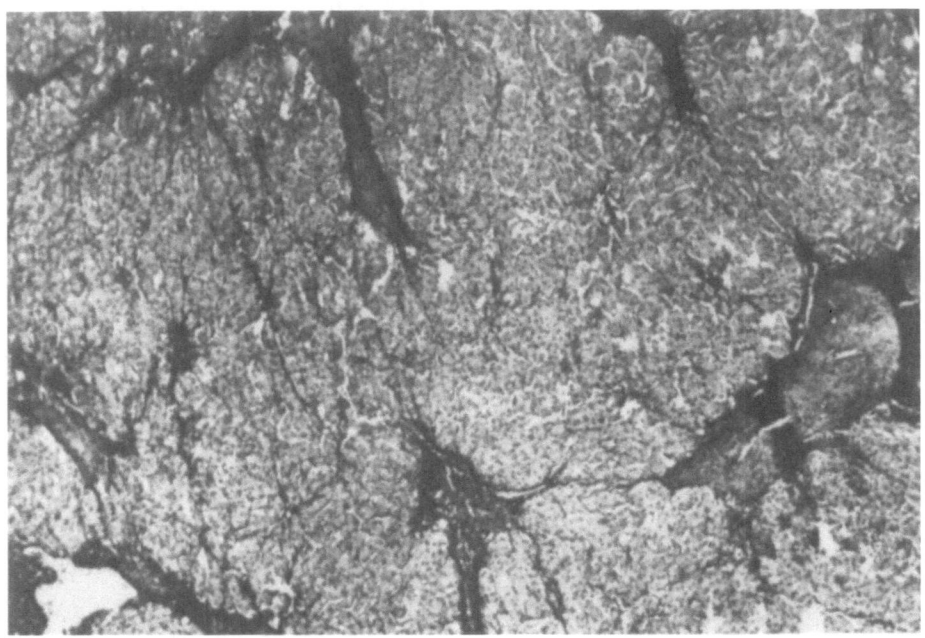

Figure 5. Chronic rejection on day 55 after liver transplantation. Marked fibrosis of periportal fields and destruction of lobular architecture through replacement of necrotic cells by connective tissue (×55).

Discussion

The results show that, similar to kidney transplantation, pretransplant blood transfusions also have a positive effect on the outcome after liver transplantation. In particular the effects of rejection on the hepatocytes have been so dampened that increases in SGOT and SGPT, otherwise seen between days 5 and 10, do not occur. Cholestasis is still observed however, manifested by rises in bilirubin, alkaline phosphatase and gamma-GT together with round cell infiltration of the portal triad and sinusoids. It can be speculated that two different types of rejection occur in man and monkeys after liver transplantation. Type one is characterised by a rapid increase in the transaminases SGOT and SGPT and causes hepatocellular damage. This type generally occurs soon after transplantation and can be positively influenced by pretransplant blood transfusions. Type two mainly involves cellular infiltration of the portal triad and results in cholestasis. This type is not influenced by preoperative blood transfusions and can occur in both the early and late course after transplantation [10]. Whereas this cholestatic type of rejection does not result in the immediate death of the animal, the fulminant hepatocellular type of rejection is fatal. If this rejection has been modified by pretransplant blood transfusions, then recurrent acute and chronic rejection will eventually cause the death of animal weeks or a few months later.

In conclusion we can say that the frequency of rejection after liver transplantation in rhesus monkeys is similar to that observed after kidney transplantation. Its course is different however as the large liver cell mass means this organ has an extraordinary regenerative capacity. Two patterns of rejection can occur. There is a hepatocellular type which can be positively influenced by immunological modifications such as preoperative blood transfusions and a cholestatic type which is not affected by pretreatment. Whether the liver is in fact an immunologically-privileged organ can be questioned. A lower susceptibility of the liver to effector mechanisms in rejection is also a plausible explanation.

References

1. Es AA van, Marquet RL, Rood JJ van et al.: Blood transfusions induce prolonged kidney allograft survival in rhesus monkeys. Lancet i:506, 1977.
2. Es AA van, Marquet RL, Rood JJ van et al.: The influence of a single blood transfusion on kidney allograft survival in unrelated rhesus monkeys. Transplantation 26:325, 1978.
3. Borleffs JCC, Marquet RL, By-Aghai Z de et al.: Kidney transplantation in rhesus monkeys. Matching for D/DR antigens, pretransplant blood transfusions, and immunological monitoring before transplantation. Transplantation 33:285–290, 1982.
4. Opelz G, Mickey MR, Terasaki PI: Blood transfusions and unresponsiveness to HL-A. Transplantation 16:649, 1973.
5. Opelz G, Sengar DPS, Mickey MR et al.: Effect of blood transfusions on subsequent kidney transplants. Transpl Proc 5:253, 1973.
6. Calne RY, Sells RA, Pena JR et al.: Induction of immunological tolerance by porcine liver allografts. Nature 223:472–476, 1969.
7. Bockhorn H: Die allogene Lebertransplantation. Res Exp Med 178:177–199, 1981.
8. Flye MW, Rodgers G, Kacy S et al.: Prevention of fatal rejection of SLA-mismatched orthotopic liver allografts in inbred miniature swine by Cyclosporine-A. Transpl Proc 15:1269–1271, 1983.
9. Neuhaus P, Neuhaus R, Pichlmayr R et al.: An alternative technique of biliary reconstruction after liver transplantation. Res Exp Med 180:239–245, 1982.
10. Pichlmayr R, Brölsch CE, Neuhaus P et al.: Report on 68 human orthotopic liver transplantations with special reference to rejection phenomena. Transpl Proc 15:1279–1283, 1983.

5. Electron microscopy of rejection in liver transplantation of the rhesus monkey

F.-J. VONNAHME, P. NEUHAUS, C.E. BRÖLSCH, W. LAUCHART
and R. PICHLMAYR

Introduction

While light microscopy remains the standard diagnostic method in liver transplantation, it is apparent that electron microscopy can contribute to a better understanding of the pathogenesis of rejection phenomena. Electron microscopic investigations after liver transplantation have been undertaken in different species [1–3], however, little information still exists about primates. Therefore it was the main purpose of our electron microscopic study to investigate with electron microscopic techniques cellular mechanisms of the hepatocytic and nonparenchymal structures involved in acute or chronic rejection after orthotopic liver transplantation in the rhesus monkey.

Materials and methods

Two groups of rhesus monkeys were transplanted, each group consisting of ten animals of both sexes. They were either untreated or they received blood transfusions before the surgical procedure. Further details on the transplantation technique are given by Neuhaus *et al.* (Chapter 4). Thirty minutes after revascularization a wedge biopsy was taken as a control of the preservation of the organ. Liver needle biopsies were obtained on days 7, 21, and 49 using Menghini needles. Small pieces of the tissue were immersed immediately into 2% glutaraldehyde in 0.1 m cacodylate buffer (pH 7.4, 340 mosm). After rinsing in cacodylate buffer the blocks were post-fixed in 1% osmium tetroxide in 0.1 m cacodylate buffer (pH 7.4, 340 mosm). The specimens were then dehydrated through a graded series of alcohol and embedded in Epon 812. Semi-thin sections were stained with toluidine blue; thin sections were contrast stained with lead citrate on copper grids and examined in a Philips TEM 201. For scanning electron microscopy the tissue was fixed in glutaraldehyde (as above). The pieces were then sliced into small parts or fractured by digital pressure. After dehydration and critical point drying the specimens were mounted on aluminium studs, coated with metallic gold, and examined in a Philips PSEM 500. Parts of the biopsies were also processed in the conventional way for histological examination.

Results and discussion

Acute rejection

Acute rejection phenomena were more pronounced in the untreated group in which six of ten animals died within 6 and 9 days after transplantation. On the contrary only two out of ten animals died from acute rejection of the organ graft in the pretreated group having received blood transfusions. All animals (n = 12) from both groups surviving for more than 22 days after transplantation were regarded as long-term survivors. The electron microscopic investigation was based on the light microscopical diagnosis which will only be summarized here.

Cellular infiltration and necrosis

Acute rejection which was more common in the untreated animals, was mainly characterized by an accumulation of mononuclear cells in the portal tracts (Figure 1). This cellular infiltrate consisted of immature and mature lymphocytes, macrophages, and plasma cells (Figure 1). In those cases of moderate acute rejection

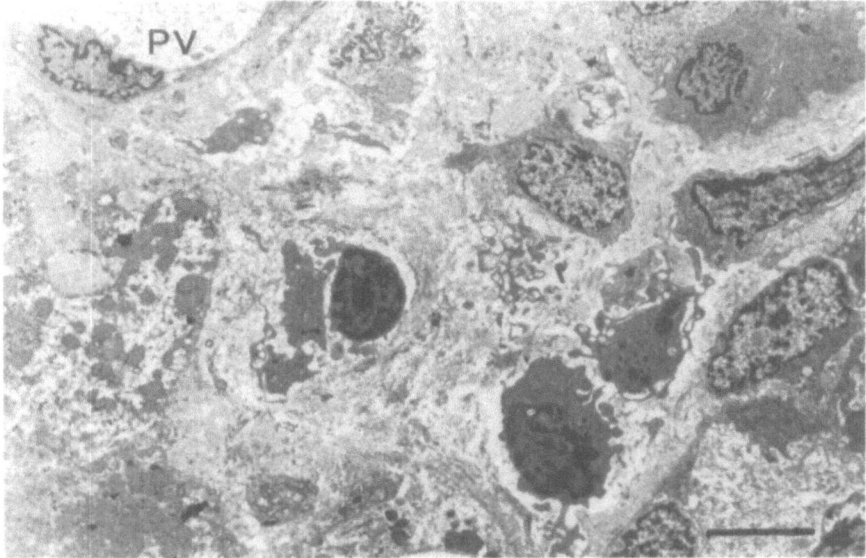

Figure 1. Mononuclear cell infiltration of a portal tract indicates acute rejection 7 days after transplantation. PV = portal vein.

these cells were diffusely distributed in the liver lobules, whereas there was a more dense accumulation in massive acute rejection. Mononuclear cells could also be found in the sinusoids and in the spaces of Disse (Figure 2). Destruction of hepatocytes occurred preferably as zonal necrosis in the centre of the lobules (acinar zone 3). Single cell necrosis could be observed as well as focal or extended massive necrosis. Simultaneously an increase in Kupffer cell number was conspicuous. They were loaden with cell debris, bile pigments, and erythrocytes. Occasionally Kupffer cells just being in the process of phagocytosis of necrotic hepatocytes were detected (Figure 3). Frequently large gaps appeared in the sinusoidal endothelium (Figure 4) which also exhibited a disruption in the centrilobular (zone 3) areas.

It can be assumed that parenchymal cell necrosis is caused by cell mediated cytotoxicity, especially if mononuclear cells are in a direct contact or lie adjacent to liver cells. However, necrosis also appeared at sites where mononuclear cells were absent. Thus our findings confirm similar observations as described in other species after liver transplantation [1, 4, 5]. Moreover during acute rejection, microcirculatory disturbances in the liver sinusoids, caused by endothelial cell damage, formation of microthrombi, and swelling of Kupffer cells may induce pericentral hypoxemia which is leading to liver cell necrosis as well as to further lesions of the sinusoidal endothelium. It cannot be distinguished if sinusoidal cell necrosis in the grafted liver is only dependent on a cell mediated cytotoxic effect or if there is an additional ischemic damage. Therefore it is difficult to regard the 'sinusoidal type' of rejection [1] as a separate entity. Furthermore the integrity of the sinusoidal endothelium seems to be less important for the graft survival, as a conspicuous absence of the endothelium occurred in rat auxiliary liver grafts for several months [2, 6].

Portal edema
Frequently the cellular infiltration was associated with a widening of the portal lymphatics and an edema (Figure 5). However, edema also occurred in the absence of mononuclear infiltrates. In this respect one has to consider that due to the ligation of the lymph vessels of the donor liver a dilatation of the lymphatics and also an edema might develop. Therefore it cannot be assumed that it is a rejection-specific phenomenon [3].

Cholestasis
In the monkey liver acute rejection was frequently associated with centrilobular (zone 3) cholestasis (Figure 6). The dilated bile canaliculi contained an electron-dense, amorphous material. A complete loss of the microvilli of the canalicular membrane occurred. In addition a thickening of the 'terminal web' of the liver cell membrane was conspicuous (Figure 6). Our findings are in accordance with other observations of intrahepatic cholestasis after transplantation of the monkey liver [7]. Cholestasis has also been described as an acute rejection phenomenon in

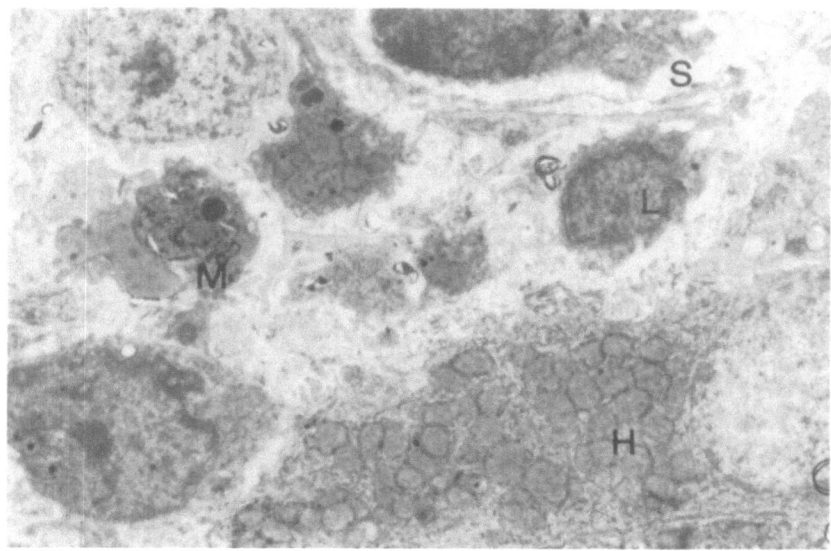

Figure 2. Lymphocytes (L) and macrophages (M) invade the space of Disse during acute rejection. S = sinusoid, H = hepatocyte.

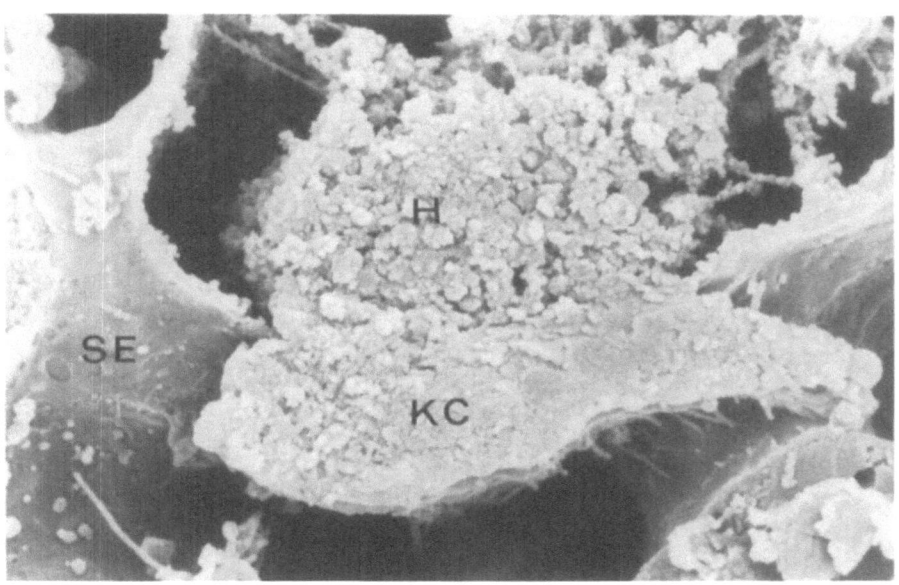

Figure 3. A Kupffer cell (KC) phagocytosing necrotic masses of a hepatocyte (H) during acute rejection. SE = sinusoidal endothelium.

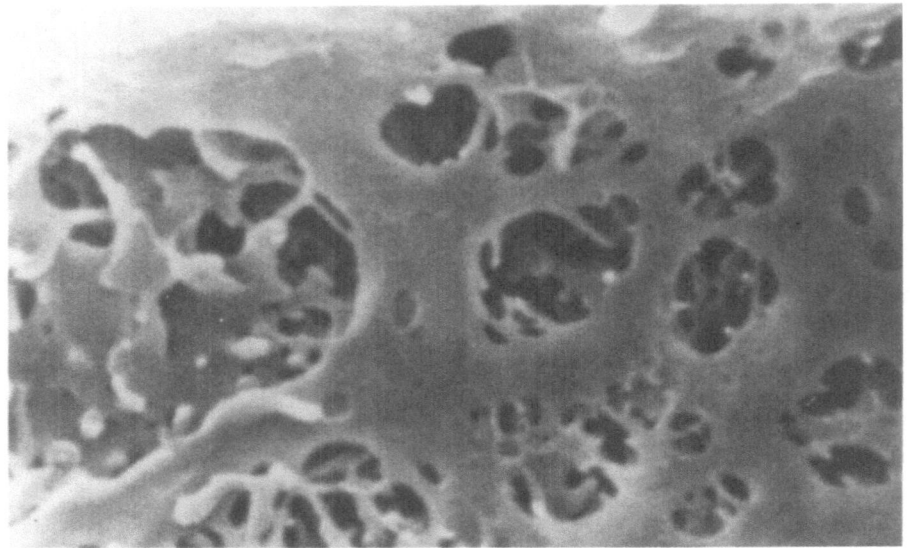

Figure 4. Large gaps in the sinusoidal endothelium indicate acute rejection.

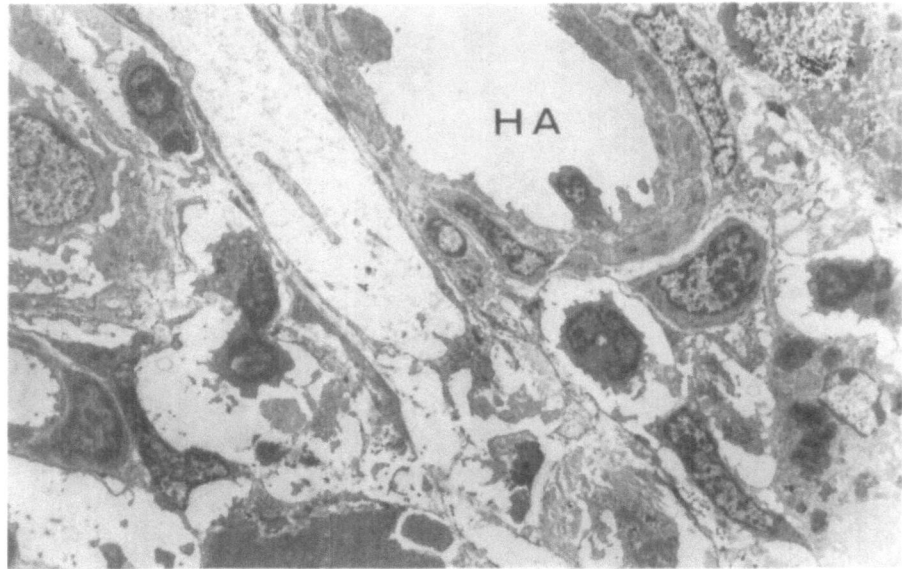

Figure 5. Cellular infiltration is associated with an edema of the portal-tract 7 days after transplantation. HA = hepatic artery.

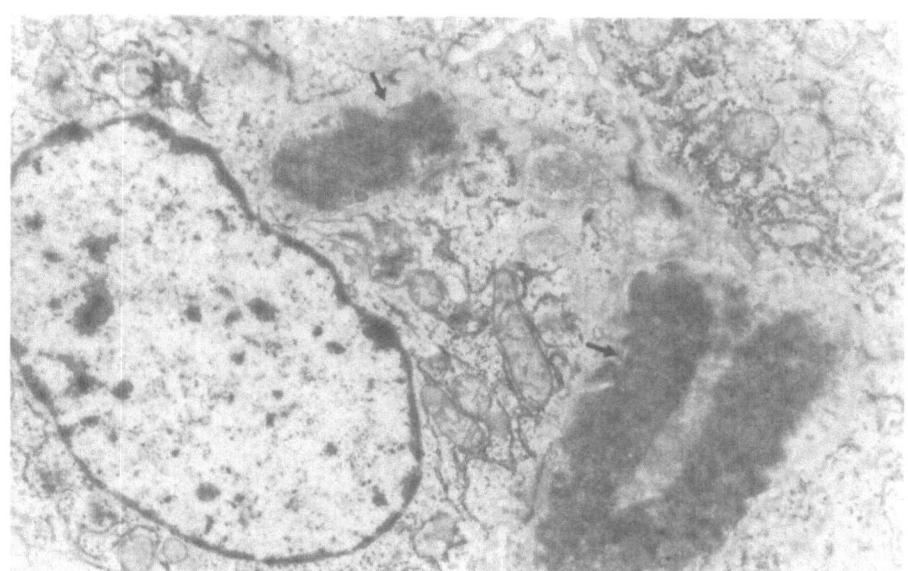

Figure 6. Cholestasis during acute rejection is characterized by dilated bile canaliculi containing electron dense amorphous material. Note the loss of microvilli of the canalicular membrane (arrows).

rats [8], dogs [1, 9, 10], and in humans [1, 11–13]. It is assumed that intrahepatic cholestasis is a consequence of cell mediated sensitivity to donor antigens. However, intrahepatic cholestasis after liver transplantation is also regarded as non-specific for allograft rejection, since foci of biliary acid necrosis and the proliferation of pseudo-bile ducts indicate a disturbance in bile flow [3].

Chronic rejection

Portal and intralobular fibrosis

In all liver biopsies of the long term survivors, taken at day 21 after transplantation, a moderate fibrosis of the portal tract could be detected which extended into the periportal areas. After 49 days portal tracts were enlarged by an increased amount of connective tissue and they were infiltrated by moderate numbers of small lymphocytes (Figure 7). The limiting plate was eroded, piecemeal necrosis occurred, and thin collagen septa extended into the liver lobule. A similarity to the histopathological feature of chronic active hepatitis was evident. Portal and periportal fibrosis are a direct consequence of chronic rejection. In contrast, the more pronounced perivenular fibrosis which was to be met in a few animals of the long term survivors, seemed to be the result of fibrous repair of former pericentral necrosis during a phase of acute rejection. Similar findings have been described by other authors [1, 3, 14].

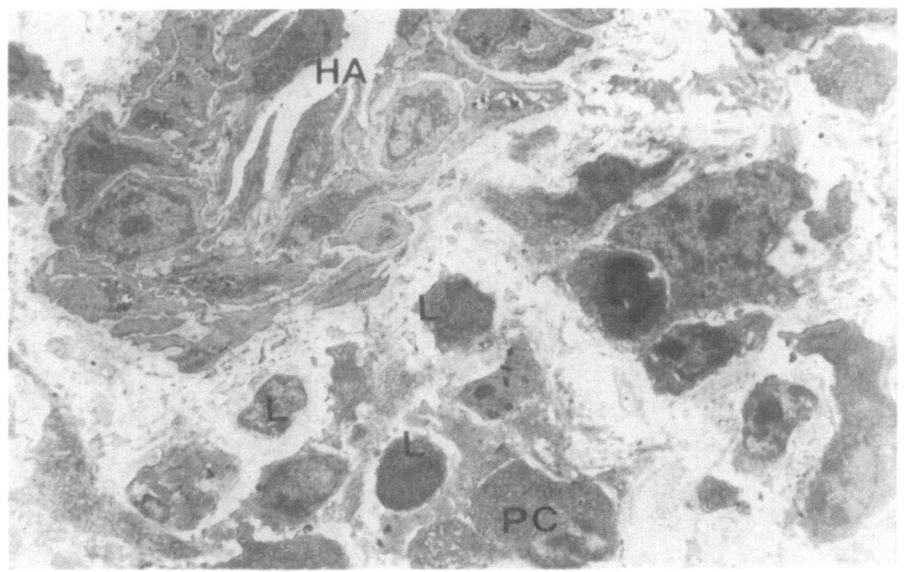

Figure 7. 49 days after transplantation small lymphocytes (L) and plasma cells (PC) infiltrate the portal tract. Lymphocytes also invade the wall of the hepatic artery (HA).

During chronic rejection hepatocyte destruction also appeared as focal or single cell necrosis (Figure 8) in the liver lobule. Electron microscopy revealed an increase in the number of perisinusoidal cells in these areas. Frequently these cells which are located in the space of Disse, showed an elongation of their subendothelial processes (Figure 8). The latter spread into the spaces previously taken by the necrotic hepatocytes. Dense connective tissue bundles were in association with the surfaces of the subendothelial processes of perisinusoidal cells. Obviously the intralobular fibrosis can be ascribed to the reaction of this kind of mesenchymal cells. A similar observation has been described for the chronic rejection of the transplanted human liver [15].

Vascular changes of hepatic arteries
During chronic rejection small branches of the hepatic arteries were also affected. The vessel walls exhibited a cellular infiltration with lymphoid cells (Figure 7). It may be assumed that this stage precedes more severe vascular injuries which might lead to a narrowing or occlusion of small hepatic arteries. The resulting circulatory disturbances in the graft may cause hypoxic damage of the parenchyma up to segmental infarction. In fact, such vaso-occlusive changes, characteristic for chronic rejection of the liver, have been observed in other species [1, 3]. It is speculated that this manifestation of rejection is brought about by circulating antibody, as an accumulation of IgG and complement could be demonstrated in the vessel wall [1].

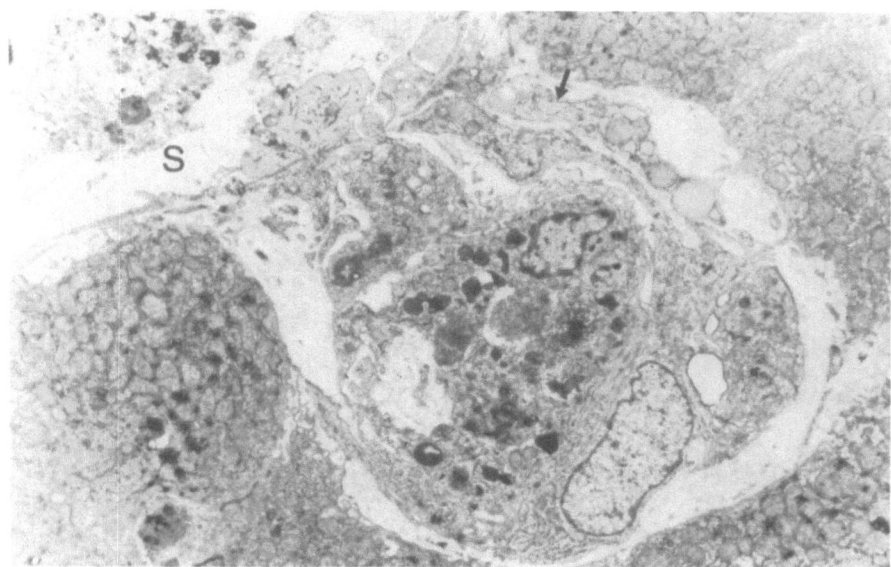

Figure 8. Single cell necrosis of a hepatocyte during chronic rejection. Note the increase of reticular fibres around the necrotic cell. A cell process of a perisinusoidal cell reveals a dilated rough endoplasmic reticulum (arrow). S = sinusoidal lumen.

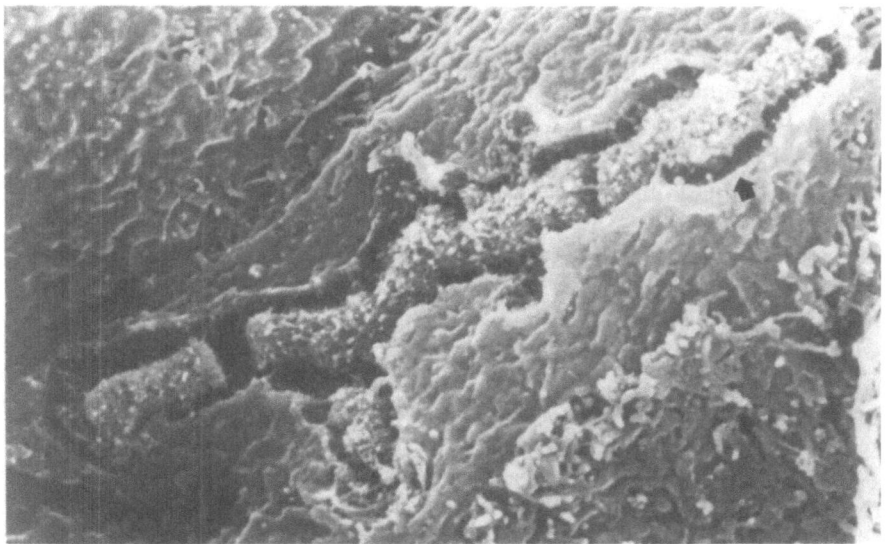

Figure 9. Intrahepatic cholestasis during chronic rejection. Inspissated bile occurs in the bile canaliculi. Note the loss of microvilli of the canalicular membrane (arrow).

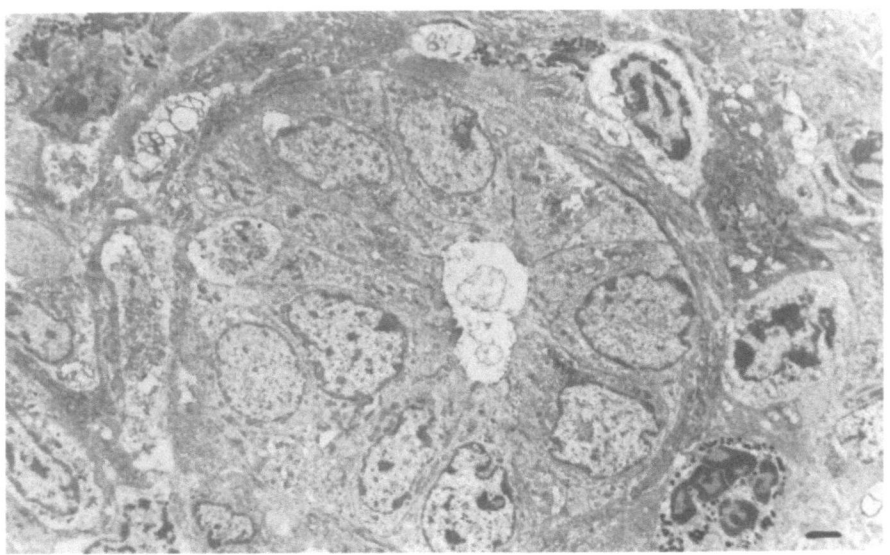

Figure 10. Bile duct 49 days after transplantation. A loss of the microvilli becomes evident. Note the periductular accumulation of lymphocytes and granulocytes.

Cholestasis

As in acute rejection intrahepatic cholestasis appeared in chronic rejection of the graft. Occasionally inspissated bile filled out the dilated canaliculi (Figure 9). Bile ducts in the portal tracts were less frequently affected. They exhibited a narrow lumen with a significant loss of microvilli. However, junctional complexes between the ductular cells seemed to be intact. An increase of lymphoid cells in the periductular tissue was evident (Figure 10). Similar findings have been reported for the transplanted human liver [1].

References

1. Porter KA: Pathology of the orthotopic homograft and heterograft. In: Starzl TE, Putnam CW (eds.) Experiences in hepatic transplantation. Philadelphia, Saunders, 1969, pp 422–471.
2. Jap P, Jerusalem C, Hess F, Heyde van der MN: Ultrastructural and histochemical investigations on long surviving rat auxiliary liver homografts. Cytobiol 5:165–180, 1972.
3. Jerusalem CHR, Jap PHK: General pathology of the transplantation reaction in experimental and clinical organ grafts. In: Altmann HW, Büchner F, Cottier H, Grundmann E, Holle G, Letterer E, Masshoff W, Meesen H, Roulet F, Seifert G, Siebert G (eds.) Handbuch der allgemeinen Pathologie VI/8. Berlin, Springer, 1977, pp 439–615.
4. Roessner A, Lie TS, Schulz DV, Bassewitz DB, Themann H: Zur Feinstruktur der orthotop transplantierten allogenen Hundeleber. Virchows Arch (Zellpathol) 9:354–370, 1971.

5. Roessner A, Lie TS, Schulz DV, Bassewitz DB, Themann H: The ultrastructure of the orthotopic transplanted allogeneic dog liver. In: Lie TS, Gütgemann A (eds.) Liver transplantation. Baden-Baden, Witzstrock, 1974, pp 131–133.

6. Warnier B, Jerusalem C, Jap P, Hess F, Heyde van de MN: The ultrastructural and histochemical aspect of auxiliary heterotopic rat liver homografts up to 22 months. In: Lie TS, Gütgemann A (eds.) Liver transplantation. Baden-Baden, Witzstrock, 1974, pp 135–141.

7. Myburgh JA, Abrahams C, Mendelsohn D, Mieny CJ, Bersohn J: Cholestatic phenomenon in hepatic allograft rejection in the primate. Trans Proc 3:501–504, 1971.

8. Jap PHK: Ultrastructural and histochemical investigations on auxiliary liver grafts in rats with some notes on the application to other species. Nijmegen, The Netherlands, Thesis, 1971.

9. McBride RA, Wheeler HB, Smith LL: Homotransplantation of the canine liver as an orthotopic vascularized graft: histologic and functional correlation during residence in the new host. Am J Pathol 41:501–519, 1962.

10. Alican F, Hardy J: Replantation of the liver in dogs. J Surg Res 7:368–375, 1967.

11. Waldram R, Williams R, Calne RY: Bile composition and bile cast formation after transplantation of the liver in man. Transplantation 19:382–387, 1975.

12. Waldram R, Williams R: Cholestasis after liver transplantation: Respective roles of rejection, hepatotoxicity, and impaired bile salt secretion. In: Gentilini P, Teodori U, Gorini S, Popper H (eds.) Intrahepatic cholestasis. New York, Raven Press, 1975, pp 93–103.

13. Starzl TE, Porter KA, Putman CW, Schröter GPJ, Halgrimson CG, Weil R, Hoelscher M, Reid HAS: Orthotopic liver transplantation in ninety-three patients. Surg Gynecol Obstet 142:487–505, 1976.

14. Williams R, Calne RY, Ansell ID, Ashby BS, Cullum PA, Dawson JL, Eddleston ALWF, Evans DB, Flute PT, Herbertson PM, Joysey V, McGregor AMC, Millard PR, Murray-Lyon IM, Pena JR, Rake MO, Sells RA: Liver transplantation in man. III. Studies of liver function, histology and immunosuppressive therapy. Br Med J 3:12–19, 1969.

15. Vonnahme FJ: The structure and functions of subendothelial processes of perisinusoidal cells in human liver disease. In: Knook DL, Wisse E (eds.) Kupffer cells and other sinusoidal cells. Amsterdam, Elsevier/North Holland, 1982.

6. Fine needle aspiration cytology and histology of liver allografts in the pig

K. HÖCKERSTEDT, I. LAUTENSCHLAGER, J. AHONEN, P. HÄYRY, C. KORSBÄCK, R. ORKO, K. SALMELA, B. SCHEININ, T.M. SCHEININ and E. TASKINEN

Introduction

In liver transplantation the diagnosis of rejection is difficult to establish by clinical findings and biochemical tests only [1. 2], and therefore needle biopsy of the liver often has to be obtained. Since the biopsy cannot be performed in every instance without danger to the patient, new diagnostic tools are needed.

Fine needle aspiration biopsy (FNAB) [3–5] has been used in human kidney transplants in Helsinki more than 5000 times. In this study the FNAB-technique has been further developed to assess intra-graft events in the pig liver transplant. The findings are correlated to biochemical tests and the morphological picture obtained by needle biopsy of the transplant.

Materials and methods

Random-bred piglets of 18–28 kg in body weight of both sexes underwent orthotopic liver transplantation using a porto-jugular shunt. The piglets were divided in three groups: I, piglets which received no immunosuppression (n = 9), II, piglets receiving 10 mg/kg/d of intravenous Cyclosporine A (CyA) on days 0–7 (n = 5), and III, piglets where an autotransplantation was performed by re-implantation of a liver which had been procured, perfused and handled as a liver allograft (except the supra-hepatic vena cava was clamped only and not cut). During the operation the piglets received 700–1100 ml donor blood, dextrose saline and plasma expanders when necessary. Kefalotin 60 mg/kg/d and Cime-tidine (10 mg/kg/d were administrated intravenously on days 0–2 after transplantation. The per- and postoperative changes in the serum electrolyte and blood glucose levels were corrected with intravenous infusions.

Fine needle aspiration biopsies and blood specimens

Fine needle aspiration biopsy of the liver was performed on days 0, 2, 4, 7, 10, 14, 21 and 28 after which the animals were killed. The method of obtaining the FNAB and processing the material has been described in detail [4, 5]. A 10–20 μl cell sample of the liver containing about 300,000–600,000 cells were taken percutaneously by suction using a 0.6 mm external diameter spinal needle. In order to adjust the in situ inflammatory events to blood background, another sample was taken from the peripheral blood. The specimens were drawn in hepesbuffered RPMI-1640 tissue culture medium containing human albumin and heparin and then cytocentrifuged onto microscopic slides using a Shandon® cytocentrifuge and finally stained with May-Grünwald-Giemsa [5]. The number of hepatocytes and endothelial cells were recorded for representativity of the liver sample.

The inflammatory white cells were visualized by the 'increment' method [5] by subtracting blood background from the FNAB differential counts. It has earlier been described that this increment gives a good picture of the inflammatory events in the kidney allograft [5]. More emphasis is given to the cell types known to be important in rejection and less emphasis on those known or suspected not to have a clear role in the rejection. The following correction factors have been used: the number of T and B blast cells have been multiplied by 1, the lymphocytes by 0.1, monocytes by 0.2 and macrophages by 1 [4]. The sum of the corrected increment values, the total corrected increment, represents the total inflammation.

Histological specimens

Transcutaneous needle biopsies or open biopsies of the liver transplant were taken on the day of operation and on days 7 [8], 14 and 28 in surviving piglets or at autopsy from those animals which died before 28 days. A light Ketamine chlorid (Ketalar®, Parke-Davies, Morris Plains, U.S.A.) anesthezia was employed. The specimens were fixed in 4% formaldehyde, embedded in paraffin and 4 μm thick sections were cut and stained with haematoxyline-eosin. Coded specimens were evaluated by one single pathologist (E.T.) only.

Blood chemistry

The reference values of s-ASAT was 8–36 U/l, s-ALAT 8–40 U/l and s-Alk. Phosph. 60–280 U/l at 37° C for man.

Statistical analysis

The two-tailed Student's t-test was used for estimating probabilities.

Results

Mortality

Three early deaths (<8 days) occurred, autopsy revealed a dense liver and ascites in all animals. One piglet died after 2 weeks of perforated gastric ulcer. All deaths occurred in the non-immunosuppressed group.

Fine needle aspiration biopsy cytology

The major cytological events in the pig liver transplant of non-immunosuppressed and sham-operated piglets are shown in Figure 1. Transplantation was followed by a prompt inflammatory episode while no inflammatory cells were recorded in the sham-operated autograft. In those animals which survived the first week (n = 6) the inflammation peaked on day 7 whereafter it declined. All inflammatory components of rejection, including blast cells, plasma cells, lymphocytes and cells of the mononuclear lineage were recorded in the inflammatory picture. This inflammation occurred earlier and was more severe in those piglets which died than in those which survived.

Administration of CyA on days 0–7 significantly depressed and delayed the first episode of inflammation (day 4, $p = 0.02$, day 7, $p = 0.06$) (Figure 2). Compared to the non-immunosuppressed animals, both the blastogenic and the mononuclear phagocyte components of the inflammatory episode were significantly suppressed.

Some typical samples in FNAB of the pig liver transplant are shown in Figure 3. No cytological changes occurred in the blood.

FNAB-correlations to biopsy histology

The characteristic findings in concomitantly obtained histological specimens were as follows: Right after the operation (day 0) some sinusoidal congestion and parenchymal bleeding was observed, probably representing the operative procedure itself since these were noted both in the autograft and the allograft. No signs of inflammation were noted in the biopsies or in the FNAB-specimens.

In the three animals which died within a week, probably in 'irreversible rejection', parenchymal bleeding and hepatocyte necrosis as well as accumulation

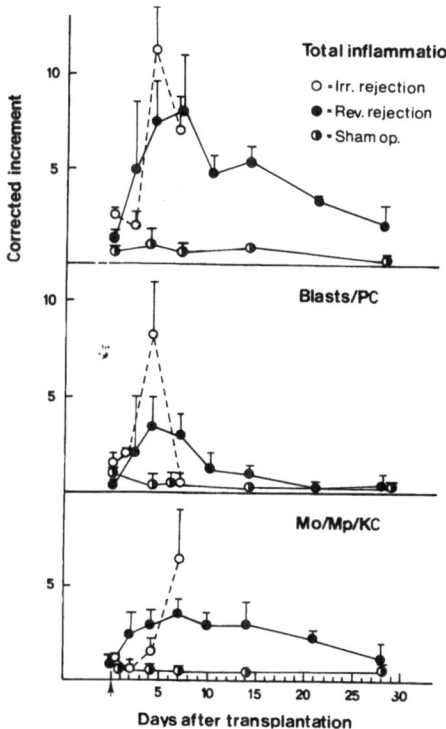

Figure 1. The inflammatory changes in the liver visualized in the FNAB with the increment method (mean ± SEM) in allografts dying during signs of acute rejection (open circles), surviving allograft recipients (closed circles) and sham-operated autograft recipients (half-closed circles). Top section: total inflammation, middle section: blast cells and plasma cells, bottom section: mononuclear phagocytes.

of leukocytes especially in the portal area were observed. This correlates rather well with the FNAB-finding of the inflammatory cells. In the surviving non-immunosuppressed piglets the inflammatory changes and hepatocyte necrosis were modest and usually only slight parenchymal changes were histologically recorded during and after the inflammatory episode seen in the FNAB. Both in irreversible and reversible rejection the inflammatory cells also tended to infiltrate the walls of the intrahepatic bile ducts.

In piglets immunosuppressed with CyA inflammatory cells were seen in the portal area while in the liver parenchyma the inflammation was less prominent. The inflammatory findings persisted both in the histological specimens and in the FNAB.

Practically no inflammation and no parenchymal cell changes were recorded in the autografts.

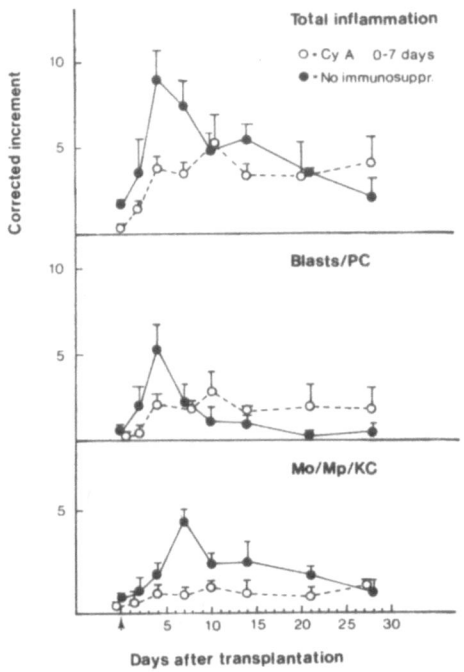

Figure 2. The intra-graft inflammatory events in non-immunosuppressed recipients (closed circles) and in recipients immunosuppressed with Cyclosporine A (open circles) (mean ± SEM). Top section: total inflammation, middle section: blast cells, bottom section: mononuclear phagocytes.

Blood chemistry

The value of s-ASAT, s-ALAT and s-Alk. Phosph. were similar in the recipients of both liver allografts and autografts (Figure 3), although the levels were somewhat higher in the allografts. The changes did not correlate with cytological or histological evidence of rejection. The highest s-ASAT and s-ALAT values were recorded on the second postoperative day, whereas s-Alk. Phosph. peaked on day 7.

Discussion

The cytological pattern of inflammation in liver allograft in the pig was very similar to that reported earlier for renal transplant rejection in both experimental animals [6] and man [5, 7]. At early stages lymphocytes and monocytes dominate with a blastogenic component consisting of (T) lymphoblasts and (B) plasmablasts. Along with advancing inflammation the frequency of blast cells de-

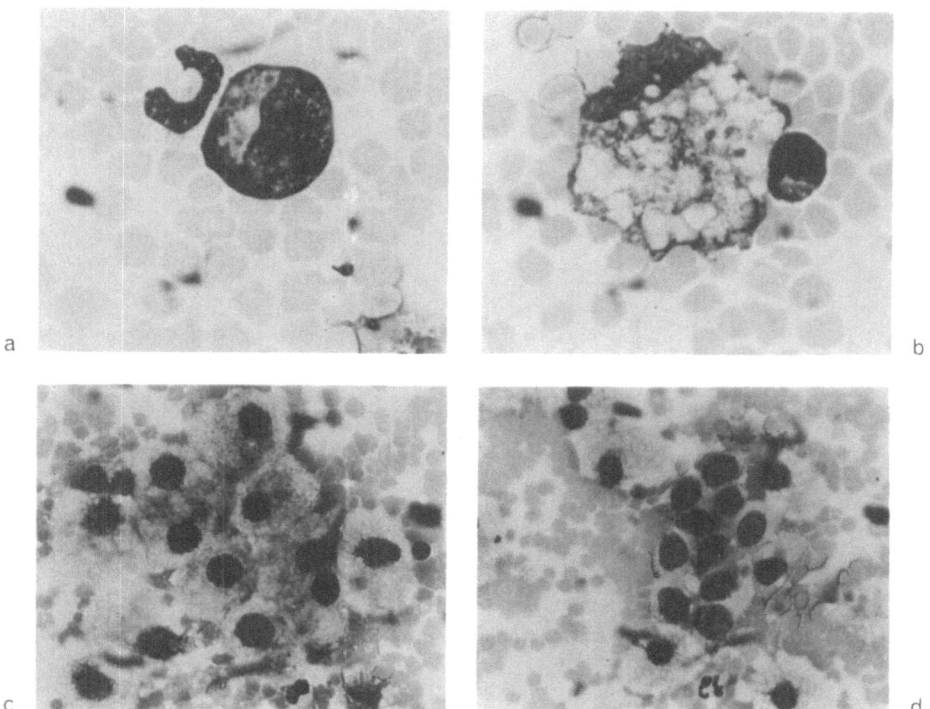

Figure 3. Some typical samples in FNAB of the pig liver transplant. (a) a plasmablast and a granulocyte (×1000), (b) a macrophage and a lymphocyte (×1000), (c) a group of hepatocytes (×400), (d) a group of endothelial cells (×400).

clines, more mononuclear phagocytes appear in the graft and the maturation of blood borne monocytes into tissue macrophages is the most significant cytological marker of irreversible rejection.

Porter [8] has described the pathological changes occurring in the liver transplant of different species. In the canine liver specific changes are seen after the third day. Mononuclear cells accumulate around the portal area and central veins and macrophages are common especially in the portal tracts. The accumulation of mononuclear cells reaches its maximum about 6 days after transplantation and is followed by centrizonal liver necrosis and death of centrilobular hepatocytes. In the porcine liver allografts the morphological changes were similar but less prominent.

In our pig transplants the histological changes were similar to those reported by Porter. Moreover, some correlation was noted between the histological and cytological findings in non-immunosuppressed animals both in those which died as well as in those which survived. A slightly increased amount of inflammatory cells was seen in those which died, especially in the portal area. The con-

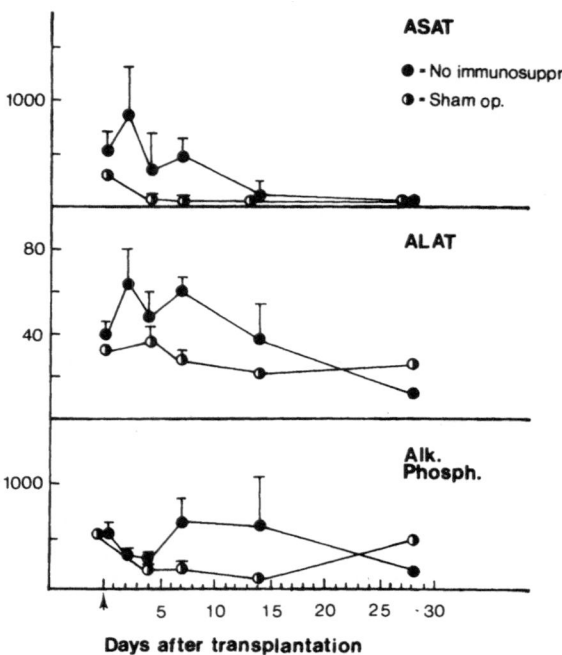

Figure 4. Biochemical markers of liver function, s-ASAT, s-ALAT and s-Alk. Phosph. (mean ± SEM) in non-immunosuppressed allograft recipients (closed circles) and in sham-operated controls (half-closed circles).

comitantly obtained cytological specimens revealed a higher degree of inflammation in those which died compared to those who survived. These differences were particularly pronounced in regard to two types of inflammation: blast cells and macrophages.

On the other hand, the correlation between the histological and cytological observations was less clear when the non-immunosuppressed animals were compared to those receiving CyA. A relatively modest cytological episode of inflammation was seen in the CyA group, but the histological findings were far more prominent resembling those of non-immunosuppressed animals. This might be explained by the fact that in the FNAB different inflammatory cells are given different correction factors according to their diagnostic significance, whereas in the histological preparation a numerical differentiation of the inflammatory cell subgroups could not be performed. It should also be noted that the inflammatory changes in the liver had no correlation with the cytological changes in the blood and only a marginal, if any, correlation to the level of three commonly used biochemical markers of liver function: s-ASAT, s-ALAT and s-Alk. Phosph.

As no complications occurred during the aspiration biopsy procedures, we conclude that FNAB and the cytological evaluation of the specimen is a useful and safe method to assess intragraft inflammatory parameters of a pig liver transplant.

Summary

We have analyzed the inflammatory changes in pig liver allografts and autografts by fine needle aspiration biopsy (FNAB) and correlated the cytological findings to transplant histology and to biochemical changes in the recipient blood. In non-immunosuppressed piglets (n = 9) the inflammatory episode of rejection occurred promptly, peaked at the end of the first week, whereafter it subsided in those grafts which were accepted by the host. The inflammatory infiltrate consisted of all major types of leukocytes including (T) lymphoblasts, (B) plasmablasts and plasma cells, lymphocytes and monocytes. Macrophages dominated the late inflammatory picture of irreversible rejection. In those piglets who lost their graft (n = 3) the inflammation peaked earlier and the total amount of inflammation was higher. In sham-operated autograft recipients (n = 3) no inflammation was recorded in the graft. Cyclosporine A (n = 5) significantly suppressed the total inflammation during the administration period of seven days, delayed the peak of both the blastogenic and the mononuclear phagocyte components. These inflammatory changes showed a fairly close correlation to biopsy histology in the non-immunosuppressed animals where irreversible rejection was characterized by hepatocyte necrosis, parenchymal bleeding and inflammatory changes in the portal tract. The changes in s-ASAT, s-ALAT and s-alkaline phosphatase (APh) bore no correlation with the episodes of rejection.

References

1. Terblanche J, Koep L, Starzl T: Liver transplantation. Symposium on the Treatment of Liver Diseases, Medical Clinics of NA, 63:507, 1979.
2. Calne RY, Williams R: Liver transplantation. Current problems in surgery. Year Book Medical Publishers, Chicago, 16:1, 1979.
3. Pasternack A, Virolainen M, Häyry P: Fine needle aspiration biopsy in the diagnosis of human renal allograft rejection. J Urol 109:167, 1979.
4. Häyry P, v Willebrand E: Monitoring of human renal allograft rejection with fine-needle aspiration cytology. Scand J Immunol 13:87, 1981.
5. Häyry P, v Willebrand E: Practical guidelines for fine needle aspiration biopsy of human renal allografts. Ann Clin Res 13:288, 1981.
6. v Willebrand E, Soots A, Häyry P: In situ effector mechanism in rat kidney allograft rejection. III. Kinetics of the inflammatory response and generation of donor-directed killer cells. Scand J Immunol 10:95, 1979.
7. v Willebrand E: Fine needle aspiration cytology of human renal transplants. Clin Immunol Immunopathol 17:309, 1980.
8. Porter KA: Pathology of liver transplantation. Transplant Rev 2:129, 1969.

Section 3

RESPONSES DURING LIVER TRANSPLANTATION

7. Liver transplantation: Pathophysiology of the anhepatic phase

J.V. FARMAN, M.J. LINDOP, F.J. CARMICHAEL and M.R. HARRISON

Introduction

The physiological changes seen in liver transplantation are the most dramatic encountered in any operation [1]. They include a sudden and prolonged reduction in venous return to the heart (while the inferior vena cava is clamped), heavy and often rapid blood loss and acute biochemical changes when the newly inserted liver is first perfused.

This paper describes the changes in cardiovascular and metabolic function seen during the operation, discusses how these arise and refers to the techniques employed to limit or manage the problems that result.

Monitoring

Continuous recording is essential during an operation where cardiovascular parameters may change so very rapidly.

Arterial pressure is recorded directly from a radial cannula and central venous pressure from a catheter in the superior vena cava. The ECG is continuously monitored. Recently we have routinely employed a Swan Ganz catheter which enables us to measure cardiac output and pulmonary artery pressure. Expired carbon dioxide concentration (sampled at the catheter mount) is continuously measured with an infra-red analyser. These signals are displayed on an oscilloscope and simultaneously recorded on a multi-channel recorder. The slowest recorder speed, 0.1 mm/min, is used in order to achieve the greatest possible data compression. Digital displays of systolic arterial pressure, mean venous pressure and heart rate are also available. Arterial blood samples are taken at intervals [2]. for analysis of serum electrolyte concentration, acid-base state, blood glucose level and clotting factors. Blood loss is assessed by swab weighing and by measuring suction bottle contents. Temperature is measured by means of an electrothermometer probe placed in the oesophagus.

Records from liver transplants in the Cambridge series were examined and a number selected for detailed analysis of cardiovascular changes.

Cardiovascular responses in the anhepatic phase

The work of Cullen [3] suggests that a fall in systolic arterial pressure is associated with reduction in the stroke volume of the heart. The application of clamps to the inferior vena cava completely cuts off the venous return flow from the lower half of the body. A reduction of carbon dioxide output occurred in the absence of any change in ventilation and before the fall in body temperature which follows insertion of the new liver [4]. We therefore concluded that these changes must be due to a fall in pulmonary blood flow (and therefore of cardiac output) during the anhepatic period. If it is assumed that the normal hepatic blood flow is of the order of 1.2 l/min via the portal vein and 0.3 l/min via the hepatic artery, and that the flow in the infra-hepatic vena cava at rest is 1.5 l/min, then the flow through the inferior vena cava will have been approximately 3 l/min. If the total resting cardiac output were 5 l/min, clamping will cause a three fifths reduction in flow. Patterson and Starling showed in 1915 the clear cut dependence of cardiac output upon venous return flow [5]. The reduction in venous pressure supports the idea that cardiac output falls as a result of the reduction in venous return. However, the changes seen were less consistent than those of arterial pressure, largely because of attempts to increase venous return by rapid transfusion of stored blood. We have usually achieved a net overtransfusion of approximately 1.5 l before cross clamping, in anticipation of these changes. However this part of the operation is often accompanied by heavy bleeding and calculated blood loss may fall behind actual blood loss at this time.

Table 1 shows the cardiovascular parameters measured in seven liver transplant

Table 1. Arterial pressure, systolic (SP) and diastolic (DP), central venous pressure (CVP), pulmonary wedge pressure (PWP), cardiac index (CI), stroke volume (SV), and systemic vascular resistance (SVR) prior to clamping and following the clamping of the inferior vena cava. (N = 7; means ± SE).

	pre-clamping	post-clamping
Arterial pressure SP mm Hg	135 ± 11	104 ± 11[a]
DP mm Hg	76 ± 6	70 ± 6 N.S.
CVP cm H_2O	10.5 ± 1.9	8.6 ± 1.3 N.S.
PWP cm H_2O	11.5 ± 2.5	6.4 ± 1.1[a]
CI l/min/m^2	5.1 ± 0.4	2.6 ± 0.2[b]
SV ml	80 ± 5	39 ± 5[b]
SVR dyne · s^{-5} · cm	790 ± 64	1443 ± 135[b]

[a] $p < 0.05$ compared to pre-clamping (Student T-test).
[b] $p < 0.01$ compared to pre-clamping (Student T-test).
N.S. not significantly different from pre-clamping.

recipients, just prior to clamping of the inferior vena cava and immediately following caval clamping. There was about a 30% fall in systolic pressure on caval clamping. Values for cardiac output were in the region of 5 l/min/m² prior to clamping, falling to around 3 l/min/m² in the anhepatic period. The heart rate is usually seen to increase after caval clamping and this is confirmed by the fall in stroke volume, which is proportionately greater than the fall in output. As would be expected, systemic vascular resistance, is enormously increased when the output falls. In case there is any doubt about the cause of the reduced cardiac output, the fall in pulmonary wedge pressure shown in Table 1 confirms that this is the result of inadequate left atrial filling pressure.

The typical response. Figure 1 shows the usual pattern of arterial and venous pressures, and expired CO_2 concentration, recorded in the theatre on a multi-channel recorder.

Prior to removal of the liver, clamps are applied to the hepatic artery, portal vein, infrahepatic vena cava and suprahepatic vena cava. When the infrahepatic

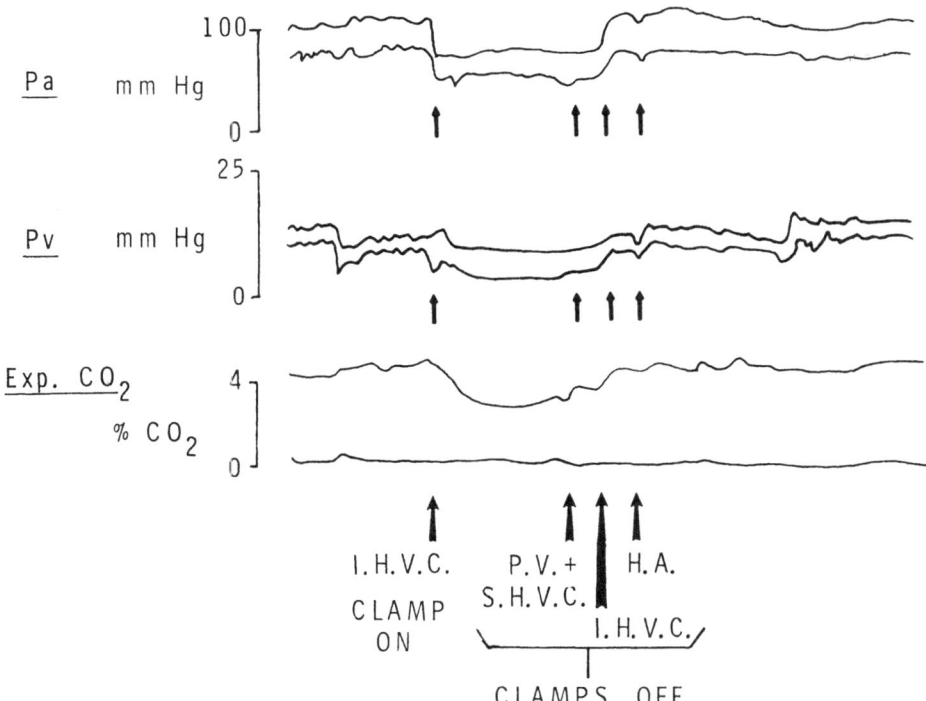

Figure 1. Tracing from a chart recording of Pa (arterial pressure mm Hg), Pv (central venous pressure, mm Hg) and expired CO_2 concentration (percent). Arrows mark the clamping of the I.H.V.C. (Infrahepatic vena cava) and the removal of clamps from the P.V. (Portal vein) and S.H.V.C. (suprahepatic vena cava), I.H.V.C. and H.A. (hepatic artery).

vena cava is clamped, there is a sudden fall in both superior vena caval pressure and systolic blood pressure. Expired CO_2 concentration also declines rapidly, in association with the reduction in cardiac output. The liver is then removed. During the anhepatic period, the arterial and central venous pressures and cardiac output remain low despite increased rates of transfusion. After insertion of the donor liver, the clamps on the portal vein and suprahepatic vena cava are the first to be removed. In some cases there is a fall in systolic blood pressure and rise in central venous pressure, while in others there is only a slight rise in both. When the infrahepatic vena cava is anastomosed and unclamped, however, there is a rise (usually large) in arterial and venous pressures and in expired CO_2 concentration. The pressures resume their preclamping levels, and there may be an 'overswing' of CO_2 excretion. Lastly, the hepatic artery anastomsis is unclamped. This may be followed by a transient fall in blood pressure, lasting only a minute or two. Arterial pressure changes are shown in Figure 2.

Budd-Chiari syndrome. The majority of the patients had no significant preoperative cardiovascular disturbances. However, patients with Budd-Chiari syndrome suffering from inferior vena caval thrombosis did not show these dramatic falls in pressure when the inferior vena cava was cross clamped. Changes in inferior vena caval flow would not be expected in these circumstances. Figure 3 shows the lack of response to clamping in one of these patients.

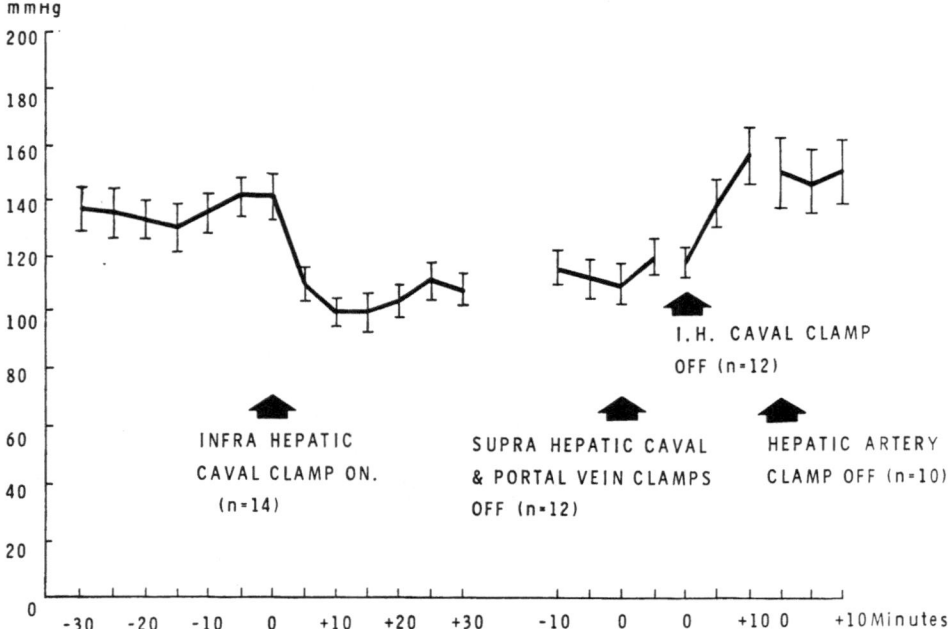

Figure 2. Systolic arterial pressures during liver transplantation (means ± SE). The timescale in each case has been zeroed with reference to the placing or removal of the clamp.

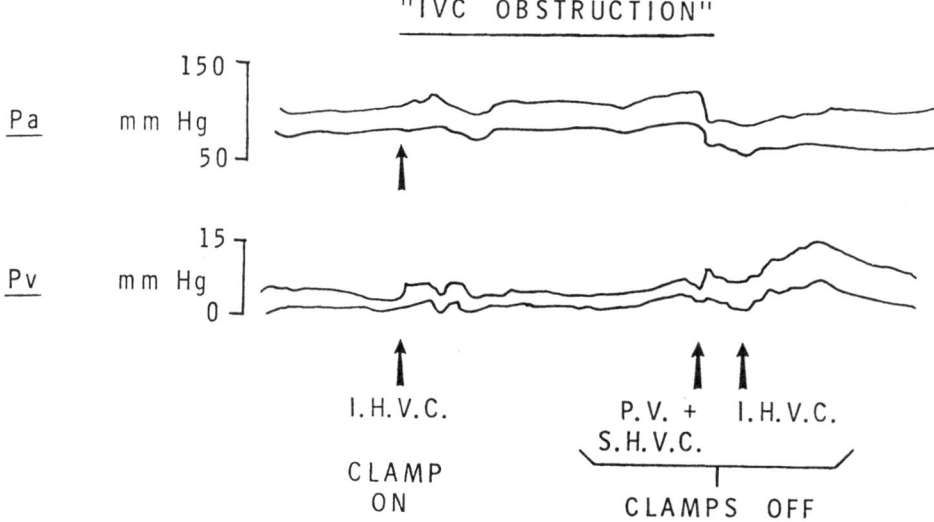

Figure 3. Tracing from a chart recording of Pa (arterial pressure) and Pv (central venous pressure), both in mm Hg, in a patient with pre-operative inferior vena caval obstruction. Placing and removing clamps caused little change in pressures although arterial pressure fell after revascularisation of the liver.

Cirrhosis. Cirrhotic patients present a complex of pre-operative cardiovascular abnormalities. Portal vein obstruction may be the main feature and several of our patients had had porto-caval shunts. We have noted that some of these patients likewise show little change in pressures when the inferior vena cava is clamped, presumably because there is little or no resulting change in inferior vena caval flow. An example is shown in Figure 4, a 37-year-old man with cirrhosis. The position is complicated by the existence of numerous anastomotic vessels in the abdominal wall which may present the surgeon with considerable difficulty. Inferior vena caval pressure may be raised as a result of the obstruction and should be measured before operation. Finally, these patients because of their poor liver function tend to develop coagulopathy which can contribute to heavy bleeding at this time. Rapid transfusion of stored blood is needed.

Metabolic responses

Potassium and hydrogen ions. As in any preserved organ the liver cells cease to function during preservation. The ionic pumps in the cell membranes no longer maintain the high concentrations of potassium and hydrogen characteristic of the intracellular environment. These ions leak out into the extracellular fluid, while presumably sodium simultaneously enters the cells. It is worth noting that pre-

PORTAL HYPERTENSION

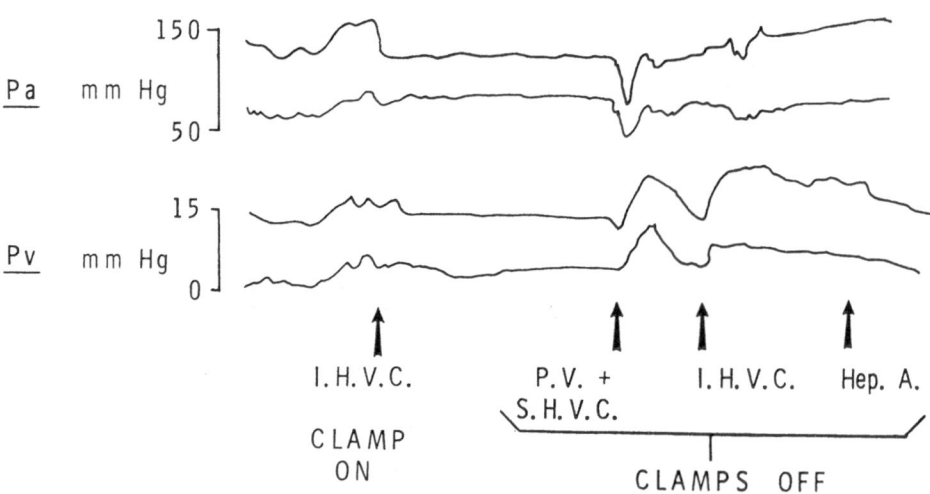

Figure 4. Tracing from a chart recording made during operation on a 37-year-old cirrhotic. There was little change in arterial pressure (Pa) or venous pressure (Pv) during the anhepatic period. Removal of the portal vein (PV) and supra-hepatic caval (SHVC) clamps was followed by a short episode of myocardial failure.

served red blood cells behave in an exactly similar way. However in the case of the liver we are dealing with an extremely large organ, weighing up to 2 kg, with an extracellular fluid volume of around 500 ml. From this it can be calculated that up to 150 nanomoles of hydrogen ions will be released when it is revascularised. In the case of potassium the extra-cellular fluid, as judged by the concentration of the effluent contains 20 mmol/l, so around 10 mmol will enter the circulation on revascularisation. We have confirmed these effects, which we believe to be responsible for the initial fall in arterial pressure seen after unclamping, by observation of the T-wave of the ECG. This can usually be seen to undergo enlargement, up to a maximum of 0.5 mv for a minute or two after unclamping as shown in Figure 5. At the same time, blood concentrations of these ions reach their maximum values [4].

Glucose. Our fear in the beginning was that the patients might become hypo-glycaemic during the anhepatic phase. In practice the glucose level rises during the operation, including the anhepatic phase. We ascribe this in part to the low metabolic requirement of a paralysed anaesthetised patient but mainly to the glucose content of the stored anticoagulated blood we give. The level tends to fall however at the end of the operation, presumably as a result of uptake of glucose into the new liver (which does show some hepatocyte glycogen depletion) and possibly due to the resumption of metabolic demand. Indeed in the early days in

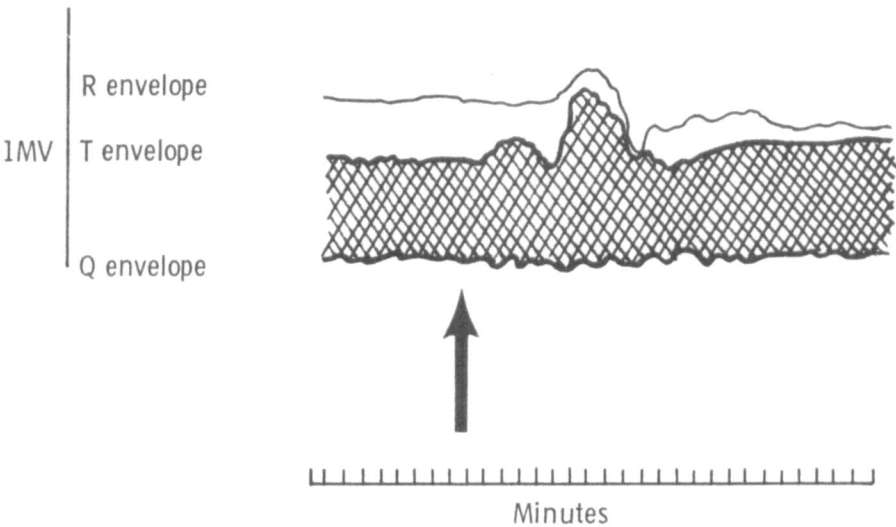

Figure 5. Tracing from a slow speed chart recording of the electrocardiogram. This shows the 'envelopes' of the R, T and Q waves, with the expansion of the T-wave after removal of the portal vein and supra-hepatic caval clamps (arrowed).

Denver two patients developed severe hypoglycaemia in the early postoperative period [6].

Temperature. A slow decline in body temperature is a common feature of long operations, especially when the abdominal contents are exposed. An additional factor in liver transplantation is the insertion of the ice-cold liver. To raise its temperature from 4°C to 37°C will therefore require 200–250 KJ (50–75 KCal). This heat must come from the recipient's body, the temperature of which will therefore fall by 1–2°C. Hypothermia will be encouraged by massive transfusion of stored blood. Unless this fall in temperature can be prevented recovery will be prejudiced.

Mitigating the pathophysiological effects of the operation

Managing of the circulation. First, the surgeon temporarily clamps the vena cava to allow the anaesthetist to judge the effect on the circulation. If the fall in arterial pressure is moderate, the surgeon then proceeds to divide the vena cava and to remove the liver. During the hepatectomy the inferior vena cava is opened; to eliminate risk of air embolus, it is important that the venous pressure is kept positive throughout this period [7]. If the fall is marked, the situation is reviewed and corrections made for any hypovolaemia or biochemical abnormality (see below). If clamping still causes profound hypotension, supportive femoro-femoral bypass is instituted before the final clamping and hepatectomy [8].

The patient loses little blood during the anhepatic phase since major vessels are visible and clamped while the cardiac output remains stable at its reduced level.

The first part of the circulation to be re-established is from the portal vein through the graft into the sub-diaphragmatic vena cava. When these anastomoses are completed the clamps are released. Despite the prior flushing of the graft with plasma, a considerable amount of cold, acid, hyperkalaemic blood passes directly into the right side of the heart. This usually causes hypotension accompanied by a rising venous pressure due to direct myocardial depression (Figure 6), although the heart may initially increase its output in response to the increased venous return. It is vital that this unclamping does not occur until the patient is absolutely stable.

Temperature control. The patients are placed on a water blanket which is maintained at 37° C. All blood and intravenous fluids are passed through a double length (4 m) Portex polypropylene warming coil [9] which lies in a warm water bath. This mitigates the fall in body temperature which inevitably occurs when the cold new liver is inserted. The patients usually return to normal by the end of the procedure.

Limiting the metabolic effects. The surgeon aims to limit the amount of handling received by the original liver and to delay the division of the hepatic artery, with the object of reducing the outflow of potassium and hydrogen ions, in the period leading up to the clamping of the inferior vena cava. The new liver must remain cold until re-vascularisation; however some measures can be taken to limit the passage of its extra-cellular fluid into the recipient. The suprahepatic cava and portal vein are anastomosed and the liver then perfused with one unit of plasma protein solution at 37° C. This will replace the major portion of the toxic fluid in the liver vasculature, which is allowed to run to waste via the temporarily

Table 2. Ionic contents of the plasma protein fraction (PPF) perfusate flushed through the donor liver and of the effluent, aspirated via the infra-hepatic cava, compared with the normal values found in arterial blood.

Fluid	Na+ mmol/l	K+ mmol/l	H+ nmol/l	Ca++ mmol/l
PPF	150	2	–	–
Effluent, Case 1	154	13.2	317	1.48
Efluent, Case 2	160	14	176	1.72
Normal values	132–142	3.4–5.0	36–45	2.0–2.6

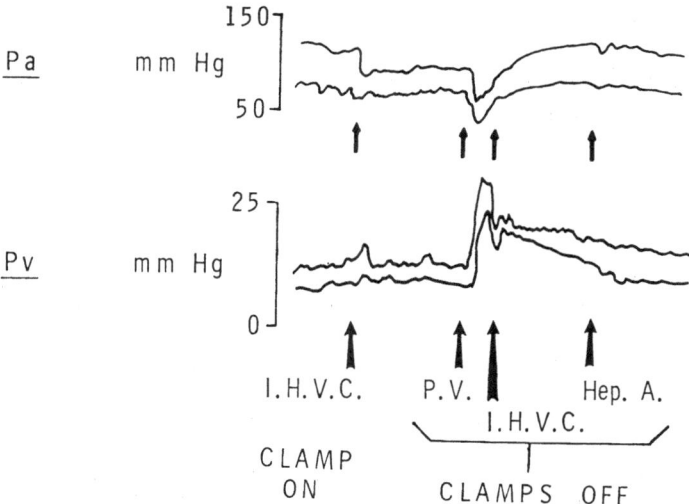

Figure 6. Tracing from a chart recording made during operation on a man with a hepatoma. When the liver was revascularised the arterial pressure (Pa) fell sharply, while the venous pressure (Pv) rose, illustrating the negative inotropic effect of the effluent from the liver.

unclamped infra hepatic cava. This manoeuvre also ensures that no air remains in the vessels of the donor liver and so prevents the possibility of air embolus. The compositions of the perfusate and the outflow are shown in Table 2.

While the surgeon concerns himself with this procedure the anaesthetist must ensure that the patient's heart is in the best condition to withstand the coming onslaught.

It is important to keep well up with any losses as they occur, but this means transfusing stored blood which is also rich in potassium and acid. Acid-base state is monitored and sodium bicarbonate is given to reduce any base deficit, while the use of calcium chloride solution counteracts the toxic effects on the myocardium of excess potassium and citrate.

Conclusions

By the employment of straightforward measures of the type described, our experience is that all patients can be brought safely through the hazardous anhepatic period. It should be emphasised however that this also depends on the careful preoperative selection of patients to exclude those with heart disease, on the use of a non-toxic anaesthetic procedure and on the availability of a skilled team of physicians, surgeons, anaesthetists, biochemists, haematologists, nurses and technicians.

70

Acknowledgments

This research was supported by a grant from the Canadian Liver Foundation, Toronto, Ontario, Canada.

References

1. Farman JV, Lines JG, Williams RS, Evans DB, Samuel JR, Mason SA, Ashby BS, Calne RY: Liver transplantation in man: anaesthetic and biochemical management. Anaesthesia 29:17–32, 1974.
2. Lines JG: Clinical biochemistry services for liver transplantation. Ann Clin Biochem 12:14–18, 1975.
3. Cullen DJ: Interpretation of Blood pressure measurements in anesthesia. Anesthesiology 40:6–12, 1974.
4. Farman JV, Mason SA: Anaesthesia for liver transplantation. In: R.Y. Calne (ed). Clinical organ transplantation. Oxford, Blackwell Scientific Publications, 1971, pp 350–372.
5. Patterson SW, Starling EH: On the mechanical factors which determine the output of the ventricles. J Physiol 48:357, 1915.
6. Aldrete JA, LeVine DS, Gingrich TF: Experience in anesthesia for liver transplantation. Anesth Analg 48:802–815, 1969.
7. Lindop MJ, Farman JV, Smith MF: Anaesthesia and intraoperative management. In: R.Y. Calne (ed). Liver transplantation. London, Academic Press, 1983, pp 121–143.
8. Calne RY, Smith DP, McMaster P, Craddock GN, Rolles K, Farman JV, Lindop MJ, Bethune DW, Wheeldon D, Gill R, Williams RS: Use of partial cardio-pulmonary bypass during the anhepatic phase of orthotopic liver grafting. Lancet, 2:612–614, 1979.
9. Smith MF: Liver transplantation. Technic, September 1976.

8. Coagulation and bleeding during orthotopic liver transplantation

G.W. VAN IMHOFF, E.B. HAAGSMA, H. WESENHAGEN,
R.A.F. KROM and C.H. GIPS

Introduction

The cause of haemorrhage during orthotopic liver transplantation (OLT) is still largely unknown. Pathological fibrinolysis and diffuse intravascular coagulation (DIC) have both been implicated, although manipulation of fibrinolysis and coagulation with antifibrinolytic agents or heparin has not been successful [1–6].

In dogs a decrease in several coagulation factors and platelets as well as excessive fibrinolysis was noted during OLT. Abnormalities could not be influenced by antifibrinolytic agents, heparin or protamine, and seemed most profound and persistent in those animals receiving injured grafts [1]. In man the same kind of pattern was found. During transplantation a more or less significant decline of platelets, fibrinogen and clotting factors, as well as a shortening of the euglobulin lysis time can be found in the anhepatic and recirculation phase [2].

The first liver transplantation in man by Starzl was complicated by haemorrhage leading to death in a few hours [3]. Pathological fibrinolysis was diagnosed on the basis of hypofibrinogenaemia, shortened clot- and euglobulin lysis times and prolongation of thrombin time. Subsequently, introduction of antifibrinolytic drugs in patients led to severe tromboembolic complications, while other patients died from haemorrhage despite such therapy [2–4]. Introduction of heparin even in small amounts led to severe haemorrhage [4, 5].

In man, like in animals, severity and duration of coagulation abnormalities seemed most of all to be related to the quality of the donor liver [2, 4, 5].

In our patients however, we had not been able to find a difference in the quality of the graft between early survivors (<7 days) and early non-survivors (>7 days) of OLT (7). This suggested that other factors might play a role in the outcome of liver transplantation, provided that the quality of the donor liver is good.

The outcome of the first nine orthotopic liver transplantations in Groningen was closely related to complications during the operation. Three out of nine patients did not survive because of severe haemorrhage during transplantation without apparent surgical cause. In order to investigate the problem of severe bleeding during transplantation, we analysed prospectively some parameters of coagulation and fibrinolysis before and during OLT in 11 consecutive patients while using a standard transfusion protocol.

Patients and methods

A cohort of 11 consecutive patients (OLT 10–20) were studied before and during transplantation.

Coagulation studies. Blood samples were taken at least on the following fixed points during transplantation to make comparison between patients possible: (1) before transplantation at the time a donor liver was announced, (2) at the actual start of surgery, i.e. recipient incision, (3) 5 min before the anhepatic phase, (4) at the end of the anhepatic phase, 5 min before recirculation, (5) 1 h after recirculation, (6) at the end of the operation.

The following assays were done according to automated standard procedures using commercially available reagents: Prothrombin time (PT) (normal 10.5–12.5 s). Activated partial tromboplastin time (APTT) (normal 25–40 s), Reptilase time (RT) (normal 11–18 s), Fibrinogen (Fibrgn.) (normal 2–4 g), Fibrin(ogen) degradation products (FDP) (normal 0–10 μg/ml). Antithrombin III (AT III) (normal 80–120%), Plasminogen (Plgn) (normal 70–130% and Antiplasmin (AP) (normal 90–130%) were assayed with chromogenic substrates. Coagulation factors (F) were done by one stage assay from frozen plasma samples within 3 weeks after OLT. Platelet counts were done routinely during the procedure, as well as at the time blood samples were taken for coagulation studies.

Blood loss and transfusion protocol. Blood loss was assessed by measuring the amount of aspirated blood from the operation field during OLT. Blood loss was replaced with red blood cell concentrates (RBC) and depending on volume need of the recipient, cryosupernatant single donor plasma. Cryoprecipitate (Cryo) was used as source of fibrinogen and factor VIII. Fresh frozen plasma (FFP) was given to compensate for other deficiencies. Based on experience in OLT 1–9 the aim was to give 1.5 donor units (U) of FFP and 4 U of Cryo every hour. For those patients expected to have severe clotting factor deficiencies, using AT III below 50% as indication, a transfusion scheme of 3 U FFP and 8 U Cryo every hour was started. Platelet concentrates (PLTS) were given only at recirculation to patients with platelet counts exceeding $60 \times 10^9/l$. To patients with counts below $60 \times 10^9/l$ platelets were given on the basis of platelet counts and blood loss, in most cases 6 U/h.

Statistics. Results were analysed with nonparametric statistical tests [8]. Differences between groups were tested with the Mann Whitney U test. For association the Spearman rank correlation coefficient and the Kendall coefficient of concordance were used.

Results

Blood loss and transfusion protocol. Cumulative blood loss during operation for individual patients is shown in Table 1. Median total blood loss was 4.4 l. Most blood loss occurred in the anhepatic phase and shortly after recirculation.

Deviations from the transfusion protocol were noted in five patients. In three patients (OLT 13, 18, 20) more was transfused due to excessive bleeding characterized by diffuse oozing. No apparent surgical cause of haemorrhage was detected. Bleeding did not seem to be influenced by transfusion of FFP, Cryo or platelets nor by tranexaminic acid (OLT 18, 20) or prothrombin complex concentrates (OLT 20). In all three patients blood loss was already markedly different from the other patients in the phase before recirculation, i.e. before the donor liver could have influenced the haemorrhage. Bleeding could finally be managed in two patients (OLT 13, 18). One patient (OLT 20) died in the operating theatre. One patient (OLT 16) received more because of prolonged clotting times in the preanhepatic phase, interpreted as insufficient substitution. One patient (OLT 15) received less substitution in order to prevent volume overload.

Coagulation studies before OLT. In general two groups of patients could be

Table 1. Blood loss during OLT 10–20.

OLT	Cumulative blood loss in l			
	Preanhepatic	Anhepatic phase	1 h after recirculation	End of operation
10	0.2	2	2.2	2.6
11	0.6	1.6	2.4	2.4
12	0.4	0.8	2.2	2.6
13[a]	*1.5*	*5.3*	*9.2*	*14.0*
14	0.4	1.3	3.8	4.4
15	2.2	3.4	4.0	5.5
16	0.4	1.8	3.0	3.6
17	0.5	2.0	4.0	5.1
18[a]	*2.7*	*14.7*	*23.7*	*42.4*
19	0.2	0.4	2.2	2.5
20[a]	*4.4*	*8.1*	*20.0*	*47.2*
Median	(0.6)	(2.0)	(4.0)	(4.4)
Range	(0.2–4.4)	(0.4–14.7)	(2.2–23.7)	(2.4–47.2)

[a] Patients with excessive blood loss due to diffuse oozing.

discerned on the basis of preoperative coagulation studies (Table 2). Patients with normal AT III activity, normal or high fibrinogen and normal or only moderately abnormal platelet counts who all had none or only minimal deficiencies of clotting factors (OLT 10, 11, 12, 14, 16). The other group of patients (OLT 13, 15, 17, 18, 19, 20) had low AT III activity, mostly low platelet counts, low or low normal fibrinogen and multiple factor deficiencies. Bleeding times were not abnormal – taking platelet count into consideration – and paracoagulation tests were negative in all patients.

Preoperative parameters of coagulation and fibrinolysis correlated significantly with total blood loss during transplantation (Table 3). However individual patients with severe bleeding could not be predicted with absolute certainty on the basis of these parameters alone because there was a considerable overlap of values between patients.

Coagulation analysis during operation. Most patients only had moderate changes in the studied parameters during transplantation. Significant changes ($p < 0.01$)

Table 2. Coagulation studies before operation OLT 10–20.

OLT	PT (10⁵–12⁵ s)	APTT (25–40 s)	Fibng (2–4 g/l)	FDP (0–10 µg/ ml)	Platelets (150–450 × 10⁹/l)	ATIII (80–120%)[a]	Abnormal
10	11.9	20	5.4	0–10	362	150	
11	11.0	30	5.1	10–20	260	158	
12	14.3	31	4.6	0–10	217	150	FV 39%
14	12.3	43	4.0	0–10	147	110	FXII 39%
16	13.3	43	2.3	0–10	90	81	FX 49% Plgn 46%
13	13.6	31	2.1	0–10	139	46	FV 36%, VII 34%, XI 40%, Plgn 39%, AP 65%
15	14.1	47	1.1	0–10	25	51	FV 38%, X 47%, XII 12%, Plgn 41%, AP 52%
17	13.4	45	1.3	0–10	35	47	FV 36%, VII 42%, IX 44%, IX 35%, XII 33%, Plgn 26%
18	13.7	36	2.5	0–10	39	60	FV 40%, VII 35%, IX 48%, XI 49%, Plgn 50%, AP 57%
19	12.9	41	1.6	10–20	39	66	FV 37%, Plgn 47%, AP 63%
20	13.6	38	1.6	0–10	62	50	FII 49%, VII 48%, XI 40%, Plgn 47%, AP 67%

[a] Normal values: factors II–XII 50–150%; Plasminogen 70–130%; Antiplasmin 90–130%.

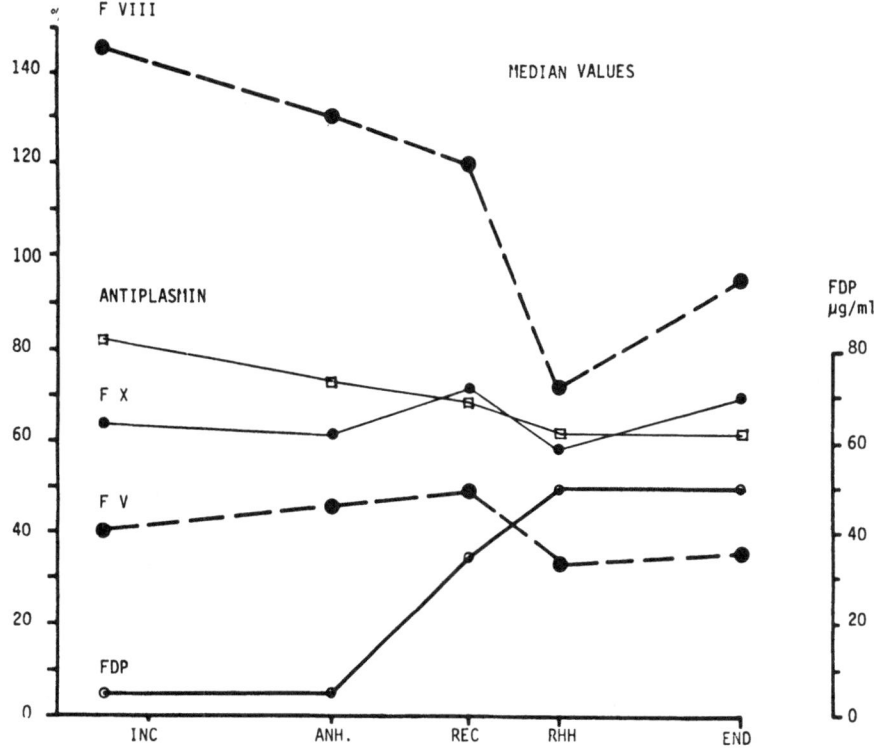

Figure 1. Significant (Kendall p<0.01) changes in coagulation during transplantation OLT 10–20. INC: incision, ANH: anhepatic phase, REC: recirculation, RHH: 1 h after recirculation, END: end of operation.

for all patients analysed together could be found for the following parameters (Figure 1). A decrease especially one hour after recirculation could be seen of FVIII:C, FV and FX. A moderate but consistent decrease of antiplasmin activity and a rise of FDP in the anhepatic phase and after recirculation were noted. Only a moderate prolongation of PT (in no patient more than 4 s from control) was

Table 3. Spearman rank correlation coefficient (in brackets) of total blood loss during and coagulation parameters before operation OLT 10–20.

p value <0.01		<0.025		>0.05	
AT III	(0.82)	Fibrinogen	(0.65)	Plasminogen	(0.52)
F II	(0.85)	F X	(0.62)	FX I	(0.51)
F VIII	(0.79)	Antiplasmin	(0.63)	F V	(0.18)
F IX	(0.74)	PT	(0.62)	F XII	(0.07)
				APTT	(0.35)
				Platelets	(0.51)

seen ($0.01 < p < 0.03$). In general, absolute values of coagulation factors were above 30–40% for all patients during transplantation. Only factor V decreased to 20% 1 h after recirculation in OLT 13, 19, 20.

Although patients with severe blood loss tended to have low levels of coagulation factors during operation, subgroup analysis failed to show significant differences during operation between patients.

Case studies. To illustrate our findings during transplantation, two patients are described. Both patients had chronic active cirrhosis, portal hypertension, varices, splenomegaly and a history of ascites as well as multiple preoperative coagulation deficiencies.

OLT 20, a 57-year-old female, was transplanted for cirrhosis. In the preanhepatic and anhepatic phase there was considerable haemorrhage, amounting to 8 l, although no specific surgical problems were encountered. Clotting times showed only a moderate prolongation from control (PT 2–3 s; APTT 10–20 s) until several hours after recirculation. Platelets and fibrinogen stayed within reasonable limits (Figure 2). Coagulation factors remained above 40% (Figure 3). Only after recirculation when blood loss was already more than 20 l a further decrease could be seen (especially FV). The sharp decline in FVIII:C activity before recirculation was also noted in the other patients, as was mentioned before. AT III activity (Figure 4) initially increased from 50% to 75% in the precirculation phase probably as a result of the transfusion of FFP and only declined at the very end of the operation. More or less the same pattern was seen for plasminogen. FDP became positive and stayed positive in the recirculation phase (not shown).

Although clotting factors, fibrinogen and platelets could be kept at levels theoretically sufficient for haemostasis untill several hours after recirculation, bleeding persisted. Finally prothrombin complex concentrates and tranexaminic acid, which was given as ultimum refugium – although at that moment the englobulin clot lysis time was not shortened – were unable to stop the bleeding and the patient died.

OLT 17, a 17-year-old girl, was transplanted also for cirrhosis. No excessive bleeding was encountered during transplantation and total blood loss was 5.1 l. Coagulation studies showed more or less the same pattern as in OLT 20 (Figures 5, 6, 7). At the end of the operation, when there was no more blood loss, coagulation factors tended to rise while Cryo and FFP were infused. No different pattern could be seen compared with OLT 20 until several hours after recirculation when there had already been massive blood loss in OLT 20. Most importantly, there was no clear difference in the pre-recirculation phase for the studied parameters while at that moment severe bleeding was already apparent in OLT 20.

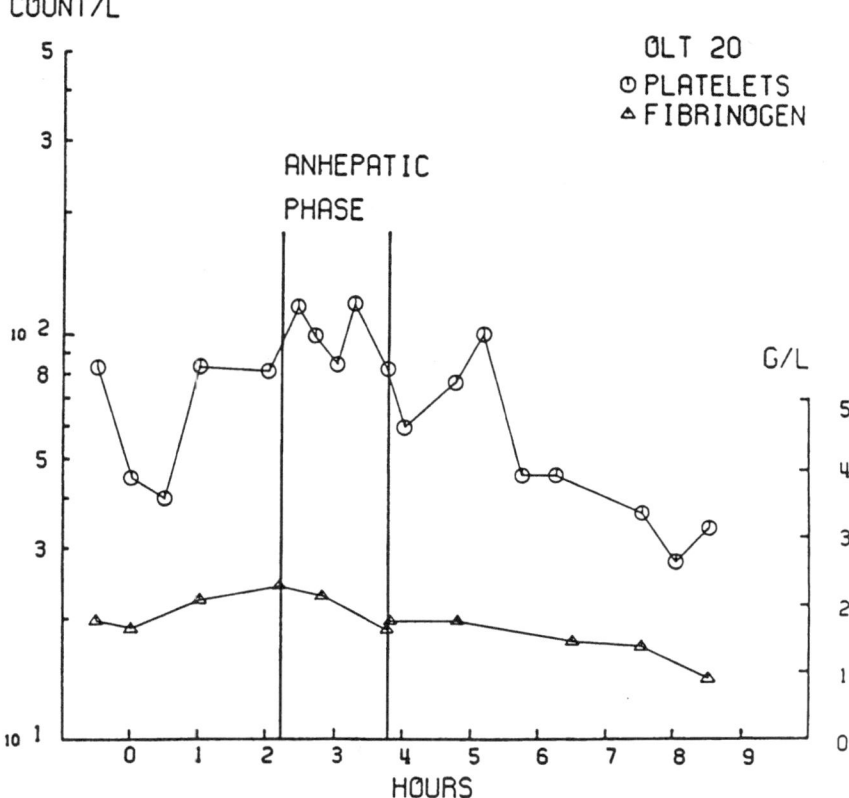

Figure 2. Fibrinogen and platelet counts ($\times$ 10⁹/l) in OLT 20.

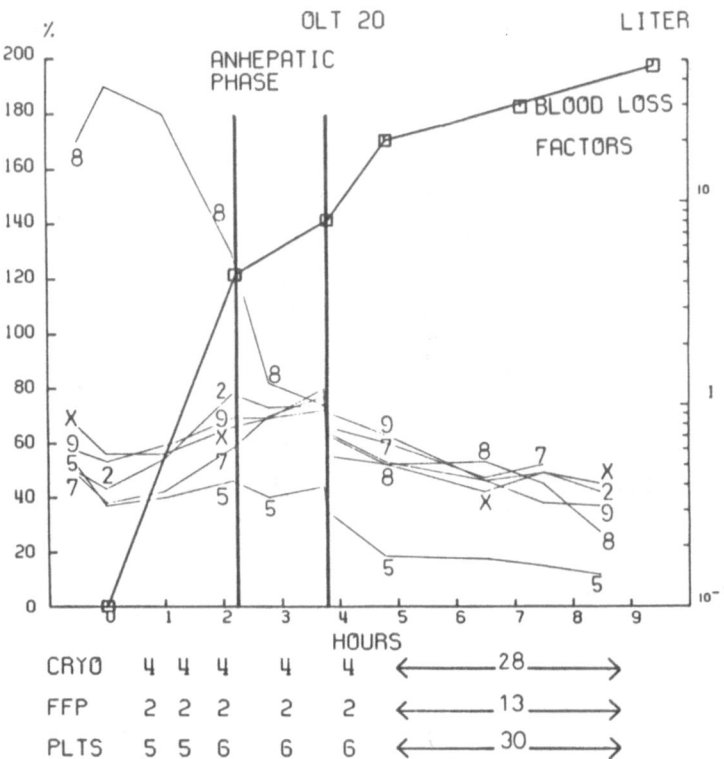

Figure 3. Blood loss and coagulation factors in OLT 20. Blood loss in squares on a logaritmic scale on right axis. Factors II–IX (2–9) and X (x) on the left axis. Transfusion of FFP, Cryo and PLTS in donor units.

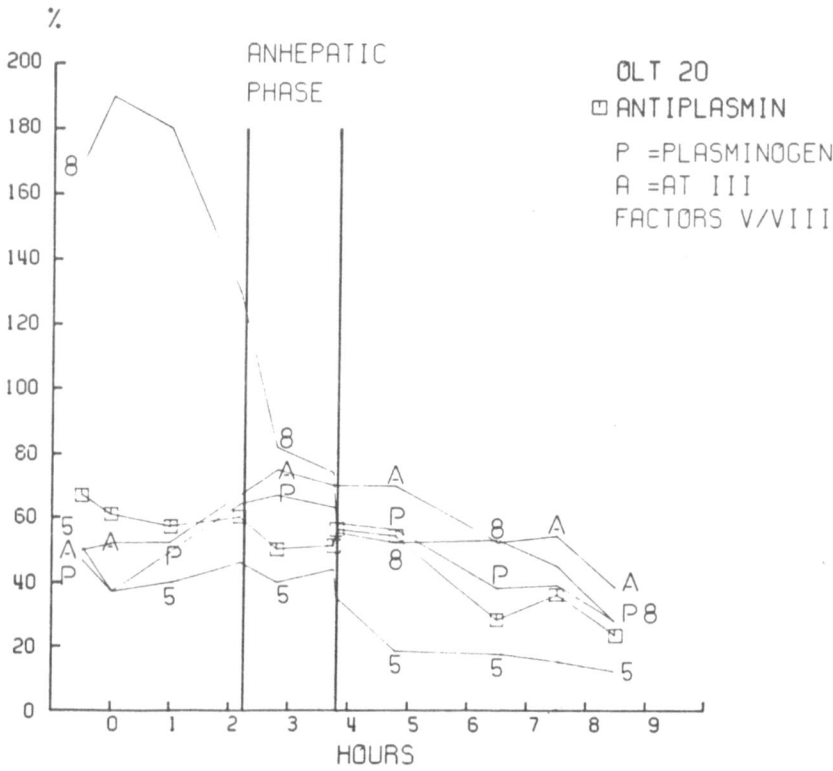

Figure 4. Factors V (5), VIII:C (8), antithrombin III (A), plasminogen (P) and antiplasmin (squares) in OLT 20.

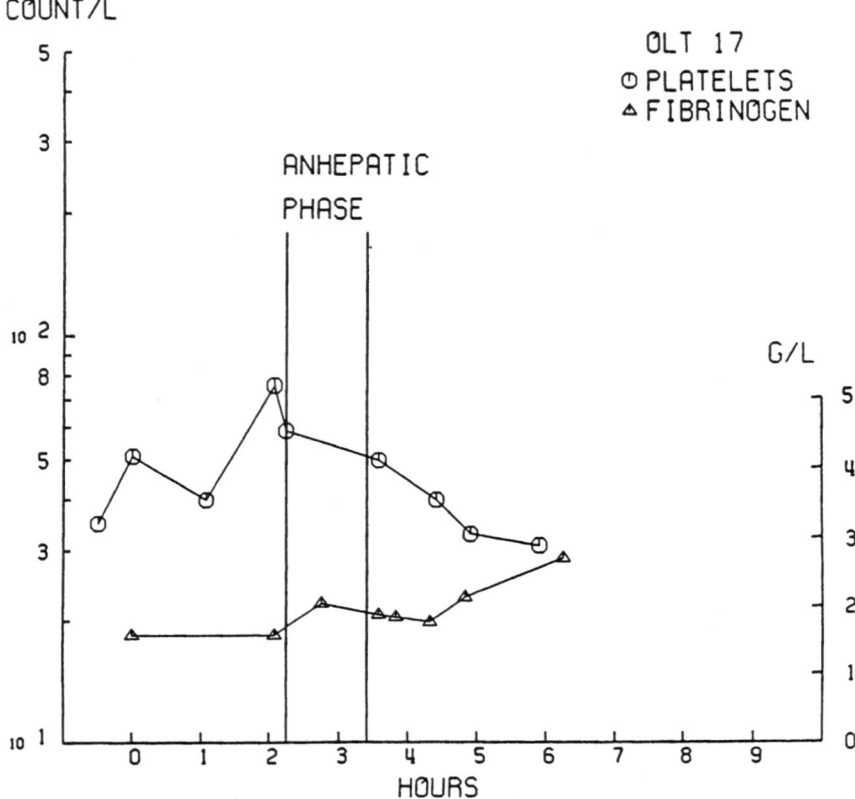

Figure 5. Fibrinogen and platelet counts ($\times 10^9$/l) in OLT 17.

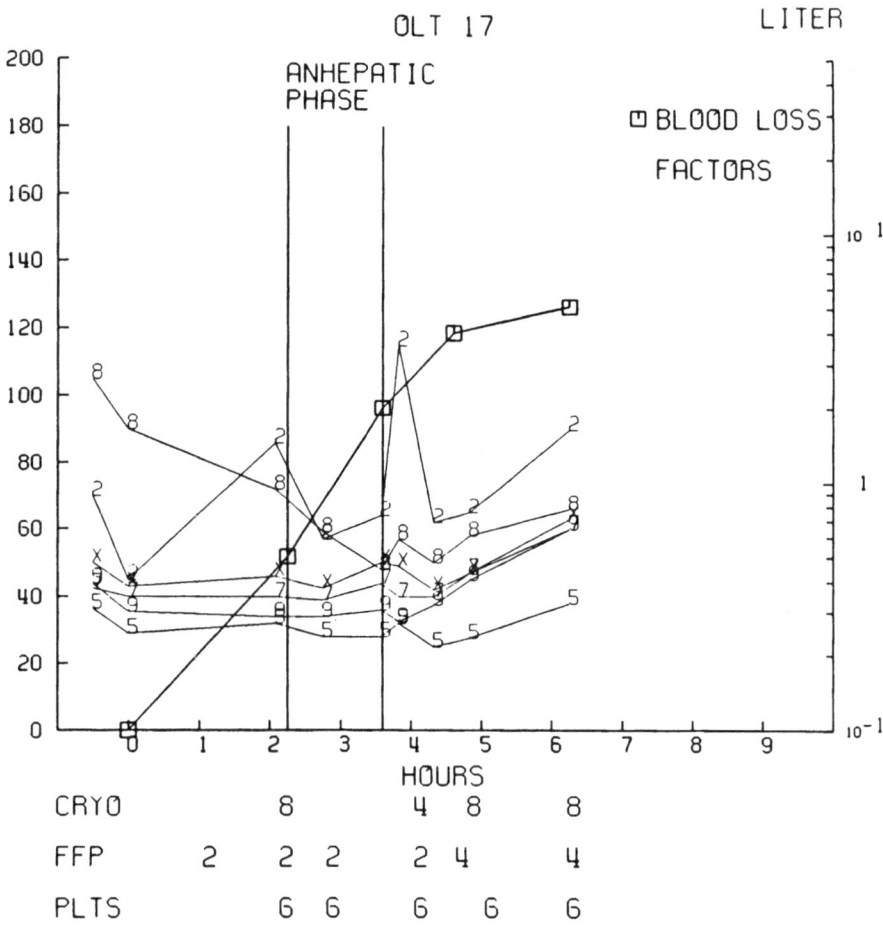

Figure 6. Blood loss and coagulation factors in OLT 17. Blood loss in squares on a logaritmic scale on right axis. Factors II–IX (2–9) and X (x) on the left axis. Transfusion of FFP, Cryo and PLTS in donor units.

82

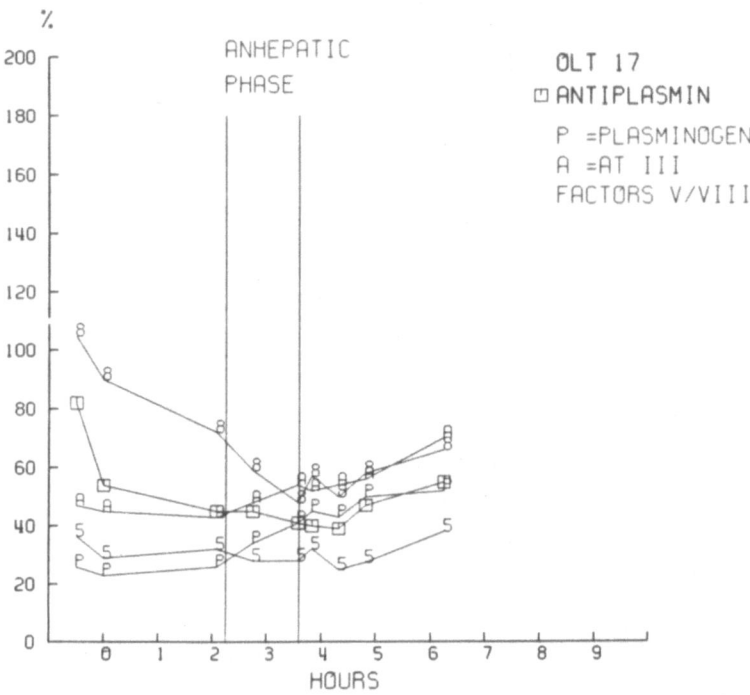

Figure 7. Factors V (5), VIII:C (8), antithrombin III (A), plasminogen (P) and antiplasmin (squares) in OLT 17.

Discussion

The aim of the study was to investigate the relation between haemorrhage during OLT and coagulation. Interpretation of changes in coagulation and fibrinolysis during liver transplantation is extremely difficult. Production of clotting factors, fibrinolytic factors and their inhibitors is often diminished as a result of hepatic failure. Thrombocytopenia is often present due to splenomegaly. The extensive surgical procedure and later on also the preserved donor liver – especially when substantially damaged – will activate the coagulation and fibrinolytic systems. At the same time there will be diminished clearance of activated factors, complexes of activated factors and inhibitors as well as breakdown products due to malfunctioning or absence (in the anhepatic phase) of a large part of the reticuloendothelialsystem. On top of this, at least in the human situation, the transfusion of blood and blood products, often as much as, or even more than the total blood volume of the recipient is complicating the interpretation of findings. For an excellent review the reader is referred to Böhmig [5].

When we started this study we assumed that interpretation of findings would be less difficult if patients received more or less the same standard treatment. However, the absolute amount of transfused bloodproducts as well as deviations from the transfusion protocol – for reasons already mentioned – probably have made our test results less specific.

Although the findings during transplantation, analyzed for all patients together (Figure 1), could be consistent with consumption coagulopathy, this remains inconclusive. An explanation for hemorrhage in OLT 13, 18, 20 solely on the basis of these test results is not possible because these did not differ significantly from results obtained in the other patients.

When excessive bleeding did occur, it was very difficult to influence. Perhaps substitution of coagulation factors during transplantation was inadequate to prevent excessive bleeding. This can not be excluded, although tests of overall coagulation like PT and APTT in our patients were only slightly prolonged during operation. In most congenital deficiencies coagulation factor activities above 40% can be considered as haemostatically safe (except maybe FVIII:C), but there is perhaps a cumulative or additive effect of multiple mild coagulation deficiencies that leads to bleeding [9]. More intensive substitution however will lead to volume problems which ipso facto can lead to more bleeding. The combination of FFP with prothrombin complex concentrates, although able to correct abnormalities in cirrhotic patients before liver biopsy [10] carries the substantial risks of thromboembolism [11] or DIC [12] as well as hepatitis [13] and does not seem to be an improvement in major surgery in severe liver disease. The use of protrombin complex concentrates in our first nine patients did not contribute to haemostasis (unpublished).

The extent and duration of surgery itself could have been the initiating event of severe blood loss in our patients. In a larger group of patients the duration of operation did not correlate with blood loss in the pre-recirculation phase [14].

Although a final explanatation for severe bleeding during transplantation still has to be found, this study reveals that excessive bleeding is already heralded before the donor liver is implanted and preoperative coagulation parameters and blood loss during operation are significantly correlated. This indicates that, provided the graft is of good quality, recipient factors play an important role in the outcome of OLT. These recipient factors need not necessarily be restricted to parameters of coagulation and fibrinolysis but are probably related to the grade of hepatic failure in a wider sense e.g. hepato renal sodium and water handling [14] (Chapter 21).

Severe bleeding not only jeopardizes the survival of the recipient but also has grave implications for the logistics of a blood bank. Selection of recipients least likely to bleed excessively and subsequently most likely to benefit from OLT therefore is of utmost importance, until more is known about the mechanisms and treatment of severe bleeding during OLT.

References

1. Pechet L, Groth CG, Daloze PM: Changes in coagulation and fibrinolysis after orthotopic canine liver transplantation. J Lab Clin Med 73:91–10, 1969.
2. Groth CG, Petchet MD, Starzl TE: Coagulation during and after orthotopic transplantation of the human liver. Arch Surg 98:31–34, 1969.
3. Starzl TE, Marchioro TL, von Kaulla KN, Hermann G, Brittain RS, Waddell WR: Homo-transplantation of the liver in humans. Surg Gynaecol Obstet 117:659–676, 1983.
4. von Kaulla KN, Kaye H, von Kaulla E, Marchioro TL, Starzl TE: Changes in blood coagulation. Arch Surg 92:71–79, 1966.
5. Böhmig HJ: The coagulation disorder of orthotopic hepatic transplantation: Sem Thromb Hemost 4(1):57–82, 1977.
6. Flute PT, Rake MO, Williams R, Seaman MJ, Calne RY: Liver transplantation in man. IV. Haemorrhage and thrombosis. Br Med J 3:20–23, 1969.
7. Krom RAF, Haagsma E, Slooff MJ, Kremer GD, Gips CH: Livertransplantation: donor, donorliver and recipient (abstract). International Congress on organ procurement. Maastricht, The Netherlands, April 14–16, 1983.
8. Siegel S: Non parametric statistics for the behavioral sciences. Tokyo, McGraw Hill, 1956.
9. Mannucci PM, Forman SP: Hemostasis and liver disease. In: Colman RW, Hirsh J, Marder VJ, Salzman EW (eds) Hemostasis and thrombosis. Philadelphia, JB Lippincott, 1982.
10. Mannucci PM, Franchi F, Dioguardi N: Correction of abnormal coagulation in chronic liver disease by combined use of fresh frozen plasma and prothrombin complex concentrates. Lancet ii:542–545, 1976.
11. Marassi A, Manzullo V, Di Carlo V, Mannucci PM: Thromboembolism following a prothrombin complex concentrate and major surgery in liver disease. Thromb Haemost 39:787–788, 1978.
12. Cederbaum AI, Roberts HR: Complications of the use of prothrombin complex concentrates in liver disease. Clin Res 21:92, 1973.
13. Wyke RJ, Tsiquaye KN, Thornton A, White Y, Portmann B, Das PK, Zuckermann AJ, Williams R: Transmission of non A non B hepatitis to chimpanzees by factor IX concentrates after fatal complications in patients with chronic liver disease. Lancet i:520–524, 1979.
14. Haagsma EB, Gips CH, Wesenhagen H, van Imhoff GW, Krom RAF: Liver disease and its effect on hemostasis during livertransplantation. Liver, 1985, in press.

9. Blood bank logistics in liver transplantation

C.TH. SMIT SIBINGA, L. ACHTERHOF, J. WALTJE, J. SWIERINGA
and P.C. DAS

Introduction

Over the past two decades transplantation of livers has been developed for patients in end-stage non-alcoholic liver disease and non-disseminated primary liver carcinoma. Both technically and immunologically, these transplants have recently come out of the experimental stage into a carefully balanced practice, limited to a few well-organized centres in the world [1].

As a result of this development, the question to be asked is: 'Do we support it or not?' This question is multi-conditional. Not only the crucial question of the transplant indication as such is of importance, but of the same magnitude are questions of socio-economic, political and logistic nature. End-stage liver disease unavoidably implies a border-line metabolic status. Protein synthesis is one of the main liver cell functions, that is dramatically impaired. Blood coagulation depends partly on the integrity of the complex enzyme-driven interaction of proteins with procoagulant activity and therefore is usually seriously unbalanced in patients meeting liver transplantation criteria [2].

End-stage liver disease unavoidably leads to anatomical abnormalities of the vessels of the porta-caval system. Portal hypertension and thin-walled dilated vessels in the upper abdominal operation area do influence the function of vascular or primary haemostasis, both surgical and physiological. Therefore excessive bleeding during the preparative, anhepatic and immediate post-anhepatic period of the operation are to be anticipated

Additionally, the necessity of an extracorporeal circuit for peroperative autotransfusion does influence the overall haemostatic capacity to a further extent, although the degree of biocompatibility of such a system might shade this problem to a certain extent [3].

For these reasons liver transplantations have gained the reputation of being very blood consuming procedures, carried out by extremely skilled and professional vampires!

Analysis of supportive haemotherapy

With respect to haemostasis and problems of bleeding of the pre, per and post-operative period, the peroperative stage can be further detailed into a preparative period, in which the recipient's liver is taken out. Once the liver is excised, the point of no return has been passed and the anhepatic period started. Now the donor's liver is carefully implanted. Vascular anastomosis of anatomically normal donor vessels and abnormal thin-walled dilated recipient vessels are needed to provide immediate and guaranteed recirculation of the implanted liver. This anhepatic stage ends at the crucial moment when the major supplying and effluent vessels are unclamped. Recirculation starts, stimulating the donor organ to refunction after the necessary period of extracorporeal preservation.

During the preparative and anhepatic period the problems of bleeding are primarily surgically defined. When unclamping the major vessels, haemostasis relies almost exclusively on platelet function and fibrin formation, provided surgical haemostasis has been done optimally. The metabolic starting point usually is minimal, and blood coagulation is already heavily impaired due to a deteriorated protein synthesis. Coagulation studies have shown decreased levels of prothrombin complex (factors II, VII, IX and X) and, to a lesser extent of procoagulant activities factor V and fibrinogen (Chapter 8) [4]. Usually, due to insufficient synthesis of balancing inhibitors, proactivators of the fibrinolytic system dominate. Antithrombin III is in most cases decreased. Platelet number and function usually are within the normal range but are affected during the peroperative preparative and anhepatic stage due to a variety of factors including the extra-corporeal circuit.

The problems of bleeding in liver transplantation therefore are multiconditional and need a carefully planned and balanced approach. Supportive laboratory control plays an important role in the eventual blood transfusion practice, to avoid both over and under transfusion with appropriate blood components.

As the impaired metabolic status of the recipient influences not only haemostasis, but also has an important effect on the detoxification rate of metabolites and substances like ammonia and citrate as well. The policy for handling the problems of massive bloodloss, shock and homeostasis needs to be carefully designed.

The need for banked whole blood therefore is questionable. The use of plasma, containing citrate as the main anticoagulant, should be restricted to those situations where the substitution of crucial procoagulant factors is indicated.

Immediately following the unclamping of the main vessels, the restoration of the donor's liver will depend on an optimal perfusion and oxygen delivering capacity of the circulating blood. This stage of the transplant operation is the only stage in which the use of younger or more 'fresh' red cells is not required. The impaired liver function, together with the extensive surgical procedure and the necessary immunosuppression postoperatively, do stress intensively the host defense mechanism, both cellular and humoral. Immunoglobulins, opsonic activity and complement factors will be needed to support the obligatory infection prevention regime [5]. In summary the supportive haemotherapy is defined by what is actually needed:

a. Volume, without causing further metabolic problems.
b. Haemostatic capacity, applying a tailor-made support with the use of concentrates of proteins and platelets.
c. Oxygen delivery capacity, where 2.3.–diphosphoglycerate (2.3 DPG) containing younger cells are the product of choice in the immediate postanhepatic stage.
d. Immune support with blood components containing gammaglobulins, fibronectin and complement factors.

From the analysis we learn that during the transplant operation the full potential of specific supportive functions is hardly ever needed at the same time. In other words, supportive haemotherapy can best be carried out according to the principles of component policy.

Component policy

Blood is a national resource, given voluntarily and non-remunerated. Access to this resource is depending on the willingness and readiness of the community to share. Once shared, the medical profession has the moral obligation to utilize the resource in the most equitable, ethical and economical way [6]. Each transfusion of blood or blood component carries potential risks, defined by the possibility for transmitting diseases like viral hepatitis and clinical cytomegalovirus infection (CMV) [7] as well as the immunologically defined risks such as haemolysis, isoimmune phenomena and graft-versus-host disease [8–10]. Component policy involves both bloodbankers and clinicians. The bloodbanker should process each unit of blood into components. He should take care for the appropriate processing and storage conditions to guarantee optimal function of individual components, whether cells or proteins. The clinician should carefully define the clinical need for transfusion, judging what actually is needed to support the patient. He should balance the indication against the unavoidable risks, jeopardizing the patient's condition. Therefore bloodbanker and clinician should closely cooperate in defining and shaping a blood transfusion protocol, especially when dealing with the complicated situation of a liver transplantation.

Preparation of the tranfusion protocol

Liver transplantations do not just happen. They are carefully planned and prepared in great detail. However, the necessary blood transfusion support is not always planned and prepared with the same dedication. The question arises whether the reputation of excessive blood consumption really reflects a carefully organized strategy based on a well-prepared analysis of the actual needs, or reveals a shortcoming in the organization within the transplant team. From the moment a liver transplantation is anticipated, the Blood Bank should be involved as an active ally in the final preparation. The involvement of the Blood Bank is twofold:

1. Preparative support. The period of time between the setting of the indication and the actual operation may vary widely. During this unpredictable period of time the necessary amount of blood components needed for the actual haemo-therapy has to be available and in stock. As the individual blood components do have different conditions for storage and vary considerably in shelf-life, the logistics for guaranteeing the actual peroperative haemotherapy support are a serious problem. Each Blood Bank has a series of clinically defined responsibilities, carried out through the organization of day-to-day logistics.

Motivation of the community to support liver transplantation by making available a special stock is one of the premises for a successful operation.

However, the unpredictability of the necessary period of time in preparation unavoidably will lead to outdating of cellular blood components. This drawback needs careful handling, both ethical and economical. Demotivation of the community should be avoided. Unreasonable increase in costs associated with such a supportive effort may complicate socio-economically and politically the motivation and willingness of the community.

2. Actual support. Once a donor liver is accepted, the operation will depend on the definite availability of blood components according to the transfusion protocol. When in the preparative period waiting for the donor liver to come, the Blood Bank should organize the necessary quantity of red cells and plasma components through a satellite liver transplantation Blood Bank. The necessary support with these more long-lasting components should not be a problem. Usually such a satellite Blood Bank contains the agreed amount of red cell concentrate units. These units enter the satellite at a shelf-life of one week and rotate back into the main stock when the third week of shelf-life is reached, so providing units of red cells with a fully acceptable oxygen delivery capacity. Plasma components can be stored deep-frozen. The real problem is in the storage and final availability of platelet concentrates. As platelet concentrates prepared and stored under the standard Blood Bank conditions have a very limited shelf-life of three days, this important blood component therefore is the limiting factor in the actual support. The use of 5-day storage platelet bags [11–12], now available on the market, has considerably reduced this major logistic concern. Still the production of platelet concentrates does require dozens of whole blood donations on a continuous basis. The recipient's Rhesus factor ultimately defines whether

Blood Bank and community will be able to provide a support over a longer period of time without exhausting its resources.

Conclusion

In good cooperation, mutual trust and respect a balance needs to be found between the logistically defined ethical situations of *availability of blood but no liver to be transplanted* and *availability of a liver but no possibility for haemotherapy support.*
We should realise that in liver transplantation blood donors outweigh indefinitely organ donors. Therefore limits have to be set and accepted, both for the regular and the exceptional situation in liver transplantation practice. The community should never be disappointed by unwarranted practices of overusage and unavoidable shortcomings in our organization. Blood transfusion logistics in liver transplantation therefore should be based on professional expertise and responsibility of the entire transplant team, to ultimately share the community's gift of life in the most equitable, ethical and economical way.

References

1. Calne RY: Recent advances in clinical transplantation of the liver and pancreas. Transpl Proc 15:1263–1268, 1983.
2. Blood coagulation and haemostasis. Thomson, JM (ed). Edinburgh, Churchill Livingstone, 1980.
3. Ten Duis HJ: Intra-operative autotransfusion. Groningen: Red Cross Blood Bank Groningen-Drenthe, 1982, Academic thesis, University of Groningen.
4. Van Imhoff GW, Wesenhagen H, Haagsma E, Smit Sibinga CTh, Krom RAF, Gips CH: Bleeding during orthotopic liver transplantation in man. In: Fondu P, Thijs O (eds). Haemostatic failure in liver disease. Dordrecht, Martinus Nijhoff, 1984.
5. Van der Waay D, Verhoef J (eds): New criteria for antimicrobial therapy: Maintenance of digestive tract colonization resistance. Amsterdam, Excerpta Medica, 1979.
6. International Society for Blood Transfusion: Socio-economic aspects of blood transfusion. Vox Sang 44:328–332, 1983.
7. Greenwalt TJ, Jamieson GA: Transmittable disease and blood transfusion. New York, Grune and Stratton, 1975.
8. Perkins HA: Immunological hazards of blood transfusion. In: Ikkala E, Nykänen A (eds). Transfusion and immunology. Vamala. Vamala Kirjapaino OY, pp 107–120, 1975.
9. Engelfriet CP, Pegels JK, Von dem Borne AEGK: Immunological aspects of transfusion therapy. In: Collins JA, Lunsgaard-Hansen P (eds). Surgical haemtherapy. Biblioteka Haematol 46:120–131, 1980.
10. Brubaker DB: Human posttransfusion graft-versus-host disease. Vox Sang 45:401–420, 1983.
11. Simon DL, Nelson EJ, Carmen R, Murphy S. Extension of platelet concentrate storage. Transfusion 23:207–212, 1983.
12. Wouthuysen E: Een onderzoek naar de houdbaarheid van bloedplaatjes concentraten in drie typen bloedzakken: Fenwal PL1240, Cutter CLX^{tm} en Biotest. Groningen: Rode Kruis Bloedbank Groningen-Drenthe, 1983.

Section 4

MICROBIOLOGY AND THE EVALUATION
OF IMMUNOREGULATION

10. Bacterial infection prophylaxis by selective decontamination in liver transplant patients: General principles

D. VAN DER WAAIJ

Introduction

Colonization resistance (CR) implies the resistance which a potentially pathogenic microorganism meets if it tries to colonize one of the three tracts with open communication with the outside world. Similarly, the biliary tree is protected to colonization from the intestine. The colonization pattern of the digestive tract – and in particular of the intestine – is therefore of great importance in liver transplantation, since most infections by (gram-negative) potentially pathogenic bacteria that develop after transplantation have their source in the intestine. The CR of the digestive tract is the result of cooperation between the host and his autochthonous microflora (1), and this is susceptible to antibiotics.

Colonization resistance of the digestive tract

Initially in animals but later on also in patients in whom 'gastro-intestinal-tract sterilisation' was attempted for infection prophylaxis, a great number of different factors have been found to influence the colonization pattern of the alimentary canal. The colonization pattern appears to be not merely the result of direct interbacterial interactions, but perhaps even more the resultant of a close cooperation between the host organism and its (anaerobic) microflora [1]. Which bacterial species and genera are involved in this complex mechanisms of interactions is not yet known in detail. It is however clear, as mentioned before, that predominantly anaerobic bacteria are involved; aerobic or facultative anaerobic bacteria may influence the growth pattern of one or several related other bacteria in the gut by producing specific bactericines. In contrast to the anaerobes they exert that activity only directly and not via the host organism. Anaerobic bacteria, which outnumber the aerobes by a factor of 10^1 to 10^5 in the colon, appear to control not only the intestinal colonization by the aerobes but also the fate of contamination with aerobic (facultative anaerobic) bacteria in the oropharynx.

Oral contamination with relative small numbers of potentially pathogenic organisms such as Escherichia coli or Klebsiella species, appears to have in general no chance to colonize the oropharynx area nor to grow out in significant numbers in the intestine [2]. On the contrary, they disappear often completely during intestinal passage as long as a normal (anaerobic) flora controls the situation. More heavy contaminations with high numbers of for example 10^6–10^{11} bacteria may 'take' for some time; one strain better than an other of the same species [3, 4]. This implies that only following heavy oral doses a 'contaminant' can be recovered from the faeces of an experimentally contaminated individual during several days to weeks after contamination. In some cases gram-negative bacilli used for experimental contamination persist for one or two days in the oropharynx. In general, however, the area is cleared within hours after contamination [2]. This relation between the number of bacteria to be swallowed by an individual required for subsequent colonization changes most drastically during treatment with some antibiotics; particularly during treatment with those that have an inhibitory effect on anaerobic bacteria [5]. The antibiotics may contaminate the bowel contents either because of incomplete absorbtion or as a result of excretion by the liver. During penicillin or tetracyclin therapy for example (oral as well as parenteral) the number of bacteria required for oropharyngeal and intestinal colonization may decrease to very small numbers provided the contaminant is resistant to the drug [6].

Clinical consequences of decrease of colonization resistance

Apart from the therapeutical, i.e. the positive effect on an inflammatory process, antibiotics may exert a negative effect for the subject treated. They may, as discussed above, disturb the symbiosis between anaerobes and their host and therewith strongly enhance colonization by resistant potentially pathogenic strains and species. Particularly in an environment with resistant strains of various gram-negative and gram-positive bacteria – as may occur in hospital wards – this may have serious implications for the patient.

Therapeutical use of certain antibiotics [7] may affect the anaerobic flora of the colon and therewith the CR of the digestive tract as was mentioned above. This may even occur following low dose antibiotic therapy and as early as two days after the start of treatment [8]. In such cases 'overgrowth' by resistant bacteria or Candida species are involved [9]; they are not necessarily exogenous in origin as they may have been present in the patient's flora at the time of onset of antibiotic therapy. These resistant strains may then grow out by the selective pressure of the antibiotic in their environment; i.e. due to excretion with gingival crevicular fluid, saliva, bile or intestinal mucus. Strains of species which are susceptible to the antibiotic(s) used are killed or strongly inhibited in growth. As far as resistant potentially pathogenic microorganisms are concerned, the condition of 'overgrowth' is in general correlated with abnormal numbers of the species concerned. A rise of several logs in the number of resistant organisms is not unusual and perhaps equally important is their abnormal localisation inside the digestive tract. Gram-negative bacilli, like resistant *E. coli, Klebsiella* or *Pseudomonas* species, may for example appear in high numbers in oral washings and persist in the oropharyngeal area for quite some time instead of only for several hours as is generally found in untreated subjects [10–12]. This is in fact a serious condition which may lead to superinfections in the respiratory tract. It even may cause a (first) infection at a site remote from the original infection for which therapy was started in the case of a granulocytopenic individual. A superinfection – which in general occurs at the site of the infection for which antibiotic therapy was performed – clinically may resemble a relapse of the initial infection. Culturing of material from the infectious process (sputum, urine, pus etc.), however, reveals in case of a superinfection a different organism: a different species or a different type of the same species. The second invader is by definition resistant to the antibiotic used for therapy and can frequently be recovered in large numbers not only from the oropharynx but often also from the faeces. This sequence of events is quite common when infections occur in either one of both tracts which have an opening adjacent to the mouth respectively to the anus, i.e. the respiratory tract and the urinary tract [13–16].

Infections in respiratory, the urinary tract or the bile bladder

Infections in the respiratory tract, in the urinary tract or in the biliary tree are often enhanced by a decreased CR of these tracts. The CR of the latter is the resultant of: (1) mucus excretion which limits bacterial colonization, (2) excretion of immunoglobulin A which would more specifically than mucus interfere with bacterial (yeast) adherence, (3) desquamation of epithelial cells which can be loaded with adhering organisms and which helps to clear the tract in concert with (4) mechanical forces as epithelial ciliar movement, flow of urine and bile and the (hydro)dynamic emptying of a urinary- and gall-bladder. These host related forces – which also exist in the digestive tract (swallowing of saliva, peristalsis, mucus secretion, cell desquamation, IgA excretion) – are in the respiratory as well as in the urinary tract fully capable of controlling the microbial contaminations. The latter are likely to occur continuously, be it in small numbers, from the direct enviroment i.e. incoming air, oropharyx flora or perianal, vaginal or preputial flora. If one of these 'host related forces' is hampered and particularly if the mechanical cleansing is interfered with, like for example in patients with bronchiectasis or an enlarged prostate, potentionally pathogenic organisms may colonize the obstructed site. If they then multiply to a sufficient number they may cause an infection. Attempts to cure the patient in such cases with an antibiotic which decreases the intestinal CR like most broad spectrum penicillines may have disappointing results as recurrences of infection are often seen. This may occur during or shortly after the start of therapy by a resistant organism for reasons described above. A change in the antibiotic therapy to another CR-suppressing antibiotic, may have success as long as no resistant potentionally pathogenic bacteria are present in the patient's (hospital) environment. After contamination with a relative small number of these resistant bacteria massive enteric colonization may occur with subsequently a good chance for infection of the tract (respiratory-, biliary- or, urinary tract) with the hampered CR. In these cases is the use of an antimicrobial drug which is active against the causative organism but which does not affect the anaerobic colonic flora of great help. Firstly, it will act at the site of infection as it has been selected for it. Secondly, it will not promote acquisition and colonization of the digestive tract by resistant organisms: i.e. will not affect the CR of the digestive tract and therefore not permit small numbers of resistant bacteria to 'take'. Only following heavy oral contaminations with resistant organisms, these may resist colonization resistance and stay for some time inside the enteric tract to form a temporary source for reinfection.

Consequence for antimicrobial prophylaxis respectively therapy in liver transplant patients

It has been made likely above that antimicrobial drugs may affect the CR of the digestive tract and therewith the potentionally pathogenic digestive tract microflora in the small intestine at and around the site of the connection with the bile duct system. The consequence of this then is that all antibiotics which are clinically in use should be – and have to some extent been – screened for their influence on the CR of the digestive tract following oral and/or parenteral application. In this respect it is obviously important to know whether the currently used antibiotics do decrease the CR following all clinical dosages or whether lower doses of a particular drug are safe as they leave the CR unaffected.

Antimicrobial drugs which do *not* affect the anaerobic intestinal flora may circumvent the CR-associated anaerobic flora for several reasons: (1) because they have a spectrum that does not include anaerobes; (2) because they do not reach the flora of the colon because they are well absorbed in the small intestine either following oral supply or after excretion with bile. Drugs of which it is known that they do not affect the CR such as nalidixic acid, polymyxins, tobramycin (in low oral doses [17]), co-trimoxazole and polyene antibiotics act along these lines. Co-trimoxazole and nalidixic acid however, should be avoided in liver transplant patients because of their potential (hepato-)toxicity.

CR-indifferent drugs which are not hepatotoxic should be given preference for therapy in case the drug also fulfills the conventional requirements for selection such as susceptibility, pharmacokinetic properties etc. An important second consequence of CR-inactive drugs is that depending on pharmacokinetic and toxicologic properties, most of these drugs can be given orally in such (high) doses that the susceptible potentionally pathogenic strains become completely suppressed and cleared from the intestinal canal [26, 27]. These drugs in fact artificially increase the CR for susceptible strains. Meanwhile this application of CR-indifferent drugs for this purpose has been called 'selective decontamination', as such treatment more or less selectively eliminates susceptible strains and species in patients.

Selective decontamination (SD) is perhaps particularly indicated in two categories of patients:

1. Patients with a localized decreased resistance to infections; transplant patients or patients with granulocytopenia. In both categories the obvious aim is: prevention of infections. Because the number of drugs screened and found 'safe' for SD is still limited, only gram-negative infections as well as Staph aureus and *Candida* infections can quite efficiently be reduced by this prophylaxis [18–21].
2. Patients in whom the use of CR-decreasing antibiotics is indicated on the basis of the susceptibility pattern of the organism isolated from the infection. In such patients SD may be indicated for two reasons: (a) to prevent recurrent infections at same site caused each time by newly acquired organisms or by organisms that have become resistant inside the alimentary canal. (b) to prevent acquisition of resistant bacteria from the environment. Otherwise, such patients may become a reservoir of organisms resistant to the drug(s) used and thus be a source of infection for other patients in the ward [22, 23]. This is particularly important on intensive treatment wards, burn units, urologic wards, oncologic departments and similar hospital area's in which susceptible patients are treated.

To clear 'patient reservoirs' with resistant organisms, which have been reported to exist in many hospitals – if not in all – we may have to consider the second application of SD more often than one may think on first impression. This is particularly worth consideration in intensive treatment wards in which compromised patients are treated.

References

1. Van der Waaij D: The colonization resistance of the digestive tract in experimental animals and its consequences for infection prevention, acquisition of new bacteria and the prevention of spread of bacteria between cage mates. In: Van der Waaij D, Verhoef J (eds). New criteria for antimicrobial therapy: maintenance of digestive tract colonization. Amsterdam Excerpta Medica (ICS 477), 1979.
2. Van der Waaij D: The colonization resistance of the digestive tract with special emphasis on the oropharynx. In: Van Furth R (ed). Developments in antibiotic treatment of respiratory infections. The Hague, Martinus Nijhoff, 1981.

3. Buck AC, Cooke EM: The fate of ingested *Pseudomonas aeruginosa* in normal persons. J Med Microbiol 2:521–525, 1969.

4. Cooke EM,Hettiaratchy ICT, Buck AC: Fate of ingested *Escherichia coli* in normal persons. J Med Microbiol 5:361–369, 1972.

5. Van der Waaij D, Berghuis-de Vries JM, Lekkerkerk-van der Wees JEC: Colonization resistance of the digestive tract in conventional and antibiotic treated mice. J Hyg 69:405–411, 1971.

6. Bernstein CA, McDermott W: Increased transmissibility of staphylococci to patients receiving an antimicrobial drug. N Engl J Med 262:637–642, 1960.

7. Wiegersma N, Jansen G, Van der Waaij D: Effect f twelve antimicrobial drugs on the colonization resistance of the digestive tract of mice and on endogenous potentia-ly pathogenic bacteria. J Hyg 88:221–230, 1982.

8. Louria DB, Brayton RG: The efficacy on penicillin regimens: with observations on the frequency of superinfections. JAMA 186:987–990, 1963.

9. Seeling MS: Mechanisms by which antibiotics increase incidence and severity of candidiasis and alter the immunological defenses. Bact Rev 30:442–459, 1966.

10. Tillotson JR, Finland M: Bacterial colonization and clinical superinfection of the respiratory tract complicating antibiotic treatment of peumonia. J Inf Dis 119:597–624, 1969.

11. Rosenthal S, Tager IB: Prevalence of gram-negative rods in the normal pharyngeal flora. Ann Intern Med 83:355–357, 1975.

12. Sugarman B, Donta ST: Effect of antibiotics on the adherence of Enterobacteriaceae to human buccal cells. J Inf Dis 140:622–625, 1979.

13. Johanson WG, Pierce AK, Sanford JP: Changing pharyngeal flora of hospitalized patients: emergence of gram-negative bacilli. N Engl J Med 281:1137–1140, 1969.

14. Spencer RC, Philip JR: Effect of previous antimicrobial therapy on bacteriological findings in patients with primary pneumonia. Lancet ii:349–351, 1973.

15. Mihara G, Stamey TA: The effect of low-dose co-trimoxazole (trimethoprim-sulfamethoxazole) on rectal and vaginal flora. In: Van der Waaij D, Verhoef J (eds). New criteria for antimicrobial therapy: maintenance of digestive tract colonization resistance. Amsterdam, Excerpta Medica (ICS 477), 1979.

16. Grüneberg RN: Co-trimoxazole: effects on the urinary and bowel flora. In: Van der Waaij D, Verhoef J (eds). New criteria for antimicrobial therapy maintenance of digestive tract colonization resistance. Amsterdam, Excerpta Medica (ICS 477), 1979.

17. Mulder JG, Wiersma NE, Welling GW, Van der Waaij D: Low dose oral tobramycin treatment for selective decontamination of the digestive tract: a study in human volunteers. J Antimicrob Chemother 13:1–10, 1984.

18. Sleijfer DT, Mulder NH, De Vries-Hospers HG, Fidler V, Nieweg HO, Van der Waaij D, Van Saene HKF: Infection prevention in granulocytopenic patients by selective decontamination of the digestive tract. Eur J Cancer 16:859–869, 1980.

19. De Vries-Hospers HG, Sleijfer DT, Mulder NH, Van der Waaij D, Nieweg HO, Van Saene HKF: Bacteriological aspects of selective decontamination of the digestive tract as a method of infection prevention in granulocytopenic patients. Antimicrob Agents Chemother 19:813–820, 1981.

20. Guiot HFL, Van der Meer JWM, Van Furth R: Selective antimicrobial modulation of human microbial flora: infection prevention in patients with decreased host defense mechanisms by selective elimination of potentially pathogenic bacteria. J Inf Dis 143:664–654, 1981.

21. Dekker AW, Rozenberg-Arska M, Sixma JJ, Verhoef J: Prevention of infection by co-trimoxazole in patients with acute non-lymphocytic leukemia, Ann Intern Med 95:555–559, 1981.

22. Seldon R, Lee S, Wang WLL, Bennett JV, Eickhoff TC: Nosocomial Klebsiella infections: intestinal colonization as a reservoir. Ann Intern Med 74:657–664, 1971.

23. Chow AW, Taylor PR, Yoshikawa TT, Guze LB: A Nosocomial outbreak of infections due to multiply resistant *Proteus mirabilis*: role of intestinal colonization as a major reservoir. J Inf Dis 139:621–627, 1979.

11. Infections complicating liver transplantation

G.P. SCHRÖTER

Introduction

I would like to describe some of the infectious problems encountered in the last 84 patients who received orthotopic liver transplants in Denver, Colorado, before the liver transplant program moved to Pittsburgh, Pennsylvania [1]. The results will show that the majority of infectious complications stemmed from the location of the liver in the portal venous circuit and the close relation of the liver to the gastrointestinal tract, which is the normal habitat of myriads of bacteria.

Material and methods

During the 5 years from 8/30/75 to 9/28/80, 92 liver transplants were performed on 84 patients in Denver. These patients included 55 adults, 29 children; 50 females and 34 males (Table 1). The average age of the children was 7.2 years ranging from 10 months to 16 years of age. The average age of the adults was 32.5 years ranging from 20 to 53 years of age.

The original liver diseases of these patients are listed in Table 2. The majority had liver failure due to chronic active hepatitis, extrahepatic biliary atresia or alpha-1 antitrypsin deficiency.

Ten of the 13 children with extrahepatic biliary atresia had undergone porto-enterostomy (Kasai operation) earlier in life.

Nine patients were HBsAg positive before transplantation including six patients with chronic active hepatitis or postnecrotic cirrhosis and one patient each with alcoholic cirrhosis, alpha-1 antitrypsin deficiency or multifocal hepatocellular carcinoma.

Standard immunosuppression included prednisone and azathioprine to which a course of antithymocyte globulin was added if the platelet counts permitted. Beginning in the spring of 1978, 27 patients also underwent thoracic duct drainage. This practice was abandoned when cyclosporine became available. Cyclosporine was used in combination with small doses of prednisone in the last fourteen patients since March, 1980 (Table 3).

All patients received a short course of antibiotics which was started before transplantation, continued intraoperatively and for 3–5 days postoperatively. Usually methicillin and ampicillin or a cephalosporin in combination with an aminoglycoside were used. The doses were calculated on a weight basis and adjusted to impaired renal function. The choice of antibiotics was influenced by preexisting colonization or infection. For instance, carbenicillin was used instead

Table 1. Liver transplant recipients (Denver: Aug. 30, 1975–Sept. 28, 1980).[a]

	Males	Females	Total #	Average age	Range
Adults	23	32	55	32.5 years	20–53 years
Children	11	18	29	7.2 years	10 mos–16 years
Total #	34	50	84		

[a] Identification # OT101–184

Table 2. Underlying liver disease of 84 patients receiving 92 liver transplants in Denver (Aug. 30, 1975–Sept. 28, 1980).

Chronic active hepatitis	26
Extra hepatic biliary atresia	13
Alpha 1 antitrypsin deficiency	10
2° biliary cirrhosis	7
Primary biliary cirrhosis	5
Sclerosing cholangitis	4
Budd Chiari syndrome	4
Alcoholic cirrhosis	5
Cholangio carcinoma	2
Hepato cellular carcinoma	2
Miscellaneous[a]	6
Total	84

[a] Glycogenstorage Disease type IV, protoporphyria, tyrosenemia, choledochal cyst, congenital hepatic fibrosis, Byler's disease.

Table 3. Immunosuppression.[a]

I.	Azathioprine + prednisone	43 patients
	± Methylprednisolone IV	
	± ATG IV	
II.	+ Thoracic duct drainage	27 patients
III.	Cyclosporine + prednisone	14 patients
	± Methylprenisolone IV	

[a] ATG = antithymocyte globulin; IV = intravenously.

of ampicillin if a patient was known to harbor pseudomonas aeroginosa. The so-called second and third generations of cephalosporins and the newer ureido penicillins and piperacillin were not available at that time.

Results

The survival of the 84 patients as of April, 1983 is shown in Figure 1. There was a very high mortality during the first postoperative months after transplantation. However the prognosis improved for patients who survived this critical period of time. Currently 28 patients are still alive from more than 2 years to more than 7 years after transplantation.

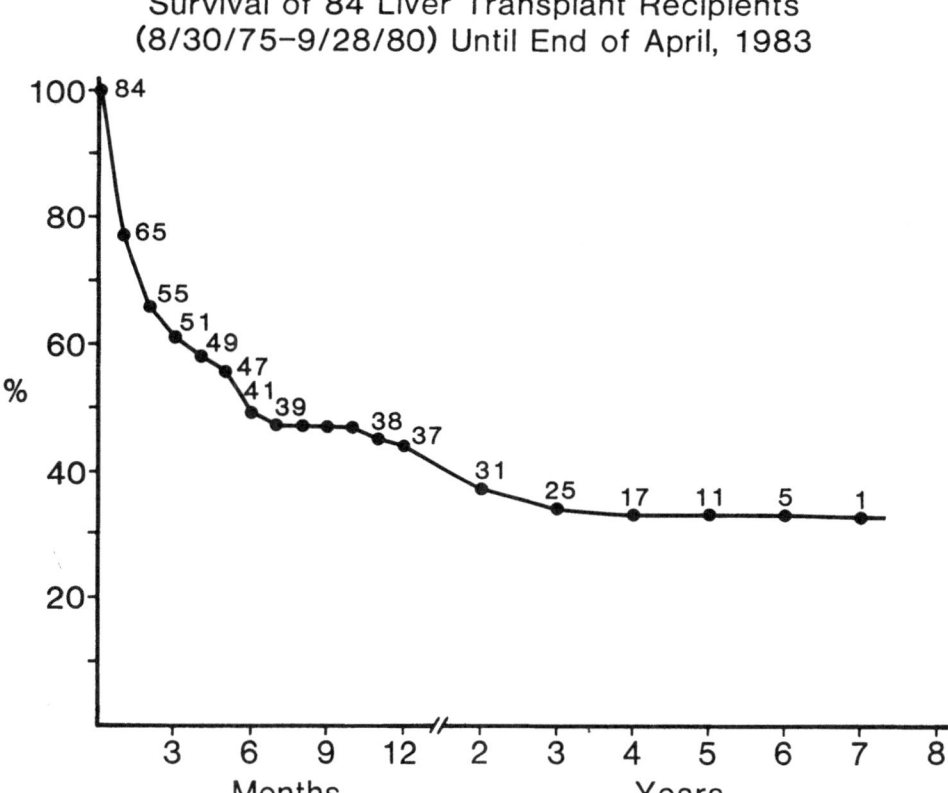

Figure 1. Survival in the Denver 1975–1980 series.

Bacteremia

Blood cultures were obtained routinely for evaluation of a fever above 38 C. The results of the cultures indicate a high incidence of bacteremia (Table 4).

Sixty-one of all 84 patients had 217 positive blood cultures but only four of the 14 patients treated with cyclosporine. Twenty-five patients had 38 blood cultures with more than one bacterial strain being isolated from the same culture. The positive blood cultures yielded a total of 152 different strains of bacteria. Twenty of these probably constitute skin contaminants. Blood cultures from 13 patients grew candida species on one or more occasions. Blood cultures from one patient yielded torulopsis glabrata.

The majority of bacteria were enterobacteriaceae, pseudomonas and enterococci but staphylococci were also common. The source of positive blood cultures was infection of the abdominal wound, peritoneal cavity, biliary tract and sometimes liver (Tables 5 & 6).

The differentiation between the origin of bacteremia from wound infection alone or with additional limited peritoneal involvement was not always clear. It remains unexplained why hardly any bacteremia could be traced to a broncho pneumonia.

Peritonitis

Twenty-five patients died with peritonitis. Complications predisposing to peritonitis in these patients are listed in Table 7. Such complications included peritoneal hemorrhage due to incomplete surgical hemostasis frequently associated with a coagulopathy in the presence of poor homograft function. Complications of biliary tract reconstruction were another common cause. In a few patients space limitation prevented primary closure of the abdominal cavity after insertion of the transplant. Other patients developed intestinal fistulae or required further operations for duodenal ulcer or hemicolectomy.

Table 4. Positive blood cultures of 84 liver transplant recipients.

Number of patients with positive blood cultures	61
Number of patients with positive blood cultures (>1 strain in single culture)	25
Number of positive blood cultures	217
Number of positive blood cultures (>1 strain in single culture)	38
Number of different strains isolated	152
Number of bacteria likely to be contaminants	20
Number of patients with blood cultures positive for Candida species	13[a]
Number of patients with blood cultures positive for Torulopsis glabrata	1

[a] Candida albicans = 10.

Table 5. Gram-negative bacteria isolated from blood cultures of liver transplant recipients and likely source.

Organism	Total	Abdominal wound	Peritoneal cavity	Biliary tract	Liver abscess	Pulmonary	Empyema	Central venous line	Undetermined
Escheria coli	17	1	8 (3)[b]	2	1	0	0	0	5 (1)
Klebsiella species	12	0	2 (1)	3	4 (1)	0	1[a]	0	3 (1)
Pseudomonas aeroginosa	11	0	7 (2)	2 (1)	0	0	0	1	1 (1)
Pseudomonas maltophilia	2	0	0	1	0	0	0	0	1
Enterobacter cloacae	3	0	1 (1)	0	0	0	0	0	2
Enterobacter aerogenes	1	0	0	0	0	0	0	0	1 (1)
Citrobacter freundii	1	0	0	0	0	0	0	0	1
Serratia marcescens	1	0	0	0	0	1	0	0	0
Aeromonas	1	0	0	1	0	0	0	0	0
Mima polymorphea	1	0	0	1	0	0	0	0	0
Proteus mirabilis	1	0	1	0	0	0	0	0	0
morganii	4	0	2 (1)	1	1	0	0	0	1
vulgaris	1	0	1 (?)	0	0	0	0	0	0
Bacteroides species	9	0	6 (3)	0	1	0	0	0	2 (?)
Clostridium species	6	0	2	0	1 (1)	0	0	0	3
Campylobacter fetus subspecies jejunum	1	0	0	0	0	0	0	0	1
Veillonella parvula	1	0	0	0	0	0	0	0	1
Total	73	1	30 (11)	11 (1)	9 (2)	1	1	1	21 (4)

[a] Also isolated from peritoneal cavity.
[b] ( ) bacteremia persistent until death.

Some patients had a combination of the aforementioned complications. The peritoneal infections frequently resulted in prolonged morbidity, acute gastrointestinal hemorrhage or death from multiple organ failure.

Two patients survived polymicrobial peritonitis associated with episodes of sepsis. Postoperative hematomata occurred in both patients and in one a bile leak and small colonic fistula also contributed to the development of infection. In both patients management included prolonged exposure of the peritoneal cavity combined with frequent peritoneal irrigation.

A third patient survived hemicolectomy in the absence of additional complication factors.

Table 6. Gram-positive bacteria isolated from blood cultures of liver transplant recipients and likely source.

Organism	Total	Abdominal wound	Peritoneal cavity	Biliary tract	Liver abscess	Pulmonary	Empyema	Central venous line	Undetermined
Staphylococcus aureus[b]	12	3	6 (2)[a]	3[c]	0	0	1	1 (AV shunt)	0
Staphylococcus epidermidis	21	5	4 (1)	0	1 (1)	0	1	3	7
Enterococcus	16	1	6 (3)	3	3 (1)	0	0	0	3
Streptococci, various types not A	6	1	1	1	1	1	0	0	1
Streptococcus pneumoniae	4	0	0	0	0	0	0	0	4 (3)
Diphtheroids	5	0	1	0	0	0	0	0	4
Micrococcus	1	0	0	0	0	0	0	0	1
Propionebacterium acnes	10	0	1	6	0	0	0	1	8
Total	65	10	19 (6)	7	5 (2)	1	2	5	28 (3)

[a] ( ) number of patients in whom bacteremia was persistent until death.
[b] Septic portal vein thrombosis 1(1).
[c] Also found in peritoneal cavity.

Table 7. Liver transplant recipients with peritonitis causing or contributing to death.

Number of patients	25
Complications predisposing to peritonitis:	
Peritoneal hemorrhage	
(usually with coagulopathy due to ischemic injury of graft, portal vein thrombosis, etc.)	7
Biliary tract complications	11
Leak cholecysto-jejunostomy	2
Cystic duct obstruction	3
Dislodged T tube	1
Leak choledocho-choledochostomy	1
Leak around T tube of choledocho-choledochostomy	1
Leak jejuno-jejunostomy	3
Inability to close peritoneal cavity	3
Surgical intervention for bleeding duodenal ulcer	2
Penetrating duodenal ulcer	1
Intestinal fistulae	3
Hemicolectomy	2
Miscellaneous	2

Complications associated with biliary tract reconstruction

The reconstruction of the biliary tract has been called the 'Achilles' heel' of liver transplantation because it is a frequent source of complications. In the Denver group of patients a cholecystojejunostomy with an anastomosis of the donor gall bladder to an already existing segment of jejunum from a previous portoenterostomy or to a newly created Roux en Y limb of jejunum was the preferred method for bile drainage in children. A choledochocholedochostomy after donor cholecystectomy splinted with a T tube or an internal stent was used in the majority of adults (Table 8). The table also lists the complications, which include obstruction at the level of the cystic duct and anastomotic leak. These complications were a major source of cholangitis or peritonitis, frequently associated with bacteremia. Persistent cholangitis in the presence of unrelieved obstruction of bile flow also was a cause of liver abscess. Correction of cystic duct obstruction by cholecystectomy and conversion of a cholecystojejunostomy to a choledochojejunostomy had a high success rate in spite of the presence of cholangitis. Some bile leaks associated with choledochocholedochostomy healed spontaneously after removal of the T tube.

These complications were not only a source of morbidity but also mortality from uncontrolled infections.

Table 8. Biliary tract reconstruction in 84 liver transplant recipients (92 grafts) and its complications.

	Total		Adults		Children	
Cholecystojejunostomy	35 (37)[a]		15 (16)		20 (21)	
Obstruction of cystic duct	8 (9)	2[b]	5 (6)	1	3	1
Leak jejunojo-jejunostomy	5	3	3	1	2	2
Leak cholecystojejunostomy	3	3	2	2	1	1
Total	16 (17)	8	10 (11)	4	6	4
Cholangitis without obstruction	4	0	1	0	3	0
Choledocho-choledochostomy	43 (47)		36 (40)		7	
Leak around T tube	11		9		2	
(with significant peritonitis						
or abdominal abscesses)	7	3	6	3	1	0
Obstruction	1	1	1		0	
Dislodged T tube	1	1	1	1	0	
Total	13	5	11	1	2	0
Miscellaneous						
Cholecystojejunostomy	4 (5)	0	2	0	2 (3)	0
Cholecystogastrostomy	1 (2)	0	1 (2)	0	0	
Cholecystoduodenostomy	1	1	1	1	0	
Total	6 (7)	1	6 (5)	1	2 (3)	0

[a] ( ) = number of grafts.
[b] = number of patients in whom these complications contributed to death.

Vascular infections of the graft

Two patients died 3 or 6 months after transplantation from vascular infection. The first patient was discovered to have a septic portal vein thrombosis due to staphylococcus aureus at the time of retransplantation (which was not successful). She had had a staphylococcal wound infection after initial transplantation. The second patient had a vasculitis due to pseudomonas aeroginosa. She had a history of cholangitis due to pseudomonas in the presence of cystic duct obstruction detected and corrected four months earlier.

Liver transplant patients with bacterial liver abscesses

Nine patients developed solitary or multiple liver abscesses containing single or multiple strains of bacteria (Table 9). Cultures demonstrated not only Gram negative enteric bacilli or enterococci but also staphylococcus aureus, staphylococcus epidermidis or hemophilus influenzae type B.

In five patients the abscesses probably developed as a complication of cholangitis. In three patients an obstruction of the cholecystojejunostomy at the cystic duct level was detected. Hepatic abscesses were discovered and drained surgically 9, 10 or 4 and again 11 months after transplantation. Obstruction of the cystic duct was recognized and corrected at surgical drainage in two patients and in one patient 14 months later. All three patients survived but in one patient in whom the biliary tract could not be reconstructed satisfactorily recurrent cholangitis eventually caused death many months later. The two other patients are currently alive, $5^1/_2$ and $6^1/_2$ years after transplantation.

In two patients liver abscesses were associated with a dislodged or obstructed T tube and contributed to death.

In two patients liver abscesses were associated with multiple infarctions of the graft. In another patient liver abscesses followed ligation of the left hepatic artery to control bleeding after erosion by an abscess in the portal area. The patient

Table 9. Liver transplant recipients with bacterial liver abscesses.

Number of patients with hepatic abscesses		9
Related to complications of biliary tract	5	
Cystic duct obstruction	3	
Dislodged T tube	1	
Obstruction by T tube	1	
Related to multiple infarcts and hepatic artery thrombosis	2	
Ligation of left hepatic artery after erosion by abscess 2° to biliary tract complications	1	
Undetermined	1	

developed the abscess after surgical conversion of a cholecystojejunostomy to a choledochojejunostomy which was complicated by persistent bile leak and peritonitis. In the final patient there was no obvious explanation for the abscess, which was surgically drained 34 months after transplantation: she is alive almost four years later.

Candidiasis

Nine patients died with disseminated candidiasis as early as 12 days and as late as 16 months after transplantation. Five of the nine patients also had bacterial sepsis. In the other four patients bacterial sepsis did not appear to be present or appeared to be controlled at the time of death.

The factors which may have contributed to invasion by candida species are listed in Table 10. They include portal vein thrombosis, peritonitis complicating biliary leaks, intestinal ulcerations and fistulae, intraaortic balloon pump for heart failure and the need for prolonged ventilatory assistance.

Five additional patients were detected to have early invasive localized candidiasis in the liver (1), kidneys (1), urinary bladder (1), peritoneal cavity (1), lungs (1) or pleural space (1) at autopsy.

Miscellaneous infections

Twelve patients died with a variety of other infections (Table 11). Two patients

Table 10. Disseminated candidiasis.

Number of patients		9
With bacterial sepsis	5	
Predisposing conditions		
Portal vein thrombosis	early 1 (2)[a]	
With bleeding esophageal varices	late 1	
Peritonitis due to bile leak	3	
Open peritoneal cavity	2	
Bleeding duodenal ulcer requiring surgical intervention	2	
Leak of pyloroplasty	1	
Penetrating duodenal ulcer	1	
Damaged graft with coagulopathy	2 (3)	
Hemicolectomy	1	
Proctitis with bleeding rectal ulcers	1	
Intraaortic balloon pump	1	
Prolonged mechanical ventilation	8	

[a] ( ) Number of grafts.

had disseminated aspergillosis discovered at autopsy. Both patients required respiratory support and one patient hemodialysis as well. One patient had received a second transplant. Both patients had been treated with amphotericin B intravenously for candida infections with positive blood cultures. No evidence of candidiasis could be found at autopsy in either patient. The candida infections were either missed, eradicated by early treatment with amphotericin B or suppressed by the superimposed aspergillosis.

Immunosuppression alone was responsible for a fatal Pneumocystis carinii lung infection of a patient recovering from Listeria monocytogenes meningitis. The single death from Pneumocystis carinii pneumonia does not reflect the true incidence of this opportunistic infection. Many patients were suspected of having the infection based on an unexplained fever and a change in arterial blood gas consisting in a fall of the arterial pO_2 or respiratory alkalosis. The suspicion prompted treatment with sulfamethoxazole and trimethoprim (plus folinic acid) whether chest x-rays showed characteristic infiltrates or not. No attempts were made to document these infections by lung biopsies.

Table 11. Liver transplant recipients dying with miscellaneous infections.

Patient #	Age/sex[a]	Infection	Other complications	Survival
OT102	50/F	Disseminated aspergillosis	Rejection of the first graft, respiratory failure, renal failure, gastrointestinal bleeding	17+56 days
OT110	53/m	Disseminated aspergillosis	Respiratory failure, peritonitis, gastrointestinal bleeding	50 days
OT104	26m/M	Pneumocystis carinii pneumonitis	Recovering from listeria monocytogenes meningitis	6 months
OT106	20/F	Undetermined	Pulmonary nocardiosis, Hydrocephalus & brain stem herniation, Cryptococcal meningitis?	15 months
OT122	29/F	Pneumococcal meningitis	Peritonitis and liver abscesses (dislodged T tube)	4 months
OT143	32/F	Pneumococcal meningitis	Abdominal abscesses and peritonitis (leaking hepatico jejunostomy)	13 months
OT128	44m/F	Acute broncho-pneumonia	General anesthesia and renal arteriogram for hypertension	5 months
OT132	16m/F	Influenza A virus with respiratory failure	Supravalvular pulmonary artery stenosis, respiratory failure	5 months
OT151	5/M	Varicella	Portal vein thrombosis	71 days
OT161	22m/F	Hepato cellular necrosis, associated with adenovirus type?		27 days
OT163	34m/F	Hepato cellular necrosis associated with adenovirus type 1		30 days
OT141	31/M	Recurrent hepatitis B virus infection with severe cirrhosis		11 months

[a] Age in years or months (m); F = female, M = male.

One patient died after treatment for pulmonary nocardiosis. She died in coma with obstructive hydrocephalus and brain stem herniation in the presence of a chronic meningitis of undetermined etiology suspect of unrecognized cryptococcal meningitis. Both infections are typical complications of immunosuppression.

Splenectomy at time of transplantation may have contributed as much as immunosuppression to the pneumococcal meningitis which developed in two patients. Both patients also had liver or abdominal abscesses and peritonitis and were described in previous sections.

Acute broncho pneumonia occurred in a small child after renal arteriogram under general anesthesia for evaluation of hypertension and cannot be attributed to immunosuppression alone.

Respiratory failure due to a respiratory tract virus infection as seen in an infant with pulmonary artery stenosis is a recognized complication of congenital heart disease of small children without immunosuppression.

A 5-year-old boy's death from varicella in spite of prophylaxis with zoster convalescent plasma after exposure emphasizes the risk of this virus for children without immunity acquired before transplantation.

One patient died 11 months after transplantation from severe liver cirrhosis. There was evidence of recurrent hepatitis B virus infection. He had recurrent HBs antigenemia and HBsAg was detected in the homograft by peroxidase stain. He was known to be HBsAg positive before transplantation and received several doses of hepatitis B hyperimmune globulin about the time of transplantation. Johnson, et al. had reported a patient without recurrence of HBs antigenaemia after such treatment [2]. Original hepatitis B virus associated disease recurred in two other transplant recipients from Denver.

Two infants died within one month after transplantation with hepatocellular necrosis associated with adenovirus (Type 1 and unknown) infection of the transplant. Adenovirus was isolated from nasopharyngeal and rectal swabs in both patients and from liver tissue in one. Numerous virus particles were demonstrated in liver tissue by electron microscopy in the latter patient.

There is suspicion that four children in the early Denver experience might also have died of liver necrosis associated with adenovirus infection.

Discussion

The results demonstrate that the majority of uncontrollable infections after liver transplantation were peritonitis with or without intraabdominal abscesses, hepatic abscesses and cholangitis.

The major risk factor for peritonitis lies in the nature of the operation. Accumulation of blood and other biological substances not normally present in the peritoneal cavity increases the chances for peritonitis after contamination. The source of bacteria is the flora of the intestinal tract. It is not clear whether the peritoneal cavity can be seeded if the intestinal tract is not entered during operation either deliberately or accidentally. It is conceivable that bacteria could migrate through an intestinal wall temporarily damaged by congestion and hypoxemia because of temporary occlusion of the portal vein during the transplant procedure. On the other hand it is easily understood how intestinal bacteria may enter the peritoneal cavity from biliary leaks or intestinal fistulae. Although some of these complications may be preventable by surgical skills, coagulopathy, tissue damage due to temporary ischemia, malnutrition or use of corticosteroids may contribute to their development. Liver transplant patients also are prone to duodenal and other ulcerations of the gastrointestinal tract.

The biliary tract always is exposed to the enteric flora if directly connected to the intestinal tract by a Roux en Y limb of jejunum and also frequently becomes colonized in the presence of a T tube even if the sphincter of Oddi is preserved. However this bactobilia gains clinical significance only if there is bile leak into the peritoneal cavity or obstruction.

Cystic duct obstruction almost always was associated with cholangitis and frequently with bacteremia. Correction of cystic duct obstruction by conversion to choledochojejunostomy usually was successful even in the presence of cholangitis.

Liver abscesses developed as a consequence of persistent cholangitis in the presence of biliary obstruction or in homograft livers with devitalized areas due to vascular thrombi, ischemic damage or rejection.

The concept of portal vein bacteremia as a cause of such abscesses is supported by clinical observations and animal experiments. However efforts to actually demonstrate transient portal bacteremia in humans have not been very successful. Blood cultures obtained from the portal vein during abdominal operations have yielded a few diptheroids and staphylocci epidermidis [3–5], but not the kind of enteric microorganism which one would have expected except in patients with ulcerative colitis undergoing colectomy [6].

Systemic immunosuppression may contribute to the lack of the host to localize infection and to the high incidence of bacteremia. One may speculate that after reestablishing of portal circulation not only bacteria but also endotoxins may enter the circulation from the altered intestine and not be cleared by the liver. Endotoxemia could affect the circulation, activate the complement system and affect the reticuloendothelial system. By these and other mechanisms it could contribute to decreased host defense mechanisms postoperatively.

Systemic antimicrobial agents at time of transplantation are used in an effort to prevent postoperative infections. Oral antimicrobial agents are started before operation for selective bowel decontamination according to the concept developed by van der Waaij [7] for the same purpose in Groningen and in other centers. It is possible that this selective bowel decontamination contributed to the low incidence of septic complications in the liver transplant recipients in Groningen [8].

The danger of superinfection with candida species has to be appreciated in all efforts to control the bacterial infections. A few of our patients died of disseminated candidiasis after the bacterial infectious complications had been controlled. Early administration of low doses of amphotericin B intravenously combined with 5-fluorocytosine appears to be the best currently available treatment for candida infections. The imidazole derivatives like miconazole or ketoconazole are less reliable because of the great variability in susceptibility of yeasts to these agents.

In bone marrow transplant recipients the combination of amphotericin B and cyclosporine has been associated with increased renal toxicity [9] including thrombosis of glomeruli [10].

The infectious complications described were seen in patients who received a liver transplant before the end of 1980. The group included only a small number of patients with cyclosporine for immunosuppression. The magnitude of septic complications may only be of historical interest because cyclosporine appears to be associated with less bacterial infections [11, 12]. The explanation for this observation may be the selective effect of cyclosporine which is limited to certain T cell populations or the need for smaller doses of corticosteroids for effective immunosuppression if used in combination with cyclosporine.

I touched only briefly on the subject of virus infections after liver transplantation. The risk of recurrent hepatitis B virus infection in the graft may be a contraindication to transplantation and may be determined by the presence or absence of active hepatitis B virus infection at time of transplantation. Persistent active virus infection correlates better with the presence of HBe antigen than HBs antigen. It has been suggested that prophylaxis with hepatitis B hyperimmune globulin may prevent reappearance of hepatitis B infection [2]. However serologic reevaluation of patients in whom such prophylaxis appeared to be effective revealed that these patients had antibodies to the e antigen but not e antigen in the circulation, suggesting that the virus infection was no longer active at time of transplantation [13].

Liver transplant patients are susceptible to acquire or reactivate infections with herpes viruses (herpes simplex virus, cytomegalovirus, varicella zoster or Epstein-Barr virus). These viruses can cause hepatic injury mimicking rejection, life threatening and even fatal infections. However the problem of such infection in liver transplant recipients is even less well defined than in kidney transplant and bone marrow transplant recipients. The observation of hepatic necrosis in the presence of adenovirus infection in children should be emphasized.

Acknowledgements

Thomas E. Starzl, M.D., Ph.D., created the opportunity for this study. The liver transplant program in Denver, Colorado, was supported by grants from the

National Institutes of Health and from the General Clinical Research Centers Program of the Division of Research Resources, National Institutes of Health.

References

1. Starzl TE, Iwatsuki S, van Thiel DH *et al.*: Evolution of liver transplantation. Hepatology 2:614–636, 1982.
2. Johnson PJ, Wansborough-Jones MH, Portman B *et al.*: Familial HBsAg positive hepatoma: Treatment with orthotopic liver transplantation and specific immunoglobulin. Brit Med J 1:216, 1978.
3. Coblentz A, Kelly KH, Fitzpatrick L: Microbiologic studies of the portal and hepatic venous blood in man., Amer J Med Sci 228:298–300, 1954.
4. Schatten WE, Desprez JD, Holden WD: A bacteriologic study of portal vein blood in man. Arch Surg 71:404–407, 1955.
5. Orloff MJ, Peskin GW, Ellis HL: A bacteriologic study of human portal blood: Implications regarding hepatic ischemia in man. Ann Surg 148:738–746, 1958.
6. Eade MN, Brooke BN: Portal bacteraemia in cases of ulcerative colitis submitted to colectomy. Lancet 1:1008–1009, 1969.
7. Van der Waaij D: The colonization resistance of the digestive tract in experimental animals and its consequences for infection prevention, acquisition of new bacteria and the prevention of spread of bacteria between cage mates. In: Van der Waaij D, Verhoef J (eds). New criteria for antimicrobial therapy maintenance of digestive tract colonization resistance. Proceedings of a symposium, Utrecht, January 1979. Exerpta Medica, Amsterdam, pp 43–52, 1979.
8. Krom RAF, Gips CH, Houthoff HJ *et al.*: Orthotopic liver transplantation in Groningen, The Netherlands (1979–1983). Hepatology 4:61S–65S, 1984.
9. Kennedy MS, Deeg HJ, Siegel M *et al.*: Acute renal toxicity with combined use of amphotericin B and cyclosporine after marrow transplantation. Transplantation 35:211–215, 1983.
10. Shulman H, Striker G, Deeg HJ *et al.*: Nephrotoxicity of cyclosporine A after allogeneic marrow transplantation glomerular thrombosis and tubular injury. N Engl J Med 305:1392–1395, 1981.
11. Dummer JS, Hardy A, Poorsattar A, Ho M: Early infections in kidney, heart and liver transplant recipients on cyclosporine. Transplantation 36:259–267, 1983.
12. Peterson PK, Rynasiewicz JJ, Simmons RL, Ferguson RM: Decreased incidence of overt cytomegalovirus disease in renal allograft recipients receiving cyclosporin-A. Transplant Proc 15:457–459, 1983.
13. Rolles K, Williams R, Neuberger J, Calne R: The Cambridge and King's College Hospital experience of liver transplantation (1968–1983). Hepatology 4:50S–55S, 1984.

12. Cytomegalovirus (CMV)-infections and hosts' immunoregulation in liver transplantation

T.H. THE, H.W. ROENHORST, R.A.F. KROM, J.M. MIDDELDORP, H.J. HOUTHOFF and CH.H. GIPS

Introduction

In organ transplantation, e.g. orthothopic liver transplantation, the graft acceptance and long-term graft survival depend on many factors, most of them being only partially revealed. Next to technical-surgical factors, host factors play an important role. These include pretransplant immunocompetence (determined by genetic background, nature of liver disease and state of health), the post-transplant immunosuppression induced by immunosuppressive therapy and complicating bacterial, fungal and viral infections.

Treatment with immunosuppressive drugs is needed for the suppression of hosts' immune reactivity against transplantation antigens on grafted organ. Effector mechanisms leading to rejection or long term allograft tolerance are controlled by immunoregulatory mechanisms based on a balanced interaction of helper, suppressor and effector lymphocytes. Immunosuppressive therapy predisposes to serious viral infections and especially to reactivation of latent cytomegalovirus (CMV)-infection [1]. In this article the influence of cytomegalovirus (CMV)-infections on hosts' immunocompetence will be underlined as an additional important factor in determining allograft tolerance.

The similarity between active CMV-infection and graft rejection and the practical implications of a rapid diagnosis of 'early' CMV-disease will be discussed.

CMV–host interrelationship

There exists a close interrelationship between CMV and its hosts' immunological defence system. Firstly, specific immunity against CMV is of importance for the control of the infection. Secondly, an active CMV-infection induces immunosuppression even in a previous healthy individual. These, virus-specific immunity and CMV-induced immunosuppression, are the two sides of the same coin i.e.

hosts' infection with this virus. It is difficult to understand how the wide spectrum of (distinct) clinical symptoms can be caused by infections with one and the same virus. At the one end of this spectrum CMV-infections are harmless but at the other end they cause life-threatening complications. The expression and severity of disease symptoms are closely related to the hosts' immune status at time of the infection.

Hosts' immunity against CMV (the one side of the coin), depends on a previous infection with this virus and is evidenced by the presence of anti-CMV antibodies. Most of the CMV-seropositive individuals have an effective virus-directed immunity [2] and can keep this CMV-infection under control, i.e. in latency. However, secondary CMV-infections can occur by reactivation of latent CMV-infections or introduction of new CMV-strains. In general, these secondary CMV-infections are considered less harmful than primary infections in CMV-seronegative individuals who also lack a cellular immunity against CMV-infections.

Suppression of hosts' cellular immunity by CMV-infections (the other side of the coin), has been studied in patients with active CMV-infection [3, 4]. The results showed that even previously healthy individuals with a 'CMV-mononucleosis syndrome' have a virus-induced suppression of their general cellular immunity. This acquired immunodeficiency is only temporarily present and is associated with an increased incidence of 'secondary infections' due to increased susceptibility to opportunistic infections [4]. The associated immunological phenomena are an increased number of circulating T-cells, inverted ratios of T helper/T suppressor lymphocytes (T4/T8 ratio) [5] and finally suppression of in vitro lymphocyte proliferative responses in short term peripheral blood lymphocyte cultures after addition of distinct mitogens, bacterial antigens (or allogeneic lymphocytes). Besides, memory responses of circulating lymphocytes against CMV-specific antigens are also prolonged absent or suppressed [3].

Interestingly, in the same individual virus-specific immunity and immunosuppression are directly related. Patients with the highest cellular immunity against CMV (high responders) showed significant less immunodepression of their general cellular immunity than the low responders. In addition, when patients were followed after 6 months at reconvalescence immunocompetence of the high responders was normalised whereas the low responders still showed significant depressed general immunocompetence. The results of these studies demonstrated the close relationship between CMV-infections and the hosts' general immunocompetence. It is likely that CMV-induced immunodepression is based on the influence (directly or indirectly) of CMV-infection on hosts' immunocompetent cells. Inverted ratios of helper/suppressor T-cells may support this assumption, besides a deficiency in the T-helper cell population is also likely. In relation to liver transplantation it is important to know that the drug-induced immunosuppression enhances the above mentioned CMV-induced suppression of hosts' immunocompetence.

Pathophysiology of CMV-diseases

One of the most intriguing questions concerns the wide spectrum of clinical manifestations in CMV-infections in different hosts. At the one end of this spectrum CMV-infections are harmless as in most individuals but at the other end the virus may cause fatal disease in some. Table 1 summarises the different stages of CMV-disease as determined by their hosts' immunostatus background. In stage I there is clinical asymptomatic (latent) CMV-infection. Hosts' immunity against CMV-antigens dominates whereas no virus-induced immunodepression is present. Stage II is characterised by clinical symptomatic CMV-disease. Both virus-directed immunity and CMV-induced immunodepression are detectable in the same patient. Recovery from this stage of disease to stage I is in allograft recipients improved by lowering or stopping immunosuppressive medication. In stage III patients have irreversible end-stage CMV-disease. Virus-specific immunity is virtually absent whereas general immunodeficiency is pronounced.

In allograft recipients some of the clinical symptoms of stage II (CMV-infection, the 'early' CMV-disease) being fever of the intermittent type, arthralgia, thrombopenia, rise of serum creatinine in renal transplantation or disturbances in liver tests in case of liver transplantation are in fact difficult to discriminate from allograft rejection episodes [1]. However, the clinical implications are great. If erroneously anti-rejection treatment is given to an actively CMV-infected recipient the danger of converting stage II to stage III (the disseminated CMV-disease) is likely and a point of no return then may be reached. In contrast, a correct diagnosis of stage II CMV-disease and lowering or even stopping immunosuppressive treatment enables hosts' immunity to combat CMV-infection. This may give the opportunity for overcoming symptomatic CMV-disease and gaining or regaining viral latency (stage I or clinical asymptomatic).

Our results and also of others in renal and liver transplantations show that even drastic lowering of immunosuppressive treatment in CMV-infected recipients were not only followed by recovery from CMV-disease but also importantly were not complicated by accelerated graft rejection. This illustrates that CMV-induced

Table 1. Pathophysiology of different stages of CMV-diseases.

Stage	Symptoms	Immunestatus	
Stage I	Clinical asymptomatic (latency)	Immunity	++
		Immunodeficiency	−
Stage II	'Early' CMV disease	Immunity	+
		Immunodeficiency	+
Stage III	'Late' CMV disease (generalised CMV with opportunistic infections)	Immunity	−
		Immunodeficiency	++

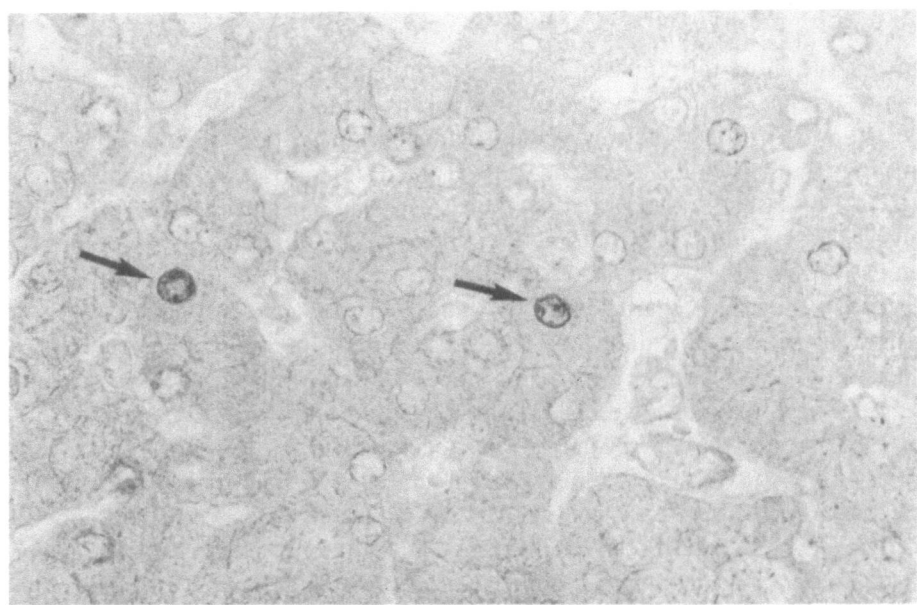

Figure 1. Immuno-histological staining of patient' liver biopsy with stage II or 'early' CMV-disease. Direct immunoperoxidase staining with labelled antibodies against CMV-EA. Positive EA nuclear staining in two hepatocytes (→). Enlargement 560×.

immunosuppression on itself is sufficient to prevent temporarily a rejection of the grafted organ.

Diagnosis of CMV-disease

The foregoing illustrates the great impact of a rapid diagnosis of early CMV-disease. Next to the clinical symptoms mentioned above, the diagnosis is made on serological tests and on tissue cultures. Indirect immunofluorescence techniques for the detection of antibodies against CMV-early and CMV-late antigens are helpful [6]. Recently, an improved CMV-ELISA technique has become available for detection of IgM antibodies against these CMV-antigens [7]. The commonly used complement fixation tests are less sensitive in the detection of CMV-latency and furthermore significant rises in antibody titres or seroconversion lag behind one to several weeks when compared o indirect immunofluorescence or CMV-ELISA tests [7].

Since CMV-isolation by culture methods asks days to weeks before having results, the direct detection of CMV-antigens offer a great advantage. Detection of CMV-early antigens in biopsy material has been described using an indirect

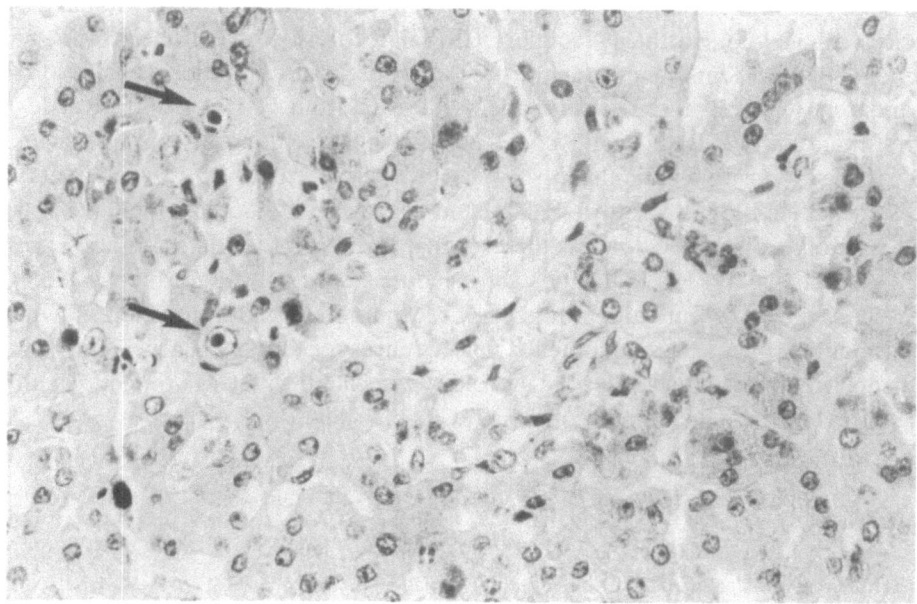

Figure 2. Histological staining (Hematoxilin Eosin) of a liver biopsy from a liver transplant patient with stage III or 'late' CMV disease. Area with confluent necrosis of hepatocytes and a minimal inflammatory reaction probably reflecting patients' immunodeficiency. Several inclusion bodies (→) are present. Enlargement 350×.

peroxidase staining method on sections [8]. Availability of monoclonal antibodies against CMV-specific antigens in the near future may improve sensitivity and specificity of in-situ detection of CMV antigens in tissue-sections.

Conclusion

1. Results from studies in patients undergoing organ transplantation stress the role of CMV-infections on the hosts' immunoregulatory mechanisms. The CMV-induced immunosuppression and drug-induced immunosuppression are both contributing to allograft tolerance.

2. Active CMV-infection can mimick allograft rejection. Frequent serologic monitoring of CMV-antibody status after transplantation by means of sensitive tests is mandatory in recognizing this situation in order to prevent conversion to stage III CMV-disease.

3. In case of active stage II or III CMV-disease lowering or even temporarily stopping of the immunosuppressive medication favours recovery by the hosts' own immunological defences, without the risk of accelerated graft rejection.

4. Pre-transplant knowledge of CMV-specific immunity in candidates for liver

118

transplantation is required as primary CMV-infections are more likely to have a serious clinical course than secondary CMV-infections. Prevention of primary infections in patients' management pre- and post-transplantation is therefore mandatory. Especially bloodcomponents derived from CMV-seropositive donors should not be used. Livers from CMV-seropositive donors should be given to CMV-seropositive patients only.

Logistics should in the future be directed to the use of blood components and livers from seronegative donors only in patients who prior to transplantation are CMV-seronegative. Rapid diagnostic procedures (serology and/or biopsy-staining) should be of great value in the early recognition of CMV-infection in liver transplant recipients with immediate consequences for therapy. Early identification and treatment may reduce the morbidity associated with CMV-infection and may prevent the development of the irreversible stage III.

References

1. Betts RF: Cytomegalovirus-infection in transplant patients. Prog Med Virol 28:44–64, 1982.
2. Schirm J, Roenhorst HW, The TH: A comparison of in vitro lymphocyte proliferation induced by cytomegalovirus infected human fibroblasts and cell-free cytomegalovirus infected human fibroblasts and cell-free cytomegalovirus. Infect Imm 30:621–627, 1980.
3. Ten Napel ChrHH, The TH: Acute cytomegalovirus infection and the host immune response. I. Development and maintenance of cytomegalovirus (CMV) induced in vitro lymphocyte reactivity and its relationship to the production of CMV-antibodies. Clin Exp Immunol 39:263–271, 1980.
4. Ten Napel ChrHH, The TH: Acute cytomegalovirus infection and the host immune response. II. Relationship of suppressed in vitro lymphocyte reactivity to bacterial recall antigens and mitogens with the development of cytomegalovirus induced lymphocyte reactivity. Clin Exp Immunol 39:272–278, 1980.
5. Carney WP, Iacoviello V, Hirsch MS: Functional properties of T lymphocytes and their subsets in cytomegalovirus mononucleosis. J Immunol 130:390–393, 1983.
6. The TH, Andersen HK, Spencer ES, Klein G: Antibodies against cytomegalovirus-induced early antigens (CMV-EA) in immunosuppressed renal-allograft recipients. Clin Exp Immunol 28:502–505, 1977.
7. Middeldorp JM, Jongsma J, Ter Haar A, Schirm J, The TH: Detection of IgM and IgG antibodies against cytomegalovirus-early (CMV-EA) and -late antigens (CMV-LA) by ELISA. J Clin Microbiol (in press).
8. The TH, Tegzess AM, Houthoff HJ, Schirm J: CMV antigenic markers in renal transplantation. In: Transplantation and clinical immunology, Vol XII. Amsterdam, Excerpta Medica, 1981, pp 26–33.

13. Immune responses to donor antigens in liver transplantation

J.M. BEELEN

Introduction

The liver compared with other transplanted parenchymatous organs is a privileged graft considering susceptibility to immunological attack.

In animals of different species a prolonged survival of the liver allograft is observed although there is progressive immune rejection. Indefinite survival without the use of immunosuppressive agents can be achieved in pig and rat. In the rat the fate of the graft proves to be strictly dependent on the donor/recipient strain combination. This model is studied extensively to clarify mechanisms responsible for the different levels of responsiveness.

In human liver transplantation ABO blood group incompatibility or a positive lymphocytotoxic crossmatch test does not induce the hyperacute rejection observed in kidney transplantation. Episodes of acute rejection commonly occur in the early posttransplant period, especially 5–14 days after surgery. In Groningen protocolled biopsies are taken the 8th postoperative day. All transplants showed a mild type of acute rejection easily reversible in spite of HLA-DR mismatches. On the other hand rejections observed during forced reduction of the immunosuppressive therapy because of the presence of viral infection occurred only in the patients sharing no DR antigens with the donor. Whether this corelation is a reflection of more intensive rejection responses or a less effective clearance of virus due to a lack of Major Histocompatibility Complex (MHC) class II compatibility needs to be clarified.

Experimental studies

In dog, baboon and monkey orthotopic liver transplantation leads to a fairly prompt rejection, although this rejection can be controlled more easily than in kidney transplantation with the use of immunosuppressive agents [1–4]. The relatively mild rejection of the liver allograft is more pronounced in the pig [5, 6].

In rat depending on the strain combination indefinite survival can be achieved. Therefore the rat model is most suitable to elucidate mechanisms involved in the induction of tolerance. Histological studies of liver grafts in two fully allogeneic strain combinations showed that in both combinations a rejection response occurred, most marked two weeks posttransplant. However in the strain combination of longterm survivors ongoing rejection was lacking, while in the other strain combination progressive rejection of the graft was seen [7]. As shown by subsequent skin grafting the state of unresponsiveness induced by liver transplantation is systemic and donor-specific. Liver grafting can even reverse a preexisting state of immunization [8].

The detected humoral response in the combinations with prolonged survival is predominantly against the class II antigens of the Major Histocompatibility Complex, while in the group of rejectors high titer antibodies to class I antigens are formed [9]. It is reported that release of soluble antigen as well as immune complexes in antigen excess can lead to specific protection of the graft [10, 11]. In the rejector strain no free soluble antigen will be present because of the high titer class I antibodies. In the long term survivors the class II antibodies themselves can function enhancing as reported in mouse and man [12, 13]. Also the soluble class I antigens and immune complexes of optimal composition can contribute to the prolonged survival.

On the cellular level tolerance induced by liver transplantation is associated with unaltered graft versus host and mixed lymphocyte culture responses. However in vitro generated cytolytic activity is markedly impaired. Also adoptive transfer assays indicate a specific deletion of clones responsible for graft rejection [14]. A comparison of the degree of survival time prolongation with that observed in the adoptive transfer experiments of Roser and Dorsch makes the involvement of suppressor cells unlikely [15].

Liver transplantation in a variety of strain combinations shows how rejection is defined by both the recipient genotype and the specific donor histoincompatibility [16]. The present understanding of immune response (Ir) gene control of allograft rejection in respect of recipient/donor combination is surveyed by Butcher and Taylor [17].

One can put forward that dosage, way of presentation and regenerative capacity may contribute to the fact that the liver is less vulnerable to immune attack than other parenchymatous organs. In this respect the Kupffer cells, cells that express both class I and class II antigens [18, 19], can process antigen [20] and become of recipient origin within 6 months posttransplant [21], deserve special attention in future investigation.

Human liver transplantation

With the use of immunosuppression in human orthotopic liver transplantation the incidence of uncontrollable rejection is low in contrast with kidney transplantation. A positive lymphocytotoxic crossmatch or ABO blood group incompatibility, in kidney transplantation causing hyperacute rejection [22–25], does not seem to influence the fate of the liver allograft.

Starzl reported two cases of liver transplantation with good early graft function, despite ABO blood group incompatibility [26]. In the first 26 liver transplantations performed in Groningen one was carried out across the ABO blood group barrier (OLT-22). In the protocolled biopsy of this patient taken the 8th day after surgery only mild acute rejection was observed normally present in biopsies in this early posttransplant period [27]. Rejection proved to be reversible without changes in the immunosuppressive regimen. Still general agreement exists that blood group incompatibilities should be avoided. A positive lymphocytotoxic crossmatch was detected in six out of the 26 transplantations. In two cases (OLT-2, OLT-4) this was due to autoantibodies. The other four patient sera contained HLA-antibodies (OLT-8, OLT-12. OLT-14 weak; OLT-26 strong) which specificity was also directed against HLA-A,B incompatibilities of the donor. Again in the protocolled early posttransplant biopsy [27] a comparable mild rejection was observed in the crossmatch positive and negative group. This outcome confirms the experiences of others [26–29]. Preexisting alloantibodies to donor incompatibilities, responsible for hyperacure rejection of the kidney allograft [30], form no contraindication in liver transplantation.

Most of the patients receive poorly matched livers because HLA-typing of the donor is done retrospectively in view of preservation time and shortage of livers. The HLA-A,B antigen system is very polymorphic so the incidence of good HLA-A,B matches is low. In Groningen 76% of the donor/recipient pairs were mismatched for 3 or 4 HLA-A,B antigens. In kidney transplantation matching for HLA-DR influence the graft outcome more than matching for HLA-A,B antigens [31, 32]. Because the HLA-DR matches system knows only limited polymorphism chances on retrospective good matches are better although only two of the first 26 grafts in Groningen were HLA-DR compatible. The mild early acute rejection was also seen in these two transplantations. Moreover this rejection episode in the group with one (n = 11) or two (n = 12) mismatches for HLA-DR was not more severe. Analysing the non protocolled biopsies [27], taken during forced decrease of the immunosuppressive therapy because of viral infection, rejection was seen in the 2 DR mismatched group (OLT-8, OLT-11, OLT-14) and in the combinations with 1 incompatible donor DR-antigen (OLT-3, OLT-5, OLT-7). However in the latter group also no HLA-DR compatibility between donor and recipient existed due to a blanc in the donor DR-typing. One can speculate if the lack of self MHC class II molecules may play a role in the occurrence of viral infection in the transplanted organ [33, 34]. The Kupffer cells deserve special attention in this respect too.

Conclusive remarks

The liver is a privileged organ considering susceptibility to immunological attack. In animal studies rejection responses proved to be defined by both recipient genotype and the specific donor histoincompatibility. In human liver transplantation HLA-DR matching does not influence the degree of early graft rejection. Reversible acute rejection as result of decrease of the immunosuppressive therapy because of viral infection is only seen in the group with no HLA-DR compatibilities. The role of the Kupffer cells in tolerance inducing responses and in handling of viral infection deserves special attention considering these cells express both class I and class II MHC antigens, can process antigen and become of recipient origin within 6 months posttransplant.

Acknowledgement

I gratefully acknowledge the assistance of Ernst Kuypers in collecting the patient data.

References

1. Starzl TE, Kaupp HA, Brock DR, Linman JR: Studies on the rejection of the homologous dog liver. Sing Gynecol Obstet 112:135–144, 1961.
2. Myburgh JA, Abrahams C, Mendelsohn D, Mieny CJ, Bersohn I: Cholestatic phenomenon in hepatic allograft rejection in the primate. Transplant Proc 3:501–504, 1971.
3. Calne RY, Davis DR, Pena JR, Balner H, de Vries M, Herbertson BM, Joysey VC, Millard PR, Seaman MJ, Samuel JR, Stibbe J, Westbroek DL: Hepatic allografts and xenografts in primates. Lancet 1:103–106, 1980.
4. Starzl TE, Marchioro TL, Porter KA, Taylor PD, Faris TD, Hermann TJ, Head CJ, Wandell WR: Factors determining short- and long-term survival after orthotopic liver homotransplantation in the dog. Surgery 58:131–155, 1965.
5. Garnier H, Clot JP, Bertrand M, Camplez P, Kunlin A, Gorin JP, le Goaziou F, Levy R, Cordier G: Liver transplantation in the pig: surgical approach. CR Acad Sci (Paris) 260:5621–5623, 1965.
6. Calne R, White HJO, Yoffa DE, Binns RM, Maginn RR, Herbertson BM, Millard PR, Molina VD, Davin DR: Prolonged survival of liver transplants in the pig. Br Med J 4:645–648, 1967.
7. Kamada N, Davies HffS, Wight D, Culank L, Roser B: Liver transplantation in the rat. Biochemical and histological evidence of complete tolerance induction in non-rejector strains. Transplantation 35:304–311, 1983.
8. Kamada N, Davies HffS, Roser B: Reversal of transplantation immunity by liver grafting. Nature 292:840–842, 1981.
9. Zimmermann FA, Butcher GW, Davies HffS, Brons G, Kamada N, Türel O: Techniques for orthotopic liver transplantation in the rat and some studies of the immunologic responses to fully allogeneic liver grafts. Transplant Proc 9:571–577, 1979.
10. Calne RY, Sells RA, Pena JR, Davis DR, Millard PR, Herbertson BM, Binns RM, Davies DAL: Introduction of immunological tolerance by porcine liver allografts. Nature 223:472–476, 1969.
11. Hutchinson IV, Zola H: Antigen-reactive cell opsonisation (ARCO) a mechanism of immu-

nological enhancement. Transplantation 23:464–469, 1977.

12. Jansen JLJ, Koene RAP, v. Kamp GJ, Hagemann JFHM, Wijdeveld PGAB: Hyperacute rejection and enhancement of mouse skin grafts by antibodies of a distinct specificity. J Immunol 115:392–394, 1975.

13. Jeannet M, Benzonana G, Arni I: Donor-specific B and T lymphocyte antibodies and kidney graft survival. Transplantation 31:160–166, 1981.

14. Davies HffS, Kamada N, Roser BJ: Mechanisms of donor-specific unresponsiveness induced by liver grafting. Transplant Proc 15:831–835, 1983.

15. Roser BJ, Dorsch SE: The cellular basis of transplantation tolerance in the rat. Imm Rev 46:55–86, 1979.

16. Zimmerman FA, Davies HffS: Response of rats to liver transplantation. In: Liver transplantation, Calne RY (ed), London, Grune and Stratton, 1983, p 40.

17. Butcher GW, Howard JC: Genetic control of transplant rejection. Transplantation 34:161–166, 1982.

18. Davies HffS, Taylor J, White DJG, Binns R: Major transplantation antigens of pig kidney and livers: comparison between the whole organ and their parenchymal constituents. Transplantation 25:290–295, 1978.

19. Daar A, Fuggle S, Fabre J, Ting A, Morris PJ: Some examples of the distribution of HLA-DR in several tissues as determined by immunoperoxidase staining. Immunol Rev 66:108 (Table 2), 1982.

20. Thomas HC, Vaez-Zadeh F: A homeostatic mechanism for the removal of antigen from the portal circulation. Immunology 26:375–382, 1974.

21. Portmann B, Schindler AM, Murray-Lyon IM, Williams R: Histological sexing of a reticulum cell sarcoma arising after liver transplantation. Gastroenterology 70:82–84, 1976.

22. Kissmeyer-Nielsen F, Olsen S, Petersen VP, Fjeldborg O: Hyperacute rejection of kidney allografts associated with pre-existing humoral antibodies against donor cells. Lancet 2:662–665, 1966.

23. Williams GM, Hume DM, Hudson RP, Morris PJ, Kano K, Milgrom F: 'Hyperacute' renal homograft rejection in man. N Eng J Med 279:611–618, 1968.

24. Patel R, Terasaki PI: Significance of the positive crossmatch test in kidney transplantation. N Engl J Med 280:735–739, 1969.

25. Wilbrandt R, Tung KSH, Deodhar SD, Nakamoto S, Kolff WJ: ABO blood group incompatibility in human renal homotransplantation. Am J Clin Pathol 51:15–23, 1969.

26. Starzl TE, Iwatsuki S, Van Thiel DH, Gartner JC, Zitelli BJ, Malatack JJ, Schade RR, Shaw BW, Hakala TR, Rosenthall JT, Porter KA: Evolution of liver transplantation. Hepatology 2:614–636, 1982.

27. Eggink HF, Hofstee N, Gips CH, Krom RAF, Houthoff HJ: Histopathology of serial graft biopsies from liver transplant recipients. Am J Pathol 114:18–31, 1984.

28. Calne RY, Williams R: Liver transplantation. Cur Prob Surg 16:1–44, 1979.

29. Iwatsuki S, Iwaki T, Klintmalm G, Koep LJ, Weil R, Starzl TE: Succesful liver transplantation from crossmatch positive donors. Transplant Proc 13:286–288, 1981.

30. Ting A: The lymphocytotoxic crossmatch test in clinical renal transplantation. Transplantation 35:403–407, 1983.

31. Ting A, Morris PJ: Powerfull effect of HLA-DR matching on survival of cadaveric renal allografts. Lancet 2:282–285, 1980.

32. Thorsby E, Moen T, Solheim BG, Albrechtsen D, Jakobsen A, Jervell J, Holvarsen S, Flatmark A: Influence of HLA matching in cadaveric renal transplantation: Experience from one Scandiatransplant Center. Tiss Anti 17:83–90, 1981.

33. Ashman RB, Müllbacher A: A T helper cell for anti-viral cytotoxic T-cell responses. J Exp Med 190:1277–1282, 1979.

34. Ada GL, Leung KN, Ertl H: An analysis of effector T cell generation and function in mice exposed to influenza A or Sendai viruses. Immunol Rev 58:5–24, 1981.

14. The use of cyclosporine in liver transplantation

S. IWATSUKI

Introduction

Cyclosporine is a metabolite isolated from culture broths of the fungi Cylindrocarpon lucidum and Trichoderma polysporum, which was discovered and characterized biochemically by scientists at the Sandoz Corporation, Basel, Switzerland. It was shown to be immunosuppressive by Borel *et al.* in mice, rats and guinea pigs [1, 2]. The drug depressed humoral and cellular immunity with a preferential and quickly reversible action against T-lymphocytes. These effects were not accompanied by bone marrow depression which frequently limits the doses of azathioprine and cyclophosphamide.

When cyclosporine was first used in patients by Calne and co-workers in 1978 [3, 4], it was hoped that no other drug would be routinely required. In their first two cases of liver transplantation, cyclosporine was used alone. However, most of their experience has been with delayed administration of the drug [5]. Aziathioprine and prednisone were used initially until renal and hepatic functions were adequate. Then, cyclosporine was begun, and the steroid dose was slowly reduced and withdrawn. The supervention of acute rejection during treatment with azathioprine and prednisone was troublesome.

In late 1979, cyclosporine became available for preliminary testing in the United States. Our initial experience in renal transplantation with cyclosporine led us to believe that the combination of cyclosporine with low-dose steroid is a more effective and safe immunosuppressive therapy than cyclosporine alone [6–8]. Since March 1980, 254 patients received orthotopic liver transplantation at the University of Colorado Health Sciences Center (14 patients in 1980) and the University Health Center of Pittsburgh before July 1984. Our experience in the use of cyclosporine with low-dose steroid in these 254 liver transplantations is briefly summarized here as an example of the use of the relatively new immunosuppressive agent–cyclosporine.

Basic formula

Cyclosporine

If there are several hours with which to prepare a recipient for liver transplantation, 17.5 mg/kg of cyclosporine is administered orally as an initial loading dose. After this, cyclosporine is usually not given until the operation is completed and the patient is moved to the intensive care unit in stable condition. At the intensive care unit, 2 mg/kg of intravenous cyclosporine is administered over 2–3 h and is repeated every 8 h. If there is not enough time for digestion of the drug before surgery, 2 mg/kg of intravenous cyclosporine is started preoperatively. When the vascular anastomoses are completed, and the recipient is hemodynamically stable and making an adequate amount of urine, the second dose of cyclosporine (2 mg/kg) is administered usually 8 h after the initial dose. This basic intravenous dose of cyclosporine (2 mg/kg every 8 h) is continued throughout the intraoperative and immediate postoperative periods.

In a few days after liver transplantation, the recipient usually can resume oral intake. Although cyclosporine is administered orally (17.5 mg/kg/day in two divided doses) as soon as the patient can tolerate it, intestinal absorption of the drug is usually poor for a few weeks. Therefore, during this early postoperative period, cyclosporine is administered orally as well as intravenously (Double-Route Therapy) in order to maintain adequate blood levels of the drug. We consider that the adequate blood level is achieved when the trough level of cyclosporine is between 800 and 1000 ng/ml of whole blood by RIA or between 150 and 250 ng/ml by HPLC measurement. When the adequate blood level of the drug is maintained by the double-route therapy, intravenous doses of cyclosporine is gradually decreased during the course of a couple of weeks and then discontinued. Often the oral dose exceeds 17.5 mg/kg/day in order to achieve adequate drug level (Table 1).

The average daily maintenance dose of oral cyclosporine at one month is 12.5 ± 4.3 mg for adults and 17.1 ± 3.9 for small children (Table 2).

Corticosteroid

Steroid therapy is begun immediately prior to the revascularization of liver graft with 1 g of intravenous methylprednisolone. After the operation, a 5-day burst of prednisone or methylprednisolone is started at 200 mg/day, and the dose reduced by daily decrements of 40 mg to an initial maintenance dose of 20 mg/day for adults (Table 1). In children, 250 mg or 500 mg of methylprednisolone is given intravenously prior to the revascularization. After the operation, a 5-day burst of prednisone or methylprednisolone is begun at 100 mg/day and the dose reduced by daily decrements of 20 mg to an initial daily maintenance dose of 10 mg/day.

Table 1. Basic formula of cyclosporine (low-dose steroid therapy).

	Cyclosporine	Steroids
Before transplant	2 mg/kg IV or 17.5 mg/kg p.o.	
Day of transplant	2 mg/kg IV q 8 hrs.	1 g of methylprednisolone IV
Day 1	(the dose may be decreased in presence of uremia, or high trough level)	50 mg of methylprednisolone IV q 6h
Day 2	(the dose may be decreased in presence of uremia, or high trough level)	40 mg of methylprednisolone IV q 6h
Day 3	3 mg/kg IV q 12h and 17.5 mg/kg p.o. in 2 divided doses	30 mg of prednisone p.o. q 6h
Day 4	(IV dose will be decreased as the	20 mg of prednisone p.o. q 6h
Day 5	intestinal absorption increases and	20 mg of prednisone p.o. q 12h
Day 6	the adequate blood level is achieved)	20 mg of prednisone p.o. q 24h
Day 7		

Further downward adjustment of steroid dosage is made in smaller children and infants.

The maintenance dose of prednisone at one month is 15 to 20 mg/day for adults and 5 to 15 mg/day for children. Further reduction of prednisone depends upon graft function.

Treatment for rejection

If rejection occurs inspite of cyclosporine and low-dose steroid therapy, principal responses are essentially the same as with conventional immunosuppressive therapy, namely to administer intravenously large doses of hydrocortisone or methylprednisolone intermittently, repeating the original 5-day burst of prednisone, and settling at a higher maintenance dose of steroid. Although cyclosporine does not permit much dosage maneuverability, because of its toxicity, it is sometimes possible to increase the doses given either orally or intravenously.

Antilymphocyte globulins (ALG, ATG or monoclonal antibodies) have been

Table 2. Daily oral cyclosporine dose (mg/kg) to avoid nephrotoxicity at 1, 3, 6, 9 and 12 months after liver transplant.

	1 month	3 months	6 months	9 months	12 months
Adults (over 40 kg)	12.5 ± 4.3	10.8 ± 6.7	8.2 ± 3.6	7.6 ± 3.5	6.7 ± 2.2
School-aged children (21–40 kg)	12.7 ± 3.1	12.1 ± 5.6	10.5 ± 2.8	9.8 ± 3.6	8.9 ± 2.7
Pre-school-aged children (less than 20 kg)	17.1 ± 3.9	17.8 ± 5.6	14.7 ± 5.3	12.1 ± 3.8	11.1 ± 2.2

used occasionally for steroid refractory rejections without convincing success.

As the success rate of the second liver transplantation with cyclosporine has exceeded 50% and the number of organ donors has been increasing, the liver grafts which require high doses of immunosuppression to maintain good function should be given up before the recipients become too ill to receive another graft. One of the factors of improved survival is certainly contributed to this early retransplant policy.

Side effects of cyclosporine

Major and minor side effects of cyclosporine include nephrotoxicity, hepatotoxicity, acidosis, hypertension, convulsions, lymphomas, gum hyperplasia, hirsutism, tremor, flusing and paresthesia. These side effects are usually dose-related and can be corrected by reducing the dose (Table 3).

Nephrotoxocity

Some degree of renal impairment was observed in approximately half of the liver recipients who were treated with our basic formula of cyclosporine-low-dose steroid therapy. However, less than 5% of the last 200 recipients required hemodialysis after liver transplantation. Most of these patients had had renal failure before transplant or were very unstable hemodynamically during the operation and/or immediate postoperative period.

Postoperative anuria or oliguria is usually of pre-renal cause in liver transplantation. However, postoperative renal failure can be exacerbated by cyclosporine nephrotoxicity. When anuria or oliguria persists despite adequate volume replacement and cardiac support, brief reduction of cyclosporine dose is recommended. After urine volume increases with the reduced dose and renal function improves, the dose is gradually increased to basic formula. If the recipient requires hemodialysis, the cyclosporine dose is usually reduced to maintain the trough level of the drug in the lower ranges (500–800 ng/ml of whole blood by

Table 3. Side effects of cyclosporine.

Major	Minor
Nephrotoxicity	Hirsutism
Hepatotoxicity	Gum hyperplasia
Hypertension	Tremor
Convulsions	Flushing
Lymphomas	Nausea, vomiting, diarrhea
Acidosis	Paresthesia

RIA) until the renal function recovers.

Mild renal impairment manifested by slightly elevated BUN and serum creatinine is commonly seen later in the post-transplant period. Intestinal absorption of cyclosporine increases with the improvement of liver function as well as that of the general condition of the recipients. Often cyclosporine dose is maintained high in the presence of mild graft rejection. Gradual reduction of the dose usually improves the renal function in these conditions.

Maintenance doses of oral cyclosporine to avoid nephrotoxocity at 1, 3, 6, 9 and 12 months are shown in Table 3. Small children and infants can tolerate higher doses of cyclosporine than adults.

Hepatotoxicity

Hepatotoxicity is an infrequent side effect of cyclosporine and is usually in mild form. It can manifest clinically both in hepatocellular injury form and in cholestatic form. Clinical differentiation of hepatotoxicity from graft rejection, virus hepatitis and mild bile duct obstruction is often difficult even after liver biopsy. Mild graft dysfunction which is refractory to anti-rejection therapy can be due to hepatotoxicity of cyclosporine. When the liver biopsy is not conclusive either for rejection or virus infection, it is worthwhile to reduce the cyclosporine dose briefly and to observe the response, particularly in the presence of adequate to high trough levels of the drug. Prolonged and intensified immunosuppression for unrecognized hepatotoxicity of cyclosporine may cause serious infectious complications. Only careful analyses of chemical and histological studies with high index of suspicion can lead to proper diagnosis of cyclosporine hepatotoxicity.

Lymphomas and lymphoproliferative lesions

The incidence of post-transplant lymphoma is probably less with cyclosporine-prednisone therapy than with conventional azathioprine-prednisone-ALG therapy (10). Epstein-Barr virus infections are usually associated with the development of these lesions. Fever, malaise and lymphadenopathy are usual clinical manifestations. Acute abdominal symptoms, such as perforation, obstruction, bleeding or diarrhea, also develop when intestinal lymph nodes are involved.

When lymphoma is confirmed by pathological examination, or even suspected by clinical manifestations, drastic reduction or discontinuation of immunosuppressive drugs (both cyclosporine and prednisone) is mandatory to overcome otherwise fatal lesions. Five of the 254 liver recipients treated with cyclosporine developed lymphomas. One patient died from airway obstruction due to tonsillar lymphoma which was unrecognized before death. Another patient had recovered from lymphoma after drastic reduction of immunosuppressive therapy, but died from necrotizing pancreatitis after the second liver transplantation for acute and chronic rejection of the first liver graft. In the other three patients, lymphomas disappeared with drastic reduction of immunosuppressive therapy. Experience in renal and heart transplant is the same as that of liver transplant [10]. The results of anti-neoplastic chemotherapy for this type of lymphoma is much worse than that of drastic reduction or discontinuation of immunosuppressive therapy. Anti-virus chemotherapy alone can not cure this lesion. Early recognition of lympho-proliferative lesions and subsequent drastic reduction of immunosuppressive therapy is the treatment of choice. Liver grafts usually suffer from rejection during this period of drastic reduction of immunosuppression, but three of the five grafts did recover from rejection with restoration of immunosuppressive therapy after lymphomas had disappeared.

External bile drainage and cyclosporine blood level

Early in the post-transplant course, a T-tube' is open to gravity drainage to prevent the leakage and secure the sound anastomosis of the bile duct. Occasionally, a large amount of bile is drained into the bag. Increases of cyclosporine blood concentrations to the toxic level after clamping the T-tube and decreases of blood

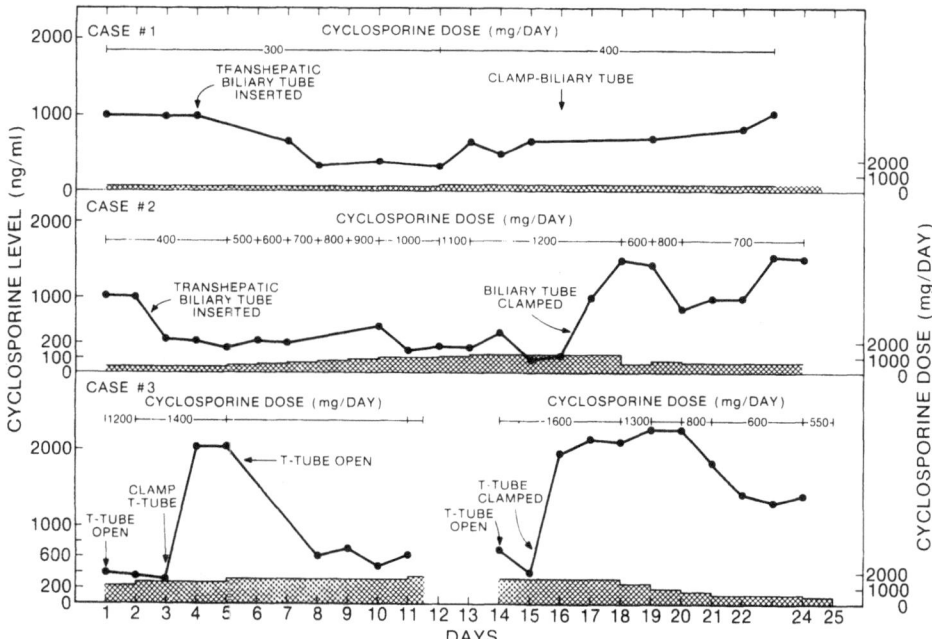

Figure 1. Three examples of changes in cyclosporine trough levels (ng/ml of whole blood by RIA) before and after external bile drainage either by a T-tube or by a percutaneous transhepatic tube.

130

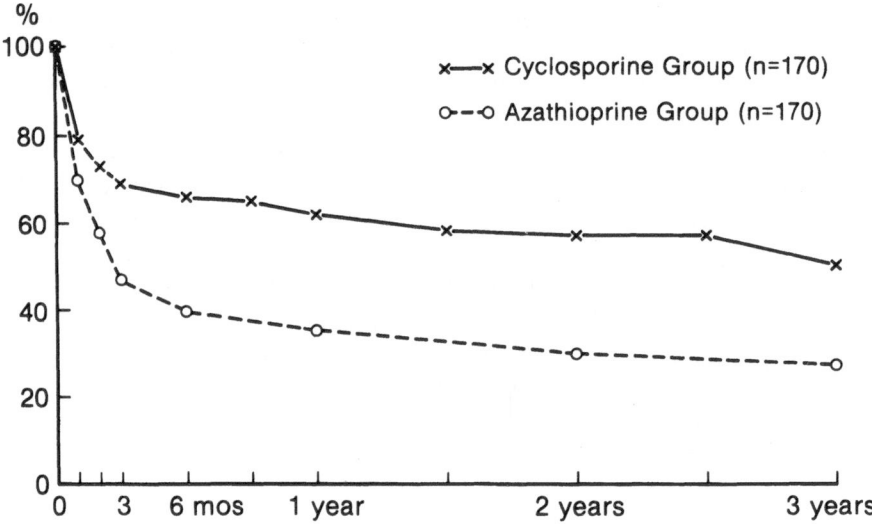

Figure 2. Improved survival after liver transplantation since the introduction of cyclosporine in 1980 at the University Health Sciences Center of Colorado and the University Health Center of Pittsburgh.

levels after opening the tube are often observed (Figure 1). There are two explanations for this observation: firstly, bile acids enhance the intestinal absorption of cyclosporine, and secondly, cyclosporine excreted into the bile in high concentration is reabsorbed by enterohepatic recirculation.

Influence of external biliary drainage upon blood levels of cyclosporine is one of the important considerations in determining the proper doses of the drug. External drainage of bile should be discontinued as early as possible in the post-transplant course in order to achieve steady blood level of cyclosporine.

Improved survival

Since the introduction of cyclosporine and low-dose steroid therapy in March 1980, the survival after liver transplantation has improved to over 70% at one year (Figure 2). Although there have been steady advances in surgical techniques, intra and postoperative care, antibiotics and other areas, this remarkable improvement could not have been achieved without the discovery of the new immunosuppressive drug–cyclosporine. The 5-year survival rate after liver transplantation will be greater than 50% in the near future.

References

1. Borel JF, Feurer C, Gubler HU *et al.*: Biological effects of cyclosporin A: a new antilymphocytic agents. Agents Actions 6:468–475, 1976.
2. Borel JF, Feurer C, Magnee C *et al.*: Effects of the new antilymphocytic peptide cyclosporine A in animals. Immunology 32:1017–1025, 1977.
3. Calne RY, White DJH, Thiru S *et al.*: Cyclosporin A in patients receiving renal allografts from cadaver donors. Lancet 2:1323–1327, 1978.
4. Calne RY, Rolles K, White DJG *et al.*: Cyclosporin A initially as the only immunosuppressant in 34 patients of cadaveric organs; 32 kidneys, 2 pancreases and 2 livers. Lancet 2:1033–1036, 1979.
5. Calne RY, White DJG, Evans DB *et al.*: Cyclosporin A in cadaveric organ transplantation. Br Med J 282:934–936, 1981.
6. Starzl TE, Weil R III, Iwatsuki S *et al.*: The use of cyclosporin A and prednisone in cadaver kidney transplantation. Surg Gynecol Obstet 151:17–26, 1980.
7. Starzl TE, Klintmalm GBG, Weil R III *et al.*: Cyclosporin A and steroid therapy in 66 cadaver kidney recipients. Surg Gynecol Obstet 153:486–494, 1981.
8. Starzl TE, Hakala TR, Rosenthal JT *et al.*: Variable convalescence and therapy after cadaveric renal transplantation under cyclosporin A and steroids. Surg Gynecol Obstet 154:819–825, 1982.
9. Starzl TE, Iwatsuki S, Van Thiel DH *et al.*: Evolution of liver transplantation. Hepatology 2(5):614–636, 1982.
10. Starzl TE, Nalesnik MA, Porter KA *et al.*: Reversibility of lymphomas and lymphoproliferative lesions developing under cyclosporin-steroid therapy. Lancet 1:583–587, 1984.

15. Pathology of infection and rejection in serial biopsies from liver homografts

H.J. HOUTHOFF, H.F. EGGINK, E.B. HAAGSMA, C.H. GIPS
and R.A.F. KROM

Introduction

Following a successful orthotopic liver transplantation (OLT) various graft syndromes may beset an uneventful follow-up. The major syndromes include episodes of acute graft rejection, viral infection with graft involvement, bacterial infection with liver abcess formation or bacterial cholangitis, obstructed bile flow in the large bile ducts, an impaired blood supply of the graft, drug reactions in the graft and chronic graft rejection. Rejection phenomena and infections of the graft being the main topics in this chapter, the other conditions will only be mentioned in relation to differential diagnostic and pathogenetic problems.

In autopsy studies of OLT recipients [1] the full-blown pathologic syndromes and their late sequelae in liver grafts have been documented. The early stages and pathogenesis of the pathologic syndromes can best be judged in studies of serial graft biopsies [2–4].

Furthermore, the recognition in a graft biopsy of early stages of rejection and their differentiation from infections may be helpful in establishing the proper diagnosis with major implications for the therapeutic regimen of the recipient: an increase in the immunosuppressive dosage may effectively treat rejection phenomena, but interferes with the recipient's ability to eliminate microbial infections.

The clinical and histopathologic presentation of the early stages of rejection episodes and infections are often modulated or masked by the immunosuppressive regimen, thus obscuring the proper diagnosis. The pathology of early stages of liver graft *rejection* in the absence of immunosuppression has been studied in experimental animals [5–7] (Chapter 3, 4 and 5). In our series the histopathology of the early and reversible stages of acute rejection in human OLT recipients could be studied in graft biopsies taken at the end of periods of forced withdrawal of immunosuppression to treat a previous viral infection [3]. The pathology of the early stages of *viral hepatitis* due to infection with cytomegalovirus (CMV), hepatitis B virus (HBV) and herpes simplex virus (HSV) in both normal and immune compromised hosts has been documented [8–11]. Together, these data could be used as guidelines for the histopathologic diagnosis of the early stages of rejection and infection.

Most important for the biopsy interpretation of early phases of graft rejection and infection, however, has been the correlation between histopathologic parameters on the one hand and liver tests, serology and clinical and therapeutic parameters on the other, supplemented with the clinical follow-up and the histopathology in a further graft biopsy. The clinical decision-making which leads to the immunosuppressive regimen employed and to any change in it for whatever reason will be directly reflected in the liver tests and in the histopathologic findings. The immunosuppression used in our centre consists of azathioprine and prednisolone, in combination. An example of this is shown in Figure 1, from which the importance of histopathologic documentation of early phases of graft syndromes can be evaluated.

The data in this chapter is mainly based on the study of serial graft biopsies in 25 OLT recipients. More than 110 planned protocolled biopsies from the grafts (before and 1 hr after OLT, on the 8th day, after 4 weeks, and at yearly intervals thereafter) have been collected and serve as a reference. Of more than 75 non-protocolled biopsies taken to document functional graft disturbances, a diagnosis of acute rejection has been made in 13 cases, viral infection was the diagnosis in 22 biopsies and bacterial cholangitis was suggested by the findings in four biopsies. In other unprotocolled biopsies an improvement of previous pathological conditions, aspecific changes in cases that were clinically suspect for one of the major graft syndromes, or a combination of syndromes were found. The methods used include light and electron microscopy and immunohistology for the detection of viral antigens, immunoglobulins, fibrin related products and lymphocytic differentiation antigens for phenotyping mononuclear subsets: a detailed description of these methods has been published elsewhere [3, 4, 9, 10, 12–18]. Also, data on the previous liver disease and the clinical follow up after OLT is presented elsewhere [19]. The criteria for the differential diagnosis of histopathologic findings have been published elsewhere, they are summarized in Table 1.

Rejection

In comparison to grafts of other organs, liver grafts are privileged as severe rejection is not a commonly occurring phenomenon [20]. In experimental studies it has been shown [21] that Major Histocompatibility Complex (MHC) incompatible liver grafts could survive for long periods depending on the recipient strain. Accordingly, in human OLT recipients MHC incompatibilities are frequently present without evidence of more prominent rejection episodes or an unfavorable prognosis under the commonly used immunosuppressive regimens. Also, allotypic antibodies to graft MHC antigens have been demonstrated in a

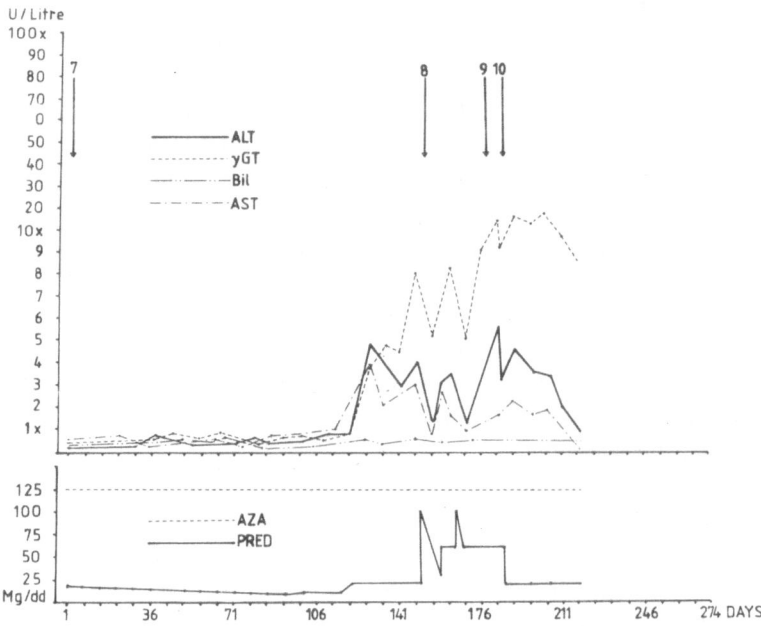

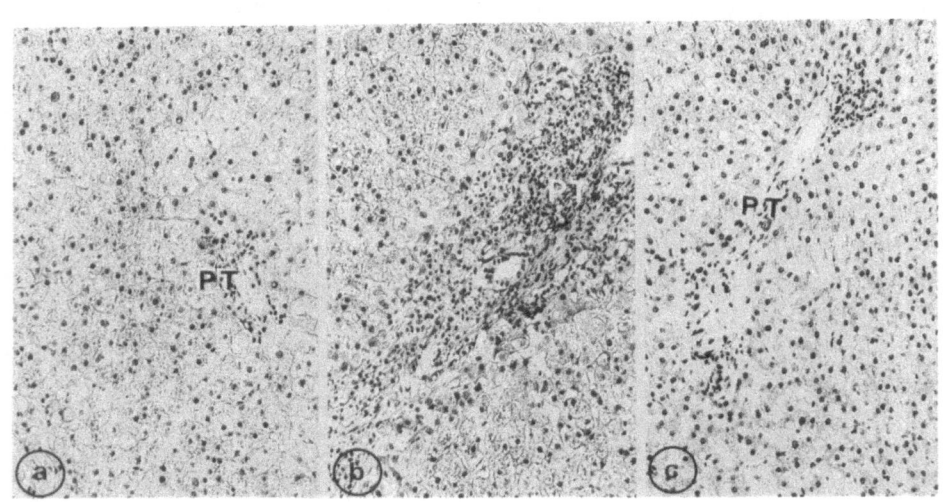

Figure 1. An episode of reversible rejection in OLT 11 is shown, during the second year after transplantation. In the graph, the time of liver biopsies (long arrows), some liver tests and the immunosuppressive regimen are presented from the 1st to the 210th day of the second year. After one year, the liver tests and the morphology in a protocolled liver biopsy (#7, shown in a) were well within the normal range. In the course of the continued decrease in the daily prednisolone dose, the serum levels of the γ-glutamyl transferase (γ-GT) and transaminases (AST, ALT) rose to approximately 4 times normal values, whereas total bilirubin (Bil) remained normal. In a non-protocolled biopsy (#8, shown in b) the portal tracts (PT) were enlarged and edematous; a dense portal infiltrate with lymphocytes, lymphoblasts and some plasma cells was present with spill-over on the periportal parenchyma and some piecemeal necrosis of liver cells. During the subsequently increased prednisolone therapy, the morphology in a biopsy (#9, shown in c) returned to normal, although the portal tracts still were somewhat enlarged and the liver tests remained elevated for some weeks. a, b, c: H&E, ×140.

Table 1. Morphologic characteristics of the major liver graft syndromes. Syndromes due to drug reactions or to infection with hepatitis B virus or non-A non-B virus have not been included in the table, since examples of these syndromes are not present in the series. +: present, ±: variable or inconspicuous, −: absent.

	Acute rejection			Viral infection	Cholangitis		Pure cholestasis	Chronic rejection	Circulation disorders
	Mild	Moderate	Severe		Bacterial	Obstruction			
portal tracts									
enlargement (edema, fibrosis)	+	+	+	−	+	+	−	+	−
inflammatory infiltrate									
lymphocytes	+	+	+	±	+	+	−	+	−
lymphoblasts	+	+	+	−	−	−	−	−	−
plasma cells	+	+	+	−	−	−	−	−	−
granulocytes	±	±	±	±	+	+	−	−	−
- with invasion of bile duct									
epithelium	±	+	+	−/±	+	+	−	±	−
periportal parenchyma	±	+	+	−	−	−	−	−	−
bile duct proliferation	−	−	−	−	+	+	−	−/±	−
prominent vascular endothelium	+	+	+	−	−	−	−	−/±	−
parenchyma									
piecemeal necrosis	±	+	+	−	−	−	−	−	−
spotty necrosis	−	−	−	+	−	−	−	−	−
bridging/confluent necrosis	−	−	+	−	−	−	−	−	+
diffuse inflammation	−	−	+	−/±	−	−	−	−	−/±
cholestasis	−	−	−/±	−	+	+	+	−	±

number of OLT recipients, but antibody dependent immune reactions have so far not been documented. Indeed, hyperacute rejection has never been observed in OLT. However, episodes of acute rejection do occur and are in most cases readily reversible [2, 3, 15], whereas chronic rejection has been observed as one of the causes of chronic graft failure [1, 22].

An episode of acute rejection is morphologically characterized by an enlargement of the portal tracts with a portal inflammatory infiltrate consisting of lymphocytes, lymphoblasts, plasma cells and some granulocytes (Figures 1, 2). As these dense and predominantly mononuclear infiltrates in the portal tracts have not been observed in any of the other graft syndromes, they are characteristic of rejection. Additional morphologic features of acute rejection were reactive changes in the vascular endothelial cells and the sinusoidal lining cells (Figure 3) and the occasional presence of some cholestasis in the liver parenchyma, but bile duct epithelial changes were minimal or absent. According to the severity of the rejection episode three types can be discerned (Figure 2), each being morphologically similar to a type of chronic active liver disease (CALD). The first type consists of the portal inflammation without evidence of involvement of liver parenchyma or bile ducts and thus conforms to chronic persistent hepatitis. A second type shows comparable features in combination with piecemeal necrosis of periportal hepatocytes, conforming to the mild to moderate type of CALD. The third type combines the features of CALD with confluent and/or bridging necrosis of the liver parenchyma and a mononuclear inflammatory reaction in the parenchyma, especially in the marginal zones of the areas with necrosis. This type, comparable to severe CALD, has only been observed after forced withdrawal of immunosuppression in relation to a previous viral infection. In our series, all three types proved to be readily reversible following an increase in the daily dose of prednisolone, as also evidenced by the disappearance of inflammation in the next graft biopsy.

Based on these morphologic findings in acute rejection the pathogenesis can be conjectured. In early stages, mononuclear cells start homing to the liver homograft and enter the portal tracts through the reactive endothelial lining of the

$\longrightarrow$

Figure 2. Morphology of successive stages of acute rejection, demonstrating the resemblance to chronic active hepatitis (CAH). (a) Initial stage, with a dense chronic inflammatory infiltrate in an enlarged portal tract. Sometimes, this is accompanied by necrosis of some periportal liver cells (arrow). The morphology is comparable to the mild type of CAH. OLT 7, biopsy #3, H&E, ×350. (b) Greatly enlarged portal tract with an extensive invasion of the periportal parenchyma by the inflammatory infiltrate (arrows). The morphology is comparable to the moderate type of CAH. OLT 7, biopsy #7, H&E, ×350. (c) Detail of the periportal parenchyma with spill-over of lymphocytes, lymphoblasts and plasma cells (arrows) and piecemeal necrosis of periportal hepatocytes. OLT 2, biopsy #10, PAS after diastase digestion, ×560. (d) Confluent and bridging necrosis of parenchymal areas (arrows). A chronic inflammatory infiltrate is present in and around the areas with necrosis and is prominent in the portal tract (PT). The morphology is comparable to the severe type of CAH. OLT 3, biopsy #6, H&E, ×140.

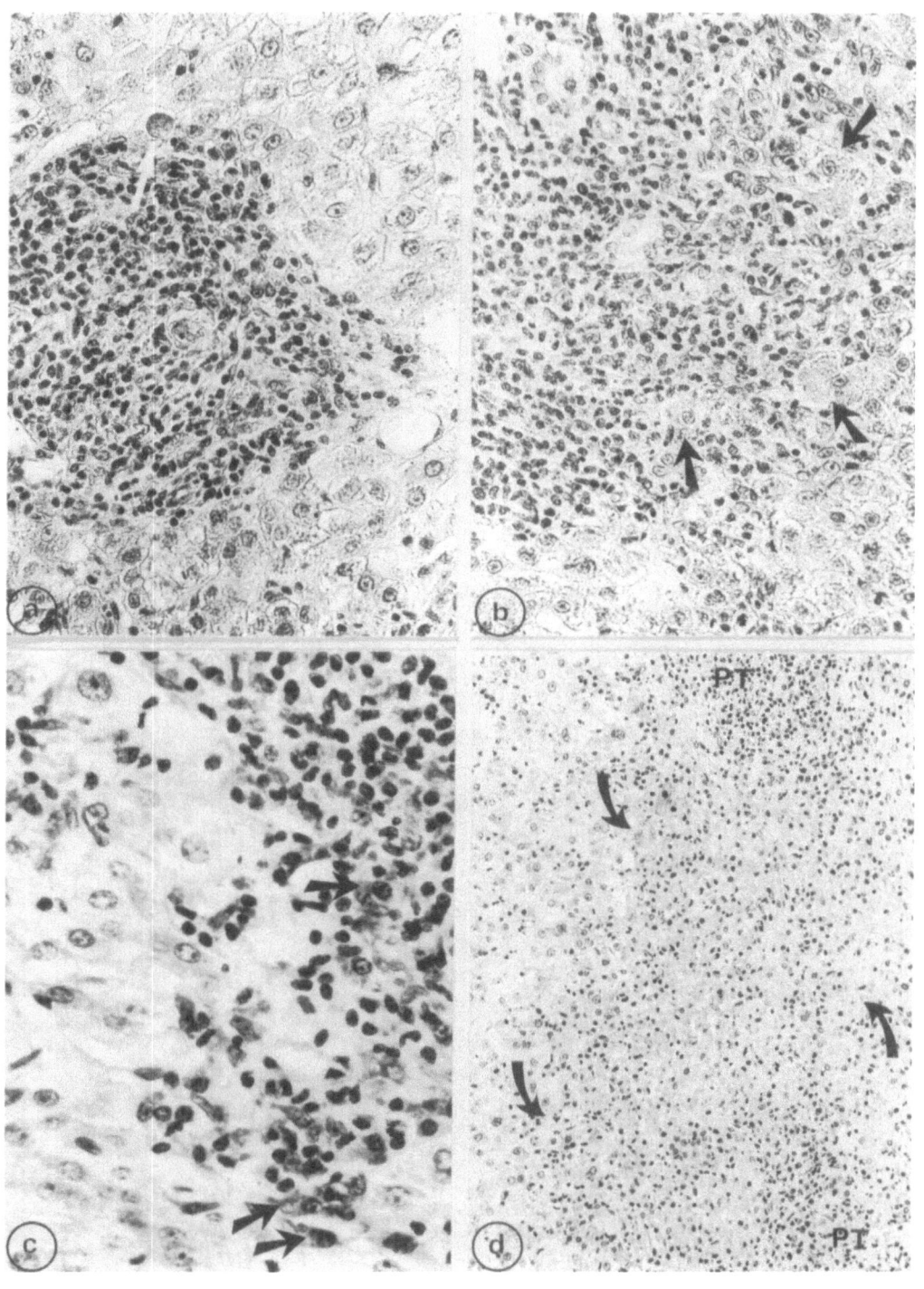

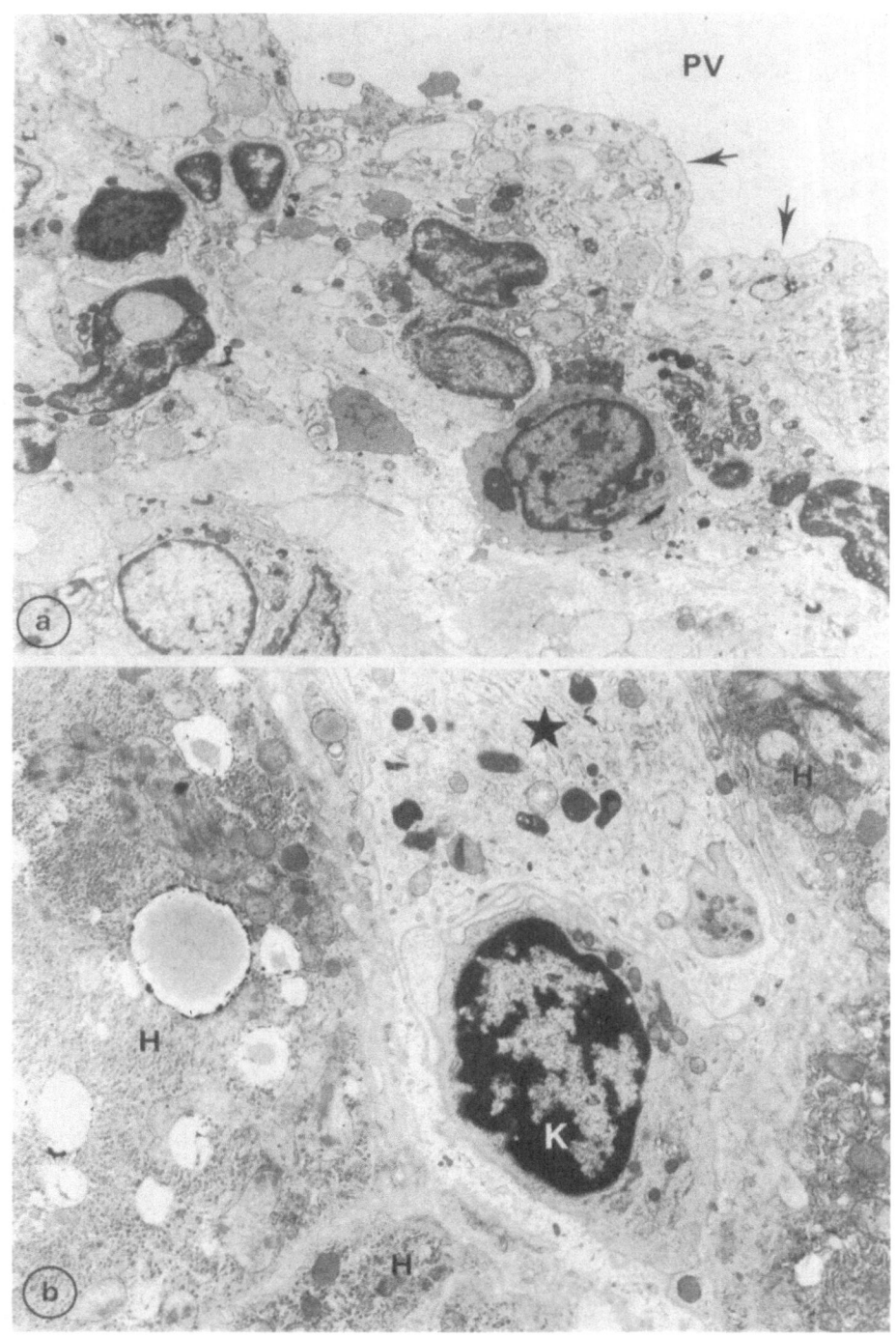

←

Figure 3. Ultrastructure of the vascular lining cells during rejection episodes. (a) In the wall of a portal vein (PV), the endothelial cells are swollen and reactive (arrows). In the portal connective tissue around the vessel wall, extravasated lymphocytes and macrophages are present. OLT 7, biopsy #3, ×5520. (b) In the wall of a parenchymal sinusoid, an activated Kupffer cell (K) with fingerlike processes is present. In the sinusoidal lumen (asterisk) cellular debris and parts of a macrophage are present. H: hepatocytes. OLT 7, biopsy #7, ×5420.

portal vessels (Figure 3a). The resulting cell mediated immune reaction is primarily directed towards the allogeneic liver cells and piecemeal necrosis can be observed (Figure 2b, c). Both T and non-B non-T lymphocytes of the cytotoxic/ suppressor phenotype (OKT 8[+]) make up a majority of the mononuclear cells, immunoglobulins as a contributing factor in the cytotoxic reaction can not be demonstrated [4, 15, 17]. In accordance with literature data on acute rejection in other organs, also in liver homografts it thus seems to be a cellular immune reaction. The reactive changes in the vascular and sinusoidal lining cells may contribute to circulation disorders in the graft, resulting in areas of confluent necrosis in cases of severe acute rejection.

The pathological changes in *chronic rejection* are more variable and the pathogenetic mechanisms are less well understood. The pathologic features of chronic rejection include (1) marked fibrosis with a sparse lymphocytic infiltrate in portal tracts, (2) intimal proliferation with foamy cells in the portal blood vessels and sinusoids with narrowing and obliteration of the vascular lumen (Figure 6a), (3) lesions of bile duct epithelial cells with infiltration of mononuclear cells into the wall and lumen of the ducts, and (4) total disappearance of the bile ducts, also known as the vanishing bile duct syndrome (Figure 6b) [1, 23]. In our series, some of the OLT recipients have the first feature in the protocolled biopsies taken at yearly intervals with an otherwise normal graft function, this is not considered to represent chronic rejection in the proper sense. In one patient the third feature has been observed in a biopsy, but both clinical and morphological changes disappeared after adjustment in the azathrioprine dose. In one of the patients that subsequently died, all features were present in graft biopsies and at autopsy. Some of the special pathogenetic problems in chronic rejection are discussed at the end of this chapter.

Viral infection

Viral infection of OLT recipients with involvement of the liver homograft occurs not infrequently, especially during the first months after transplantation. Characteristically, the pathologic changes are similar to those in viral hepatitis in immune compromised hosts in general; they include patchy acidophilic degeneration of individual hepatocytes and an inconspicuous mononuclear infiltrate in the parenchyma and portal tracts (Figure 4), including cells of the natural killer

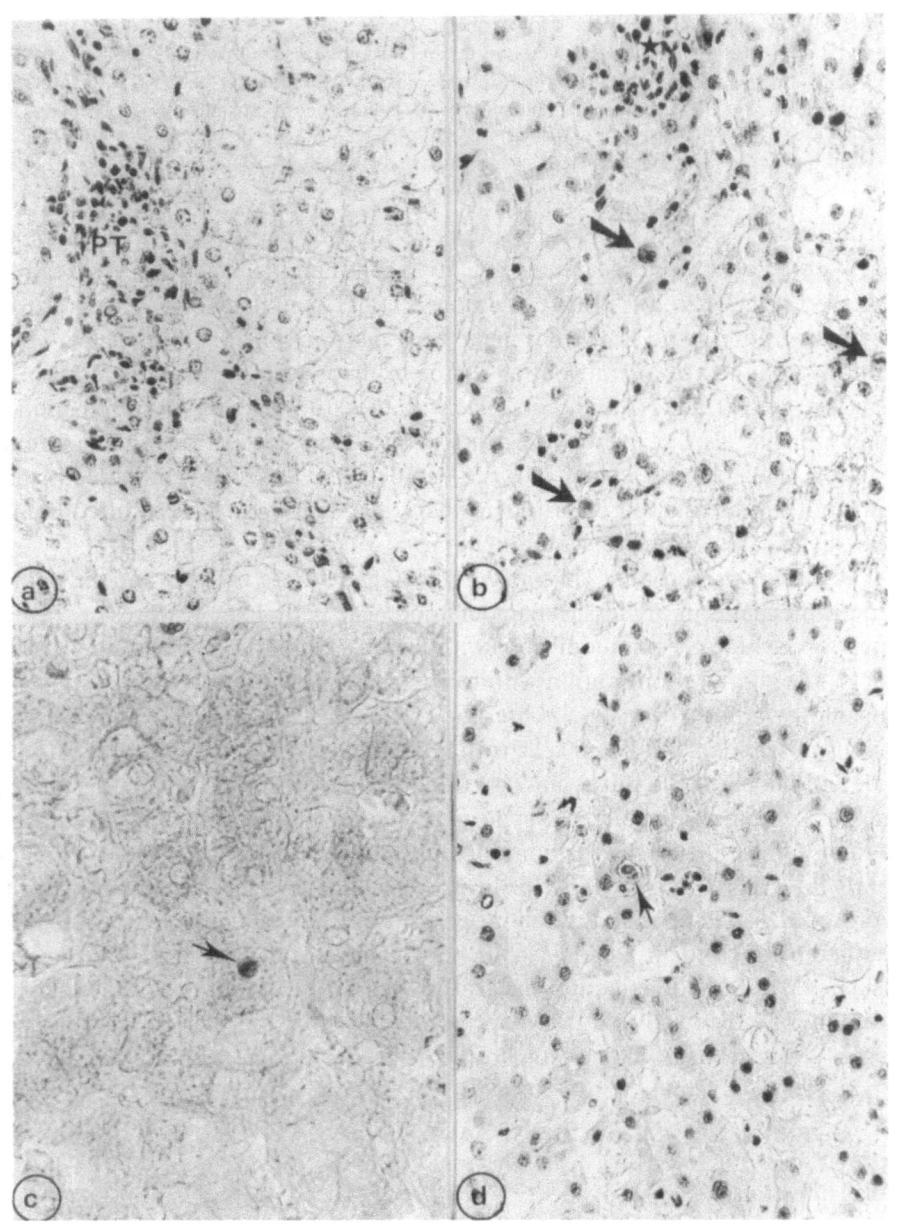

Figure 4. Morphology of viral infection in liver grafts. The morphology closely resembles viral hepatitis in immune compromised hosts in general. (a) In the portal tracts (PT) the inflammatory infiltrate is inconspicuous with only some lymphocytes and granulocytes. OLT 2, biopsy #4, H&E, ×350. (b) In the liver parenchyma, spotty necrosis with acidophilic degeneration of hepatocytes (arrows) are present, sometimes accompanied by a sparse lymphocytic infiltrate or a lymphohistiocytic nodule (asterisk). OLT 2, biopsy #3, H&E, ×350. (c) During the early and reversible stages of viral infection, viral inclusion bodies of cytopathogenic effects are not found. However, viral antigens may be demonstrable in liver cell nuclei (arrow), as in this case for CMV early antigen. OLT 2, biopsy #7, anti-CMV EA+LA+ serum in a two step reaction, ×560. (d) During the late stages of viral infection, inclusion bodies are present. Here, a CMV inclusion body (arrow) is shown. The lymphocytic infiltrate in the liver parenchyma is inconspicuous. OLT 14, biopsy #11, H&E, ×350.

phenotype (Leu 7+) [14]. During the early stages of viral hepatitis, these changes are not accompanied by demonstrable cytopathogenic effects of the virus in light microscopy, nor by the regular presence of viral particles in electron microscopy. Thus, ground glass hepatocytes or sanded nuclei in HBV infection and viral inclusion bodies in CMV or HSV infection are absent. As in these viral infections the initial pathologic changes in the graft are similar and morphologic landmarks of the virus are absent, the specific virus implicated in each case can only be demonstrated by the use of immunohistologic techniques for the detection of 'early' antigens (Figure 4c). Although serological studies usually also prove the viral etiology, antibody formation may be delayed during immunosuppression. In our series, CMV and HSV infections with graft involvement proved to be reversible during these early stages by a decrease of the immunosuppressive regimen in most cases.

If a viral infection during these early stages can not be treated effectively, a chronic viral infection of the graft may occur. During the late stages of viral infection, degeneration of individual liver cells is usually more pronounced and bile duct epithelium may also be involved, especially in CMV infection (Figure 6c). Characteristically, during these late stages of cytopathogenic effect of the virus is usually prominent (Figure 4d), viral particles can be detected in electron microscopy, and in immunohistologic studies structural viral antigens are abundantly present. Therapeutic measures usually fail to eradicate the viral infection during these late stages and the chronic infection may contribute to a poor prognosis. In our series two chronic viral infections of the graft have been documented, one with a HBV infection [11] and one with a CMV infection.

It has been conjectured [24] and afterwards demonstrated [9], that in HBV infection of otherwise normal hosts the very early stages of uncomplicated acute hepatitis mimick the various forms of chronic hepatitis before the classical picture of acute hepatitis evolves and leads to full recovery. The only difference between the very early stage and chronic hepatitis B is the abundant expression of viral antigens in the latter. In our opinion, other forms of chronic viral hepatitis (e.g. CMV) may also represent the unresolved early stages of acute hepatitis. Thus, in patients with a lack of cell mediated immunity [10, 14], the very early stage persists as chronic hepatitis, the only change being the development of cytopathogenic effects as an expression of the deficient elimination of virus infected hepatocytes. This also appears to occur in viral infection of liver homografts [3, 15, 22].

As the early stages of viral infection in liver homografts offer the histologic landmark of patchy liver cell degeneration, a liver biopsy may contribute to the diagnosis of viral hepatitis during this still reversible phase of the infection.

Bacterial infection

Bacterial cholangitis and septicaemia may both result in pronounced portal pathology with or without cholestasis in the parenchyma. The pathology in liver grafts [3] closely resembles that in non-grafted livers [25]. The main characteristics are an enlargement of the portal tracts, proliferation of marginal bile ductules, dilated ductules with sometimes inspissated bile in their lumen, and a portal inflammatory infiltrate with a predominance of granulocytes (Figure 5a). The late sequelae of bacterial infection of the graft include abcess formation; here too the morphology of an abcess wall with granulation tissue and fibrosis is similar to abcess formation in non-grafted livers.

The increased number of bile ductules in an enlarged portal tract is an early phenomenon in bacterial cholangitis and is therefore of diagnostic importance. Indeed, in some of our cases the histopathologic diagnosis of bacterial infection preceded a positive bacterial culture from bile. Apart from bacterial infection and large duct obstruction, proliferation of marginal bile ductules has not been observed in other graft syndromes [1, 3]. It is therefore an important histopathologic landmark in the differential diagnosis of graft syndromes.

Differential diagnostic problems

If the histopathologic changes in a graft biopsy can not be interpreted in accordance with a known pathogenetic mechanism, only a descriptive morphologic diagnosis or a differential diagnosis can be made. The less is understood of the

Figure 5. Morphology of cholestatic syndromes in liver grafts. Incidentally, some cholestasis may also accompany an episode of severe acute rejection and circulation disorders with confluent necrosis. (a) Proliferation of marginal bile ducts (arrows) and bile plugs in the distended lumen of a bile duct (arrowhead) are characteristics of the cholangitis accompanying large duct obstruction or bacterial cholangitis, as in this case where staphylococcus epidermidis was cultured from the bile. OLT 8, biopsy #5, H&E. ×140. (b) Bile plugs (arrows) are present in the distended bile canaliculi in this case of pure parenchymal cholestasis. Essentially, no inflammatory infiltrate is present in the parenchyma or in the portal tracts (see 5c). OLT 4, biopsy #3, H&E, ×350. (c) Same biopsy, showing a normal portal tract without enlargement or inflammatory infiltrate. The endothelial lining of the vessels (asterisk) also appears to be normal. OLT 4, biopsy #3, H&E, ×350.

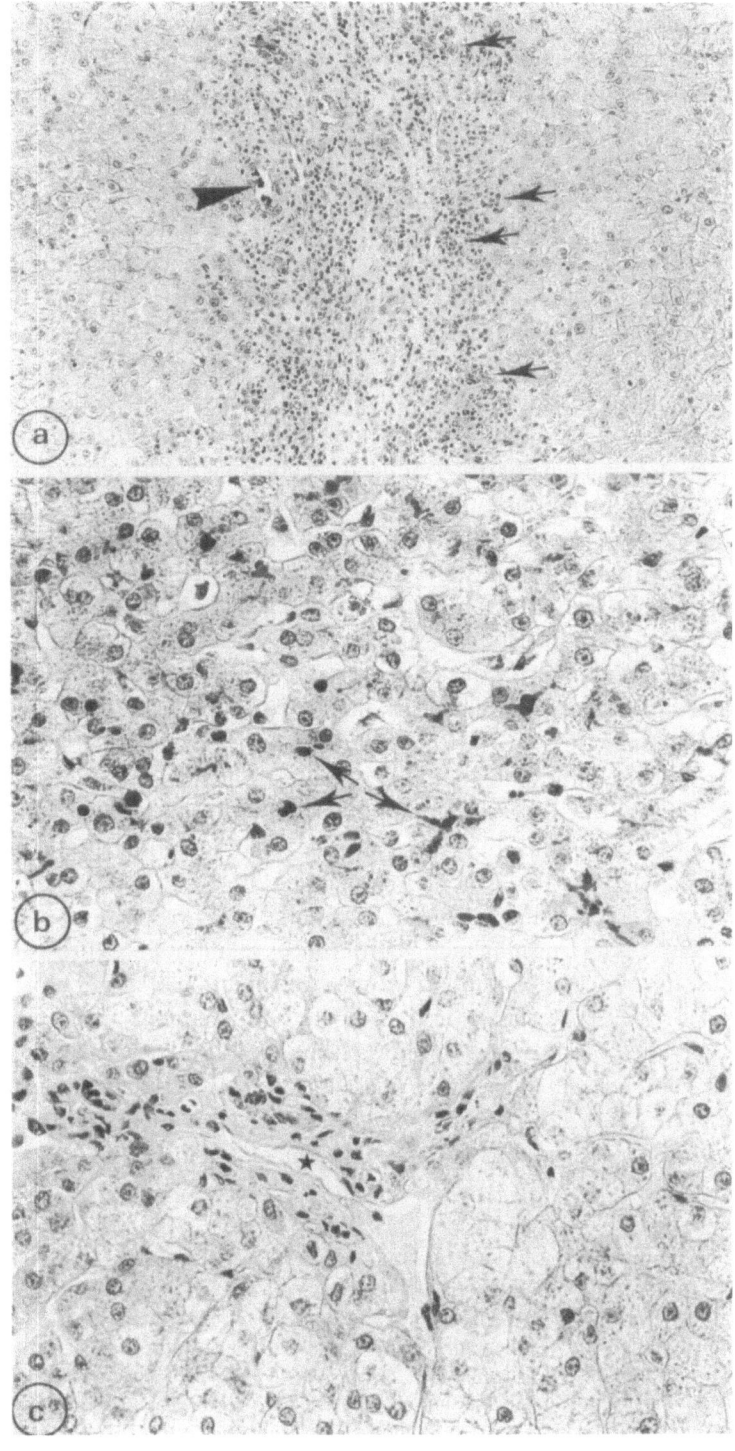

potential mechanisms involved, the longer the list of possible etiologies in the differential diagnosis will be. Here some examples of these as yet unsolved problems are given, that belong to either one of two groups, i.e. (1) nothing is known about the pathogenesis and (2) more than one pathogenetic mechanism may be involved in the formation of the pathologic syndrome.

A pure parenchymal cholestasis, as shown in the Figure 5b and 5c, definitely belongs to the first group. It has been observed in OLT recipients with a declining graft function [3]. Although rejection as a possible mechanism originally came on the first place [5], no cellular or humoral immune mechanism has been detected so far. Also, endothelial damage or circulation disorders in the graft are absent, so that any evidence for rejection as a pathogenetic mechanism is lacking at present. Although a rejection phenomenon still has not been ruled out completely, other possible explanations include hormonal and/or metabolic imbalanced, a cholestatic type of drug-induced reaction, or a nutritional disorder in relation to gastrointestinal malfunction.

The syndrome of chronic rejection may belong to the second group. In the differential diagnosis of chronic rejection, other pathogenetic possibilities are chronic viral infection or recurrence of the original liver disease, especially PBC. In chronic and therapy-resistant viral infection of a liver graft, we have now several examples in our series of the rapid formation within 6 months of a full-blown chronic rejection [22]. The pathologic syndrome included intimal proliferation of larger graft vessels with obliteration of the vessel lumen, proliferation of macrophages in the sinusoids and vanishing, bile ducts in a majority of the portal tracts (Figure 6). It is known that in non-grafted livers damage of bile duct epithelium may occur in the course of a chronic CMV infection [10] or a chronic active hepatitis due to a non-A non-B virus infection [25, 26]. Pathology of bile duct epithelium has also been described as a regularly occurring feature of chronic rejection [1, 20]. As a virus may induce differences in antigenic expression of the infected cells, it is conceivable that in chronic viral infection of a liver graft this has implications for the expression of graft antigens with recipient-graft interactions and the occurrence of chronic rejection. It may be difficult to demonstrate or exclude a viral infection in the absence of demonstrable viral particles or a chronic inflammatory infiltrate. The participation of chronic viral infection in the pathogenesis of chronic rejection thus remains to be elucidated in more cases, primarily

Figure 6. Chronic rejection, vanishing bile ducts and chronic CMV infection were ultimately present together in one of the problem cases. Three details of the pathology in the liver graft of OLT 14 at autopsy are shown. (a) Hepatic artery in large portal tract. The arterial lumen (asterisk) is nearly occluded by the accumulation of foamy macrophages in the intima. Elastin Van Gieson, ×140. (b) Enlarged and fibrotic portal tract. Bile ducts are absent, some lymphocytes may indicate their former location (arrows). In the parenchyma, the sinusoids contain many macrophages (arrowheads). H&E, ×140. (c) CMV inclusion bodies were present in the liver parenchyma (see 4d) and in the largest intrahepatic bile ducts (arrow) that still were present. H&E, ×350.

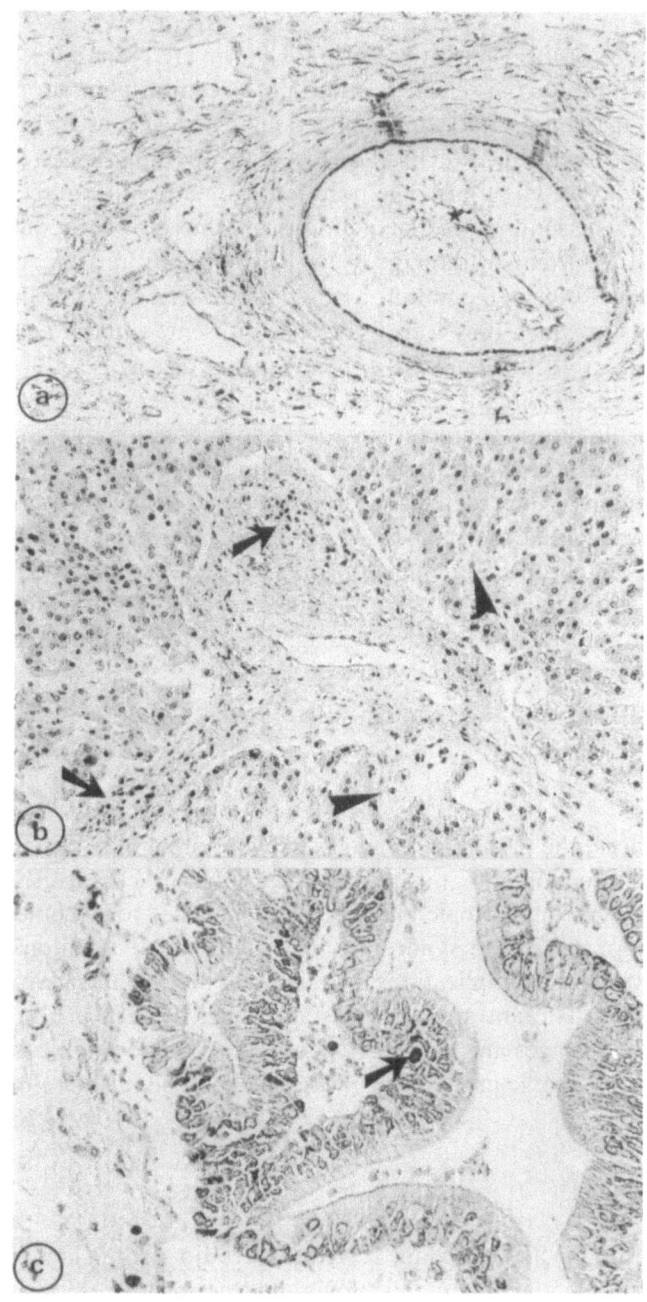

by the use of immunohistologic techniques for the demonstration of viral antigenic determinants.

The recurrence of PBC in liver grafts of long term OLT survivors has recently been reported [27]; for the selection criteria of liver transplantation in patients with PBC this may have important implications. However, as chronic rejection may mimick the recurrence of PBC in the graft one must be cautious in the interpretation of the symptoms. The portal inflammatory infiltrate and the bile duct lesions may be similar in both conditions and thus also occur during chronic rejection in OLT patients without previous PBC. After a free interval following OLT, a recurrence of liver membrane auto-antibodies has been documented in all OLT recipients in which they were previously present, without any relation to graft functioning, rejection episodes or recurrence of disease [13, 17]. And finally, in one OLT recipient with previous PBC and the persistence/recurrence of auto-antibodies, in one biopsy characteristic focal bile duct lesions were present. The pathologic changes disappeared after an adjustment in the daily dose of azathioprine, which might be interpreted as an indication that a rejection episode was the underlying pathogenetic mechanism. Thus, in the differential diagnosis between chronic rejection, chronic viral infection and recurrence of the original disease in PBC patients with a liver graft, a careful comparison of more long term survivors will be needed to establish the proper diagnosis, differential diagnostic criteria and pathogenetic mechanisms in each case.

Conclusion

In most instances, the pathologic changes in liver homografts during viral infection, bacterial infection and graft rejection episodes are characteristic and constitute separate histopathologic entities. Graft biopsies to document the early stages of each of these graft syndromes may thus provide additional diagnostic information with major implications for the direct therapeutic measures and the prevention of the late and therapy resistant stages of each of the syndromes. During these late stages and especially in chronic rejection, the contribution of the various pathogenetic mechanisms still remains to be further elucidated.

Acknowledgements

Mrs. Sippie Huitema and Mrs. Jane E. Atmosoerodjo assisted in the preparation and interpretation of the immunohistologic and electron microscopical specimens and thus contributed much to this chapter and to the papers on which this chapter is based. Mr. Hilbrand Wierenga prepared the photomicrographs. Mrs. Anneke O. Boer typed the manuscript. They are all kindly acknowledged.

References

1. Fennel RH, Roddy HJ: Liver transplantation. The pathologist's perspective. Pathol Ann 2:155–182, 1979.
2. Hofstee N, Houthoff HJ, Gips CH, Krom RAF, Kootstra G, Arends A: Rejection versus viral infection in orthotopic liver homograft recipients: histopathology of serial liver biopsies. Liver 2:137 (abstract), 1981.
3. Eggink HF, Hofstee N, Gips CH, Krom RAF, Houthoff HJ: Histopathology of serial graft biopsies from liver transplant recipients. Am J Pathol 114:18–31, 1984.
4. Eggink HF, Houthoff HJ, Huitema S, Gips CH, Poppema S: In situ analysis of mononuclear cell infiltrate in liver biopsies of patients with orthotopic liver transplantation. In: Protides of the biological fluids, Proceedings of the 13th Colloquium, 1982, pp 441–444.
5. Porter KA: Pathology of liver transplantation. Transplant Rev 2:129–170, 1969.
6. Herbertson BM: Pathology of liver transplants. In: Calne RJ (ed) Clinical organ transplantation, Oxford, Blackwell, 1971.
7. Kamada N. Davies HffS, Wight D, Culank L, Roser BJ: Liver transplantation in the rat: biochemical and histological evidence of complete tolerance induction in non-rejector strains. Transplantation 35:304 (abstract), 1983.
8. Yamada G, Feinberg LE, Nakane PK: Hepatitis B. Cytologic localization of virus antigens and the role of the immune response. Hum Pathol 9:93–109, 1978.
9. Houthoff HJ, Niermeijer P, Gips CH, Arends A, Hofstee N, van Guldener M: Hepatic morphologic findings and viral antigens in acute hepatitis B. Virchows Arch Pathol Anat Histol 389:153–160, 1980.
10. Ten Napel CHH, Houthoff HJ, The TH: Cytomegalovirus hepatitis in normal and immune compromised hosts. Liver 4:184–194, 1984.
11. MacDougall BRD, Johnson PJ, Williams R, Strunin L, MacMaster P, Calne RY, Bronkhorst FB, Katchaki JN, Brandt KH, Houthoff HJ, Piers DA, Schuur KH, Krom RAF, Gips CH: Liver transplantation in a 27-year-old female with familial HBsAg-positive hepatocellular carcinoma. Neth J Med 21:101–116, 1978.
12. Eggink HF, Houthoff HJ, Huitema S, Gips CH, Poppema S: Cellular and humoral immune reactions in chronic active liver disease. I. Lymphocyte subsets in liver biopsies of patients with untreated idiopathic autoimmune hepatitis, chronic active hepatitis B and primary biliary cirrhosis. Clin Exp Immunol 50:17–24, 1982.
13. Eggink HF, Houthoff HJ, Huitema S, Gips CH, Poppema S: Liver membrane autoantibodies and the pathogenesis of liver diseases. J Hepatol 1:S49, 1985.
14. Eggink HF, Houthoff HJ, Huitema S, Wolters G, Poppema S, Gips CH: Cellular and humoral immune reactions in chronic active liver disease. II. Lymphocyte subsets and viral antigens in liver biopsies of patients with acute and chronic hepatitis B. Clin Exp Immunol 56:121–128, 1984.
15. Gouw ASH, Houthoff HJ, Eggink HF, Huitema S, Gips CH, Poppema S, Krom RAF, Beelen JM, The TH: Immune status of liver homografts during the first months after orthotopic liver transplantation. In situ analysis of immunologic parameters in graft biopsies during major transplantation syndromes and a normal follow-up (in preparation).
16. Eggink HF, Houthoff HJ, Poppema S: T-cell subsets in liver diseases. Gastroenterology 86, 4:780–781, 1984.
17. Eggink HF, Houthoff HJ, Huitema S, Gips CH, Poppema S: Liver membrane autoantibodies and the pathogenesis of liver diseases. A serologic and immunohistologic study in patients with acute and chronic hepatitis, including cases before and after orthotopic liver transplantation in: Eggink HF, Academic Thesis Groningen 1984.
18. The TH, Tegzess AM, Houthoff HJ, Schirm J: Cytomegalovirus antigenic markers in renal transplantation. Transplant Clin Immunol 12:26–33, 1982.
19. Krom RAF, Gips CH, Houthoff HJ, Newton D, van der Waaij D, Beelen J, Haagsma EB, Slooff

MJH: Orthotopic liver transplantation in Groningen, The Netherlands (1979–1983). Hepatology 4:61S–65S, 1984.

20. Starzl TE, Iwatsuki S, van Thiel DH, Gartner JC, Zitelli BJ, Maltack JJ, Schade RR, Shaw BW, Kakala TR, Rosenthal RJ, Porter, KA: Evolution of liver transplantation. Hepatology 2:614–636, 1982.

21. Zimmerman FA, Davies HffS, Knoll PP, Gokel JM,Schmidt T: Orthotopic liver allografts in the rat: the influence of strain combination on the fate of the graft (submitted for publication).

22. Gouw ASH, Houthoff HJ, Beelen JM,The TH, Eggink HF, Huitema S, Gips CH, Krom RAF: Chronic rejection in liver homografts: persistent CMV infection. J Hepatol 1: S57, 1985.

23. Calne RY, Williams R: Orthotopic liver transplantation: the first 60 patients. Br Med J 1:471–476, 1977.

24. Desmet V: Chronic hepatitis (including primary biliary cirrhosis). In: Gall EA, Mostofi FKC (eds). The Liver. International Academy of Pathology Monographs, No 13 Baltimore, Williams & Wilkins, pp 286–341, 1972.

25. International Group: Histopathology of the intrahepatic biliary tree. Liver 3:161–175, 1983.

26. Poulsen H, Christoffersen P: Abnormal bile duct epithelium in chronic aggressive hepatitis and cirrhosis. A review of morphology and clinical, biochemical and immunologic features. Hum Pathol 3:217–225.

16. Fine needle aspiration biopsy inflammatory profile. An evaluation in a liver transplant patient

K. HÖCKERSTEDT, I. LAUTENSCHLAGER, J. AHONEN, B. EKLUND,
P. HÄYRY, A. KAUSTE, C. KORSBÄCK, R. ORKO, K. SALMELA,
B. SCHEININ, T.M. SCHEININ and E. VON WILLEBRAND

Summary

We have studied a liver transplant by frequent fine needle aspiration biopsies (FNAB) and transplantation aspiration cytology. The patient was a 21-year-old woman with chronic active hepatitis, she died 80 days after the transplantation in sepsis and probably of prolonged graft rejection. Three episodes of inflammation were recorded during the postoperative course. These three episodes all coincided with clinical evidence of transplant failure. The first episode of inflammation consisted mainly of mononuclear phagocytes and was devoid of any lymphoid blastogenic component. Concomitantly both clinical and cytological evidence of cholestasis were present. The second and third episodes were typical blast dominated 'rejections'. In addition, deposits of Cyclosporin A (CyA) were observed by direct immunofluorescence in the liver FNAB. The deposits correlated roughly to the level of CyA administration but not necessarily to the blood level of CyA. We conclude that FNAB of a liver transplant is a safe procedure that can be performed repeatedly without danger to the graft or to the recipient. It seems to be possible to record inflammatory episodes of 'rejection' from these cytological specimens.

Introduction

The first liver transplantation in Helsinki was performed in December 1982. The liver graft was studied by repeated fine needle biopsies (FNAB) and based on earlier experience with kidney grafts [1, 2] and pig liver grafts (see Chapter 6), some new findings could be observed. In addition to the inflammatory episodes of rejection, particular attention was paid to the transplant parenchymal cells, cholestasis and deposits of Cyclosporin A in the liver transplant.

Patient and methods

Patient

The recipient was a 21-year-old woman with chronic aggressive hepatitis in a steady down-way course. Right before the operation her clinical condition had rapidly worsened, she could only drink fluids and was even too tired to sit up. The s-albumin was 24 g/l, s-bilirubin 310 μmol/l, P + P 21%, prothrombin time 32% and Factor VII was 22% of normal.

Donor

The donor was a 36-year-old man with intracerebral hemorrhage. The liver and the kidneys were procured for transplantation. In retrospect we learned that the donor had a history of heavy drinking a week before his death. The liver was perfused in situ with buffered Ringer's lactate solution and after removal preserved with Eurocollins solution.

Operation and clinical course

The recipient's operation followed the guidelines set by Calne using the gallbladder conduit technique [3]. After re-establishment of liver circulation the patient had a 20-min cardiac arrest due to high potassium serum levels. During resuscitation the liver became severily congested, but regained normal appearance after successful resuscitation. The patient recovered well postoperatively but the transplant never quite regained normal function. Thus, protein rich pleuritis and ascites were continuously present and consequently amino acids and glucose had to be infused during the whole postoperative period.

During the second week a typical post-transplant jaundice developed. Because the bile ducts of the transplant were not visualized on T-tube cholangiography a laparotomy was performed. The ducts appeared normal and a new T-tube was positioned.

Although the patient was free of infection at transplantation, Klebsiella pneumoniae and Staphylococcus aureus were found in her nose and throat already from the first postoperative day onwards. Because of sepsis and suspicion of intra-abdominal abscess on CT-scan a second laparotomy was performed on the 58th day. No abscess was found, but the sepsis continued and the patient died on the 80th postoperative day.

Immunosuppression

The basic immunosuppression was methylprednisolone (M. Pred.) 0.5 mg/kg/day and azathioprine (AZA) 2–3 mg/kg/day during the first six days. Thereafter Cyclosporine (CyA) 6–10 mg/kg/day was instituted instead of AZA. During the first rejection the dose of M.Pred. was elevated to 2–3 mg/kg/day and CyA to 17 mg/kg/day (orally or i.v.) until the rejection subsided. The second rejection was treated by elevated doses of CyA to 15 mg/kg/day (i.v) but the M.Pred. was increased to only 1 mg/kg/day due to septicemia.

Fine needle aspiration biopsy and transplant aspiration cytology

FNAB of the transplant were performed at 1–3-day intervals from the moment of operation. The method of performing the biopsy, processing the specimens and reading the results of the aspiration cytology have been described in detail [4]. (See also Chapter 6.)

Cyclosporine A deposits were demonstrated in acetone-fixed smears by rabbit anti-CyA antiserum (Sandoz) and by direct immunofluorescence as previously described [5].

Biopsy histology

The biopsy specimens were fixed in 10% formalin, embedded in paraffine, cut to 4 μm thick sections and stained with hematoxylin-eosin.

Results

The profile of inflammation

The inflammatory profile, as total corrected increment, is given in Figure 1. The patient underwent three episodes of inflammation during the postoperative course of 80 days. The first episode commenced shortly after the transplantation on day 12, the second on day 28 and the third on day 62. The major inflammatory cell sub-components are also demonstrated in Figure 1. The first episode of inflammation contained no lymphoid blast cells but only a few monoblasts and monocytes. The dominating cell types in the second and in the third episode were lymphoid blast cells and plasma cells, although also lymphocytes, early mono-blasts, monocytes and tissue macrophages were recorded in these specimens (Figure 2).

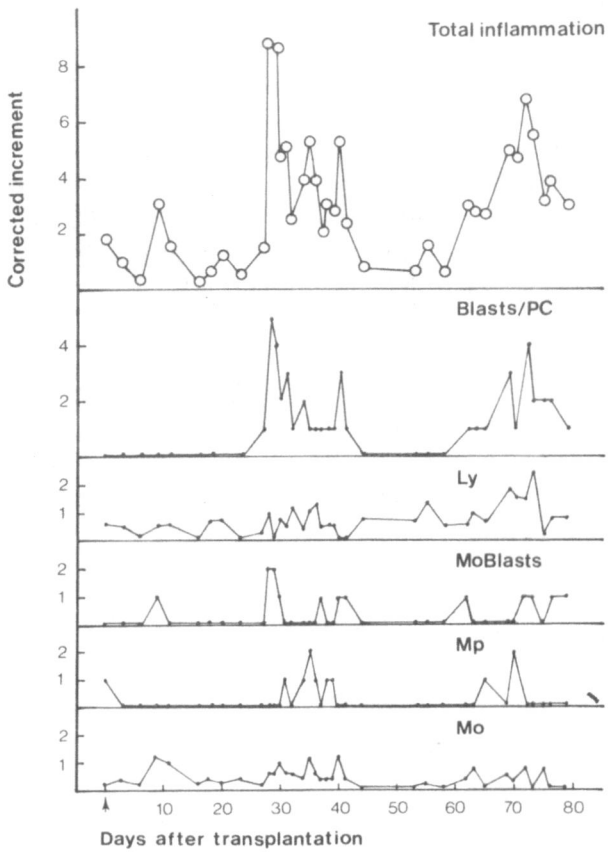

Figure 1. Top section: the inflammatory profile given as corrected increment. Three inflammatory episodes were seen during 80 days after the transplantation. Following sections: the major inflammatory cell components, shown from the second section downwards: lymphoid blasts and plasma cells, lymphocytes, monoblasts, macrophages and monocytes.

Correlation to biopsy histology

Open biopsies of the liver transplant were obtained at the end of operation, in the relaparotomy performed on day 12 and at autopsy on day 80.

In the specimen taken at operation fatty liver, some fibrosis and weak periportal inflammation were documented. In the specimen obtained on day 12 the most significant change was cholestasis with minimal inflammation in the portal area and around the biliary tree. There were no signs of fatty liver any longer.

At autopsy, fibrosis, cholestasis and residual inflammation together with parenchymal necrosis were recorded.

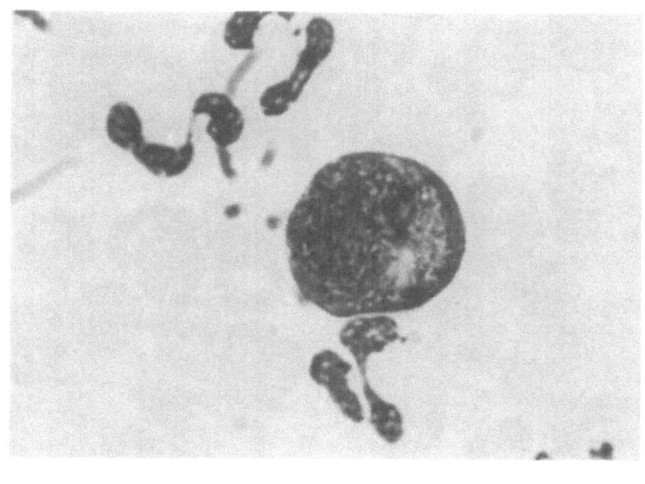

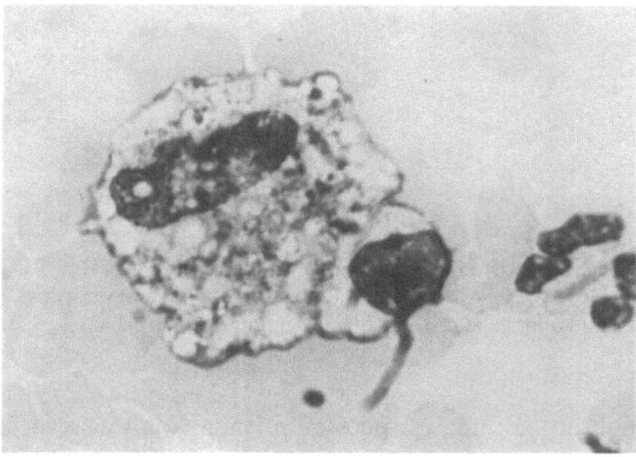

Figure 2. Inflammatory cells in the FNAB: (a) A plasmablast and neutrophile granulocytes, (b) A macrophage or a Kupffer cell.

Parenchymal cell changes in aspiration cytology and correlations to blood chemistry

Correlations of the three episodes of inflammation to cytological findings of cholestasis and to the major parameters of blood chemistry are recorded in Figure 3. All episodes of inflammation including the one without any blastogenic component, were associated with cytological evidence of cholestasis. During the two episodes of blastogenic inflammation severe degenerative changes were noted in the liver parenchymal cells (Figure 4).

154

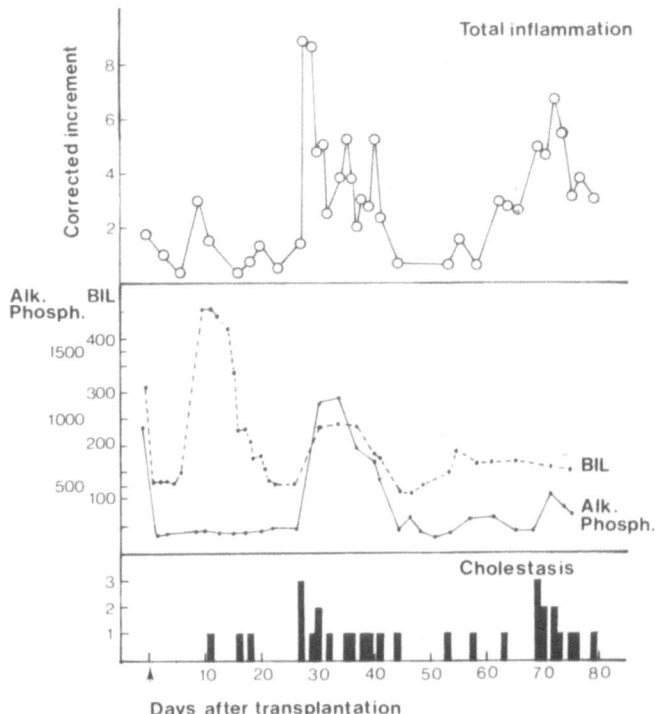

Figure 3. The biochemical markers of hepatocyte function and the cytological evidence of cholestasis during the postoperative course of 80 days. From the top section downwards: total inflammation, s-bilirubin and s-Alk.Phosph., and presence of bile deposits in the hepatocytes.

No association of the three episodes of inflammation was recorded with the levels of s-ASAT and s-ALAT as they remained normal after the first week. The initially high s-bilirubin and s-Alk.Phosph. values declined rapidly after the operation (Figure 3). During the first episode of inflammation which displayed cytological and histological evidence of cholestasis but lacked any blastogenic component, the level of s-bilirubin (but not s-Alk.Phosph.) increased rapidly. Both biochemical markers of hepatocyte function were elevated during the second episode of inflammation but neither s-bilirubin nor s-Alk.Phosph. responded during the third (Figure 3).

On the other hand, when s-Alk.Phosph. was elevated around days 30 and 70, a clear picture of cholestasis was noted in the hepatocytes in the FNAB.

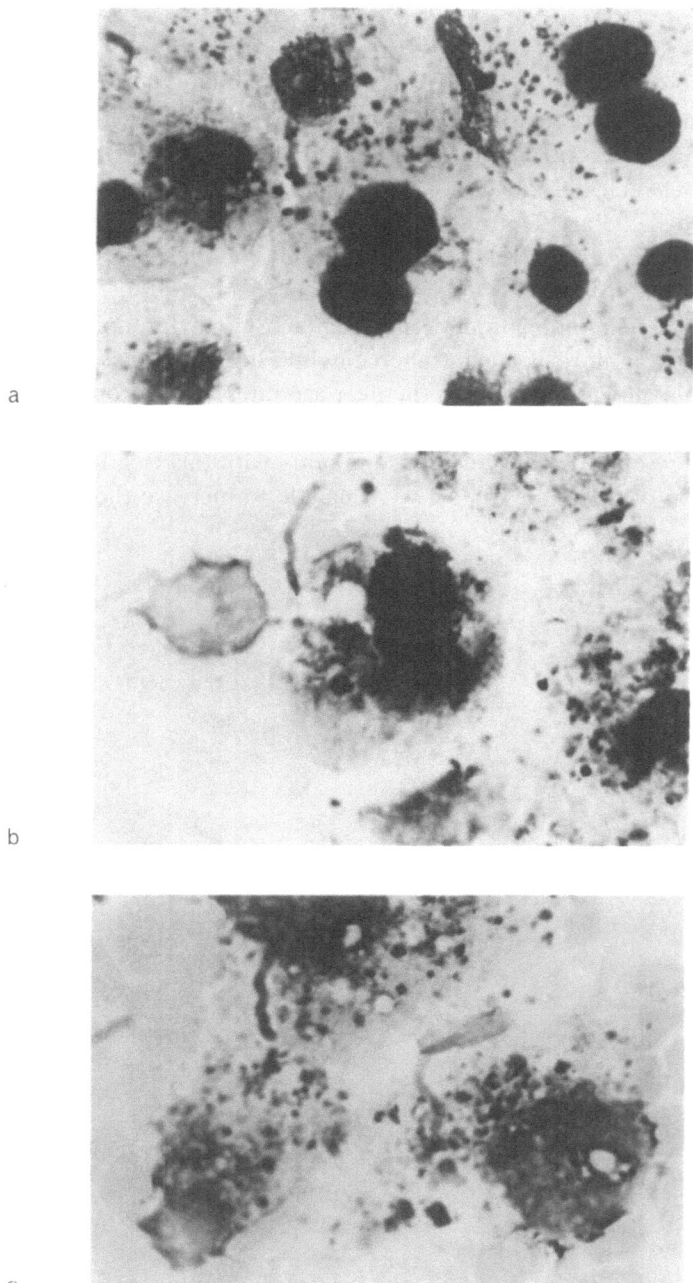

Figure 4. Parenchymal cell changes in the FNAB: (a) A group of normal hepatocytes – the dark granules are hemosiderin, (b) Bile deposits seen as dark droplets in the hepatocytes, (c) Vacuolized and badly degenerated, necrotic hepatocytes with evidence of cholestasis.

156

Correlations of the episodes of inflammation to immunosuppressive drug therapy and to deposits of Cyclosporine A in the liver transplant

CyA deposits (Figure 5) in the transplant correlated roughly to the dose: CyA deposits were noted particularly when high intravenous doses (10–17 mg/kg/d) were used during the second and third episodes of inflammation. The blood level of CyA varied between 490 and 885 ng/ml during the low dose regimen (6–10 mg/kg/d) and between 225 and 1750 ng/ml during the high dose regimen (10–17 mg/kg/d). There was no clear correlation between the blood level of CyA and the deposits seen in the aspiration cytology of the transplant.

The first episode of inflammation was not treated by methylprednisolone as the clinical condition was more like an intrahepatic cholestasis and since no lymphoid blast cell component was recorded in the liver aspirates. The second episode of inflammation was treated by an elevated oral dose of MP and additional CyA. The inflammatory episode subsided concomitantly with this treatment. During the third episode of inflammation we were unable to increase the dose of MP

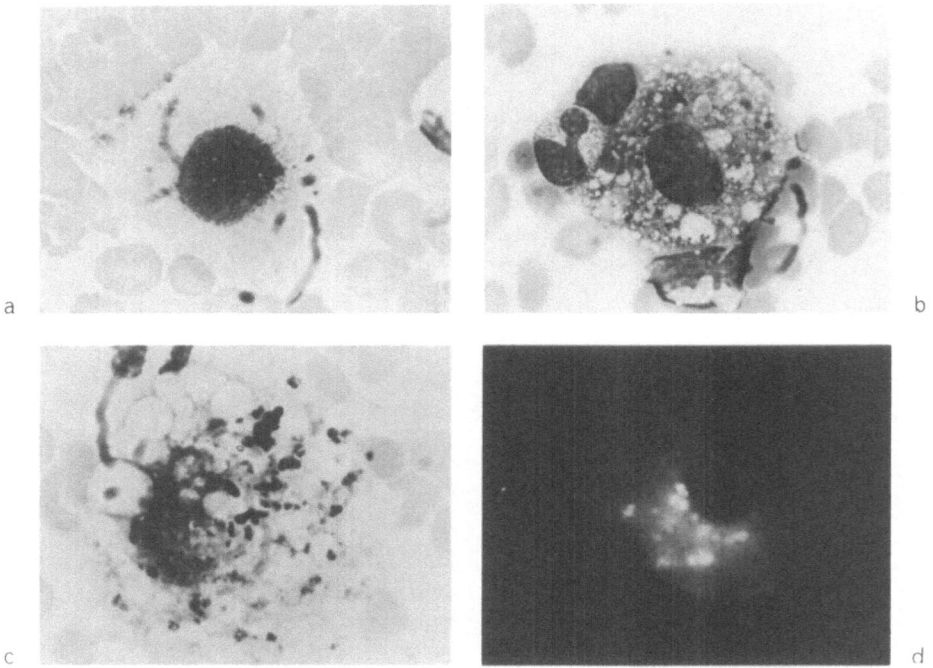

Figure 5. Morphological changes in the hepatocytes coinciding with CyA deposits and demonstration of CyA by immunofluorescence. (a) A normal hepatocyte, no CyA deposits seen by immunofluorescence. (b) Vacualization in a hepatocyte. (c) A badly vacuolized hepatocyte coinciding with large amounts of CyA in immunofluorescence analysis. (d) CyA deposits in a hepatocyte visualized by indirect immunofluorescence.

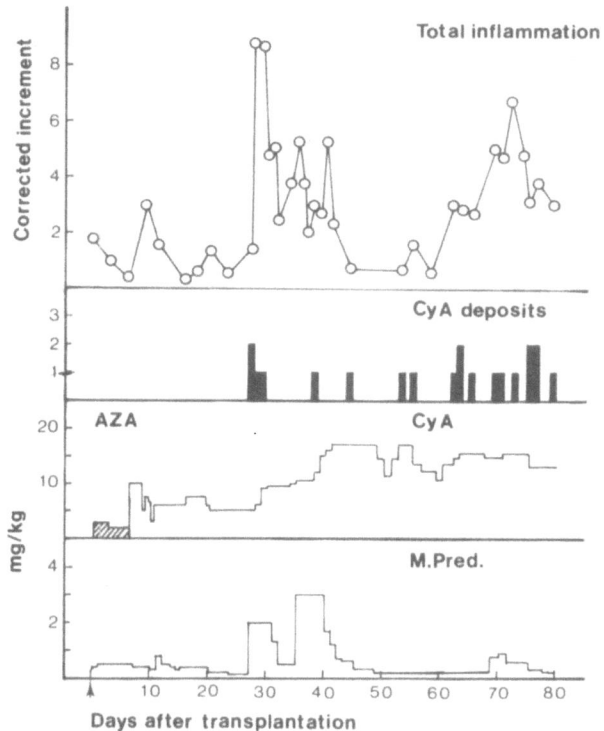

Figure 6. The immunosuppressive drug therapy and presence of CyA deposits in the liver transplant. From top section downwards: total inflammation. CyA deposits (scores 1–3); the dose of azathioprine and Cyclosporine A, the dose of methylprednisolone.

because of septicemia. Instead, the dose of CyA was raised, but rapid increase of CyA deposits in the liver transplant precluded this approach, too. The patient died on day 80 after the operation.

Discussion

Based on our experience on liver transplants in the pig and the current experience in man, it may be concluded that repeated FNAB can be performed on human liver transplants safely, without risk to the transplant or the transplant recipient, and that both the inflammatory events and, to a lesser extent, certain parenchymal changes may be evaluated from these specimens. It has not escaped our attention that the whole postoperative time was characterized by bacterial infections and repeated septic periods. It seems, however, that the clinical and bacteriological evidence of infection did not correlate with the periods of inflammation observed in the FNAB.

Two inflammatory patterns were noted in this patient: one consisting of mononuclear phagocytes without any lymphoid blastogenic component and another which represented a typical blastdominated episode of 'rejection', closely resembling the acute cellular rejection of renal transplant in man [1, 2]. The first episode of inflammation thus lacked the typical cellular signs of acute rejection, also clinically the patient displayed a typical intrahepatic cholestasis often seen at this stage. This may be considered to be related to liver ischemia during the preservation period and operative manipulation. Furthermore the resuscitation and the enormous enlargement of the liver during this time must have had deleterious effects on its function. The second and third episode of inflammation, instead, represent in our opinion typical acute episodes of rejection.

References

1. Häyry P, v Willebrand E: Monitoring of human renal allograft rejection with fine-needle aspiration cytology. Scand J Immunol 13:87–97, 1981.
2. Häyry P, v Willebrand E, Ahonen J, Eklund B, Lautenschlager I: Monitoring of organ allograft rejection by transplant aspiration cytology. Ann Clin Res 13:264–287, 1981.
3. Calne RY: Hepatic transplantation. In: Wright R, Alberti KGMM, Karran S, Millward-Sadler GH (eds). Liver and biliary diseases. WB Saunders, London, 1979, pp 1180–1190.
4. Häyry P, v Willebrand E: Practical guidelines for fine needle aspiration biopsy in human renal allografts. Ann Clin Res 13:288–306, 1981.
5. v Willebrand E, Häyry P: Cyclosporin A deposits in renal allografts. Lancet II:819–912, 1983.

17. Radionuclide techniques in the follow up of liver-transplanted patients

H. CREUTZIG

Introduction

Nearly 60 years have passed since radioactive materials were first used as tracers in man: in 1927, Blumgart and Weiss used radon gas to study cardiovascular hemodynamics of patients with heart diseases [1]. Some thirty years ago Vetter *et al.* first estimated the liver blood flow with gold-198, an artificial radionuclide [2], while Stirrett *et al.* used the same radionuclide for imaging of the regional distribution of intrahepatic RES in man [3]. Today newer scintigraphic devices as well as other radiopharmaceuticals are used, but there are no new ideas in general.

Since 1978 we investigated more than 80 patients in the routine follow-up with radionuclide techniques after liver transplantation and we will summarize our findings in this chapter.

Radionuclide techniques

Liver blood flow

After intravenous administration of microparticles there is a three-step interaction with macrophages: (i) attachment at the receptor of the macrophage membrane, (ii) phagocytosis, and (iii) intracellular degration of the material [4]. The uptake measurement of labelled millimicrospheres enables the regional in vivo assessment of phagocytic properties of the hepatic RES [5].

The attachment takes place at specific receptor sites and is dependent on capillary blood flow only [6]. This flow may be calculated from the clearance rate or the regional hepatic uptake. Direct comparison of this technique with the indocyanine green (ICG) method showed a close correlation for the estimated liver blood flow (ELBF) both in animals [7] and men [8].

The radionuclide technique is simple, safe and can be done in the intensive care unit as well as in the diagnostic department: the patient is positioned under a normal scintillation camera linked to a dedicated computer. After i.v. injection of Technetium-99m labelled human serumalbumin millimicrospheres (37 MBq) the accumulation into the liver is recorded for 20 min in 15-s increments. Time activity curves are generated for the right and the left lobe, and the half-time of these uptake curves assessed. The ELBF can then be calculated with the following formula: $ELBF = k \times BV/E$, where BV is the blood volume and E the hepatic extraction efficiency [9]. The BV in transplanted patients can differ from one examination to the other, therefore BV must be measured before every examination. The extraction efficiency has not been assessed in liver transplants, it might differ from that in normals or cirrhotics. Therefore we recommend in the transplanted patient the calculation of the individual k-value and its intraindividual comparison only [10]. The interobserver variation is below 10%, the reproducibility excellent [10].

Relative arterial and portal blood flow

A noninvasive scintigraphic method for determining the portal venous fraction (PVF) of total hepatic flow was described by Biersack *et al.* [11]. After modifying their technique, we have developed a more accurate and reproducible method for assessing PVF [12].

The study is done immediately after the measurement of ELBF without moving the patient. A 500 MBq Technetium-99m DTPA bolus in 0.5 ml is injected into a peripheral vein, preferably the basilic. The uptake is measured in 0.2 s increments for up to 60 s. Representative regions over the left ventricle, right lung, lower abdominal aorta, right hepatic lobe without the kidney region, right kidney, and spleen are selected (Figure 1) and time activity curves generated. Pulmonary as well as the radioactivity from the ELBF measurement is subtracted.

To analyze the corrected hepatic curve, three points have to be identified: the time when radioactivity enters the organ (A); second, the time radioactivity was maximal in the spleen or the kidney, indicating the beginning of the portal phase (B), and the beginning of the recirculation (C) (Figure 2). Then the integral from A to B is calculated (I). The count rate at B is subtracted from the hepatic curve, and the integral from B to C is calculated (I). The portal fraction of hepatic perfusion is $I/(I + I)$). In normals it is about 70% of total hepatic flow, while in compensated cirrhotics it falls to about 50% and comes to near zero in decompensation [13]. The technique has been well established in cirrhotics both preoperatively in selecting shunt procedures (in patients without PVF a porto-caval shunt will not reduce hepatic flow) and postoperatively in evaluating the results of shunting [11, 12, 14, 15].

There are, however, some limitations in this technique. A sufficient bolus

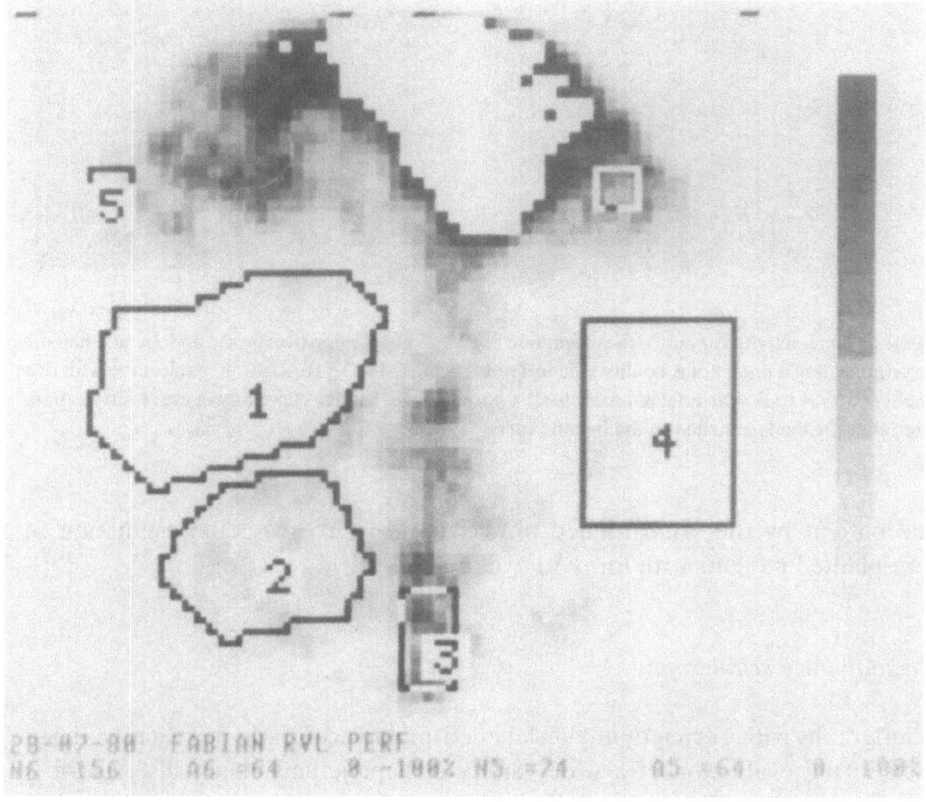

Figure 1. Estimation of Portal Venous Fraction (PVF) by radionuclide angiography. Regions of interest for time-activity-curves: (1) = right hepatic lobe, (2) = right kidney, (3) = Aorta abdominalis, (4) = spleen, (5) = lung, (6) = left ventricle.

quality is needed: the mean transit time in the aorta must be shorter than the expected arterial phase in the liver, i.e. less than 7 s. This will be dependent on the input function (injection technique) as well as on the pump function of the heart. We therefore calculate for each study the ejection fraction (EF) using the first pass of the bolus through the left ventricle; if the EF is lower than 30%, the bolus is so much fragmented, that the calculation of PVF will be impossible. In the postoperative course the estimation of the EF gives additional information about the outcome: all cirrhotics with an EF lower than 28% at the third day after grafting died later on at the intensive care unit. Another main problem is the reproducibility of the study. In repeated investigations there is a good correlation [12], if the calculation is done by the same operator. The interobserver variation is much greater, especially in patients with low PVF there might be a difference up to 30–50% between two observers. We therefore recommend the follow-up of

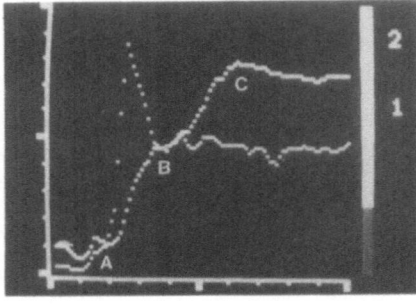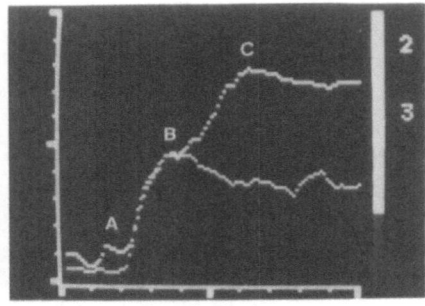

Figure 2. Time-activity curves for the estimation of PVF. Left: Region over Aorta abdom. and hepatic curve indicating a good bolus quality (Mean Transit Time (MTT) 5 s). Right: hepatic curve with two distinct parts A to B = arterial phase, B to C = portal phase. Kidney curve (lower curve left) as pure arterial perfusion is matched to the hepatic curve.

one patient by the same trained physician [10]. Otherwise the estimation in transplanted patients with low PVF will be useless.

Hepatobiliary scintigraphy

Scintigraphy with Technetium-99m labelled imidodiacetic acid derivates has been used in the evaluation of a wide variety of hepatic and biliary diseases; it is capable of yielding dynamic and limited morphological information on the function of the liver and biliary tract. In a large proportion of cases, transplant failure is due to complications, involving the bile-duct-to-bowel anastomosis [16]. Bile leakage can be detected by cholescintigraphy before the onset of clinical symptoms [17, 18].

The study is done with the patient in the same position as described above. Modern mobile gamma cameras can be used even in small intensive care units. After i.v.injection of 200 MBq Technetium-99m labelled HIDA or a similar radiopharmaceutical static anterior images are obtained at 5 min intervals until 30 min; delayed and multiple oblique views are added until the liver has completely cleared from the labelled bile.

The hepatic uptake and biliary excretion of the radiopharmaceutical is dependent on the hepatocyte function: with serum bilirubin levels of more than 20 mg/100 ml (300 μmol/l), no hepatic uptake and no excretion via the bile is seen. A new radiopharmaceutical (IODIDA) will enable a scintigraphic image in icteric patients with bilirum levels up to 35 mg/100 ml (550 μmol/l). The imaging of biliary leakage needs a sufficient bile flow: less than 0.5 ml/h of bile extravasation is not detectable by scintigraphy [17].

Scintigraphy of other organs

Sometimes it might be useful to image other organs like the kidneys (exclusion of vascular complication in acute renal failure), the lung (confirmation or exclusion of ventilation/perfusion abnormalities, endothelial metabolic dysfunction [19] or altered microvascular permeability [20]) or to do a white blood cell scan for the localization of an infection.

Normal course after grafting

The postoperative course of blood flow reveals two distinctly different patterns: in tumor patients with normal portal flow ELBF and PVF stayed normal from the second day after transplantation (first time of measurement) with a k-value between 0.8 and 1.2 and a PVF of 60–70%. In end-stage cirrhotics the ELBF is about 60% of normal at the second day after transplantation and gets normal within 10–14 days. The portal fraction is initially very low (about 20%) and will never reach normal values. Few of the cirrhotics measured had an uncomplicated postoperative course, in these the portal fraction was not higher than 50%. One to two years after transplantation ELBF decreases to 65–85% of its initial value. This might be due to removing Kupffer cell population in the graft by host's cells or to histologically not detectable slow rejection.

In children with biliary atresia there is a different course: six to ten days after transplantation ELBF and PVF are normal. This correlates well with the better postoperative outcome in this subgroup.

In bilio-bilary anastomosis, both end-to-end or side-to-end, the normal outcome is a functional stenosis. This will not alter biliary flow and needs no special treatment. In jejunal interposition the 'blind loop syndrome' can be confirmed by scintigraphy.

Acute rejection

In acute rejection (AR) the ELBF dropped dramatically 20 to 30 hours before the expression of liver enzymes [10]. In two patients with uncontrollable acute rejection there was no uptake of colloid in the graft with activation of lung RES, indicating a complete loss of ELBF. In controllable rejection the ELBF decreased to 1/2 or 1/3 of initial postoperative values, while in tumor patients with initially normal PVF a purely arterial perfusion was a constant finding in AR; after successful treatment the normalization of PVF was more rapid than any other finding (Figure 3). After AR the initial plateau of ELBF values was never reached; we interpret this as a sign of irreversible damage of some Kupffer cells even in normal histology (Figure 4).

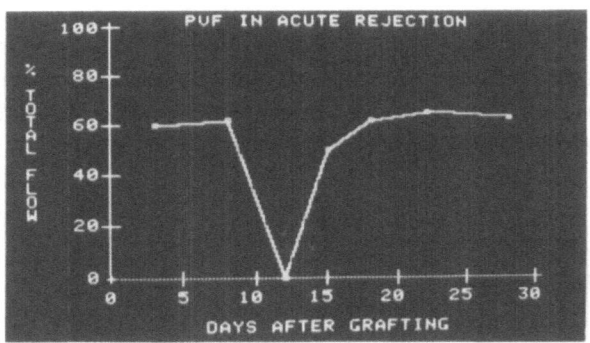

Figure 3. Course of portal venous fraction of total hepatic flow in a patient with acute rejection.

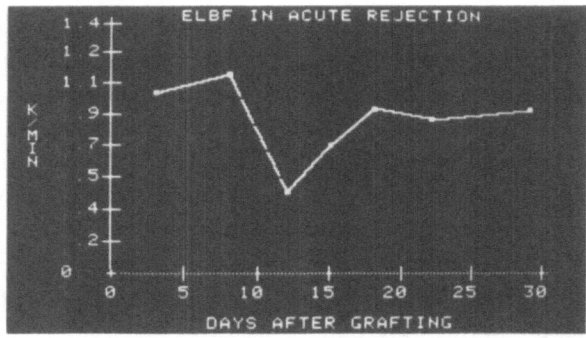

Figure 4. The estimated liver blood flow in the same patient.

Acute rejection can be detected with radionuclide techniques earlier than with other methods [21], the differentiation between AR and vascular complications however (see below) might be difficult.

No normalization of PVF and no increase in ELBF after AR with a further decline is a sign of a subacute (or chronic) rejection with a fatal outcome for the transplant (Figure 5). All patients without improvement of ELBF within 10 days after AR died because of progressive multiple organ failure some weeks later. The scintigraphic signs of a subacute rejecton are a strong indication for an elective retransplantation.

In the later follow-up (some years after grafting) all of our patients had a moderate decrease of ELBF without any clinical or enzymatic sign of impaired liver function. This might indicate a subclinical slow progressive rejection, but this is still in discussion.

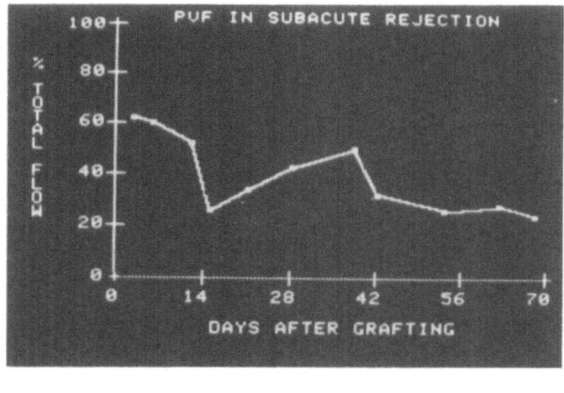

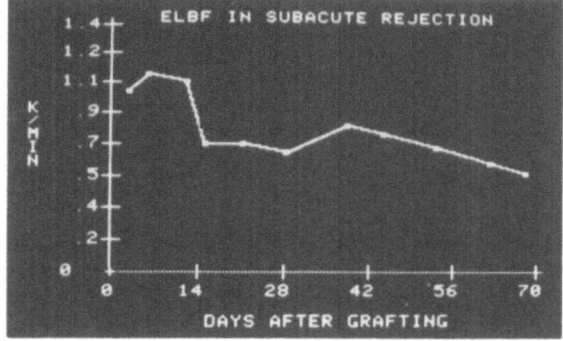

Figure 5. Portal venous fraction of total hepatic flow and estimated liver blood flow in a patient with subacute (chronic) rejection.

Vascular complications

The occlusion of the portal vein will decrease PVF and also ELBF. The differentiation to AR might be impossible in cirrhotics; in our three patients with this disease there was only one correct diagnosis.

In occlusion of the A. hepatica communis, there is a decrease of ELBF with a complete lost of ELBF some days later (Figure 6). This is an indication for an emergency retransplantation. Thrombosis of smaller intrahepatic arteries led to a necrosis with a circumscript lost of radionuclide fixation (Figure 7).

Biliary tract complications

In transplanted patients bile leakage (BL) may occur without or with minimal clinical symptoms. As cholescintigraphy is both sensitive and specific for the

166

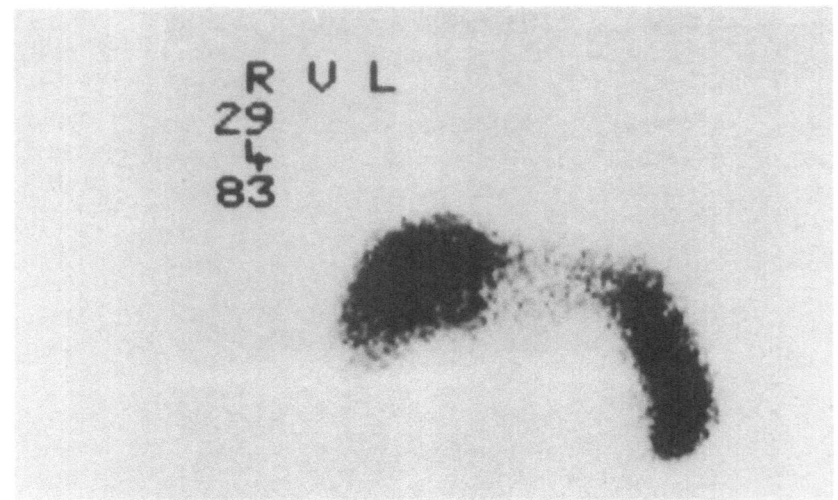

a

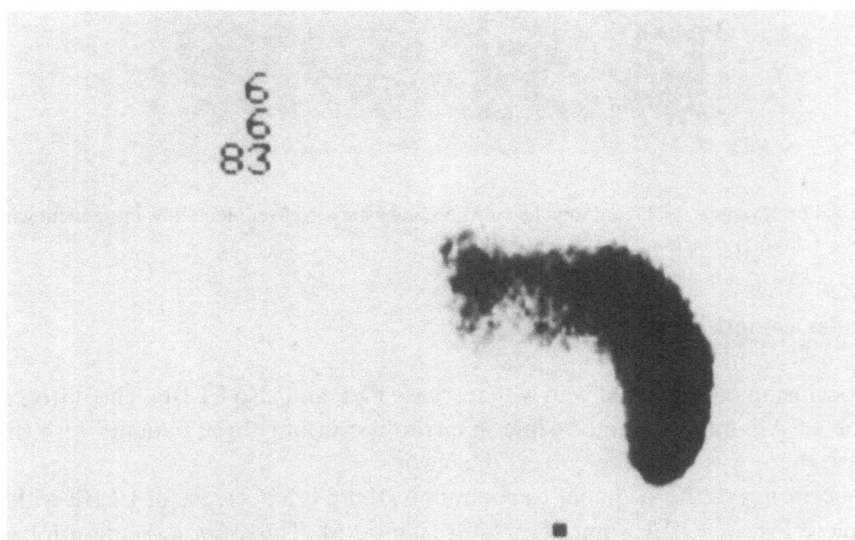

b

Figure 6. Scintigraphy as an indicator of regional hepatic blood flow in a 3-year-old infant with biliary atresia: (A) 2 days after transplantation normal hepatic uptake, normal ELBF; (B) 5 weeks later (acute fever, acute rejection?): normal perfusion of left lobe, no perfusion right lobe: occlusion of right A. hepatica; (C) another 6 weeks later after some episodes of acute fever and liver function impairment: no hepatic uptake, no ELBF; occlusion of A. hepatica communis, angiographically confirmed. Emergency retransplantation of one lobe; (D) 6 days after retransplantation normal uptake in the lobe, normal ELBF.

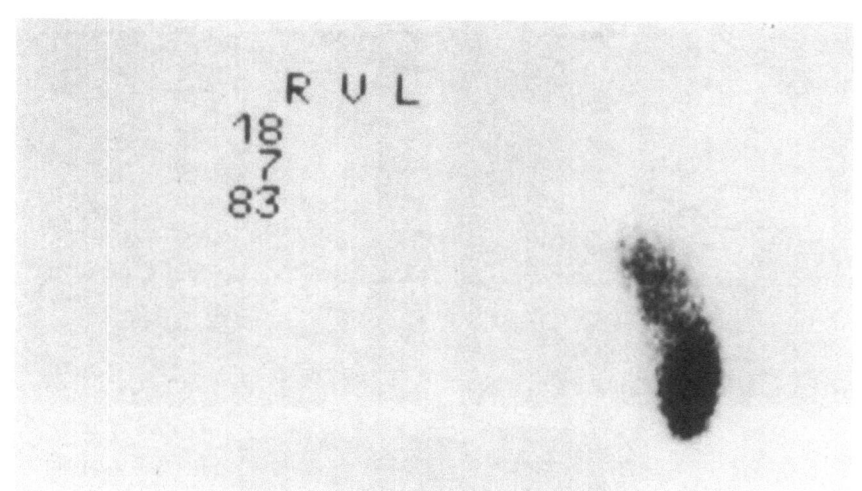

c

d

168

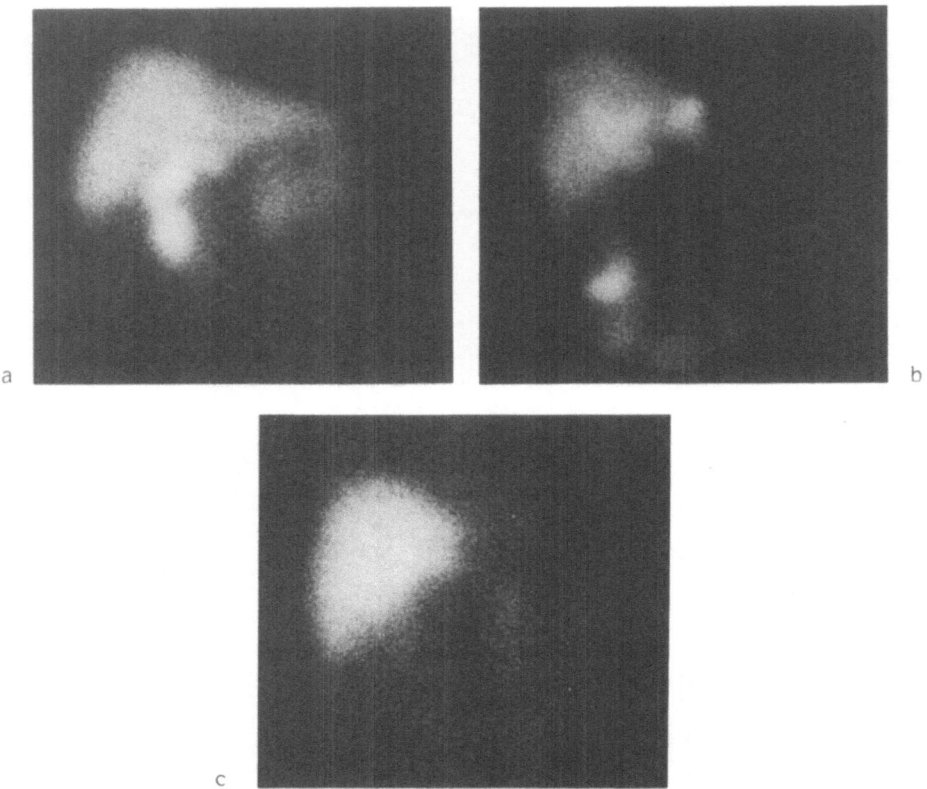

Figure 7. Cholescintigraphy in a 4-year-old infant with biliary atresia: (A) 6 days after transplantation and 30 min p.i. normal hepatic uptake and rapid excretion of labelled bile into jejunal loop; (B) 3 weeks later (emergency examination because of abdominal pain, acute fever): 30 min p.i. (left): no uptake in the left lobe, delayed excretion. 45 min p.i. (right): excretion into the small intestine and refilling of the lesion in left lobe. Scintigraphic diagnosis: Occlusion of the left A.hepatica with subsequent necrosis, bile leakage. Confirmed by emergency relaparatomy.

detection of BL [17], nearly half of the 227 cholescintigraphic studies in our transplanted patients were done to confirm or exclude this diagnosis (Figure 8). There are four distinct scintigraphic patterns of BL: the intrahepatic lesion with or without refilling of labelled bile, the intrahepatic lesion with extrahepatic accumulation (Figure 7) and the extrahepatic form with extrahepatic accumulation (Figure 8) [22]. The study must be done and interpreted carefully; initially in one patient the extrahepatic accumulation was misinterpreted as normal intestine bile uptake [17]. The scintigraphic sign of BL is an indication for an emergency surgical intervention.

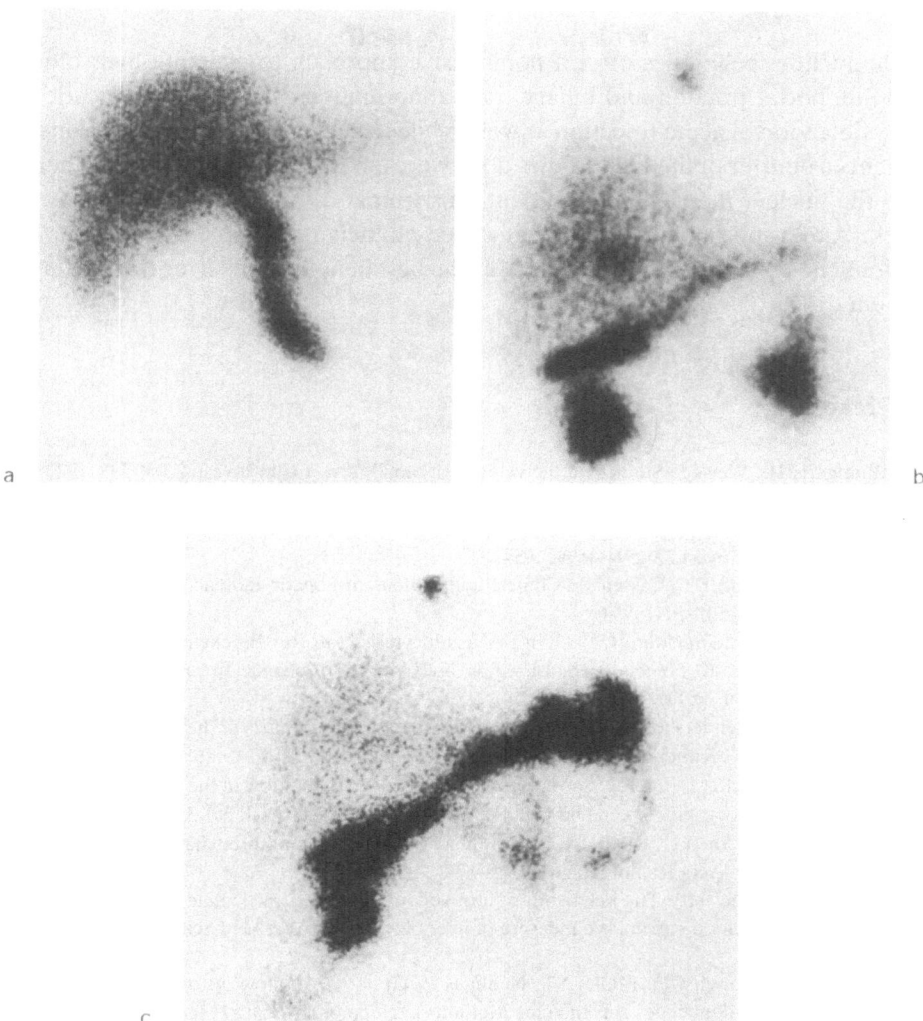

Figure 8. Cholescintigraphy in a 36-year-old patient with cirrhosis: (A) at day 6 after transplantation and 30 min p.i. normal hepatic uptake, normal excretion; (B) at day 24 after transplantation and 30 min p.i. (emergency examination because of acute fever, lower back pain): uptake in both kidneys as sign of hepatic insufficiency, extravasation of labelled bile at the side of anastomosis with distribution around the lower edge of the graft; (C) same study, 10 min later: the labelled bile has reached the left upper epigastrium and the stomach. Scintigraphic diagnosis: bile leakage with diffuse distribution within the upper abdomen. Confirmed by emergency relaparotomy.

Conclusions

Radionuclide techniques offer a noninvasive approach to estimate liver blood flow, its portal fraction and biliary tract abnormalities. They are diagnostic in early detection of acute rejection as well as bile leakage. In our liver transplanted patients a quarter of the 1326 studies done were emergency examinations. Therefore the nuclear medicine department must run at 24 h a day and seven days a week. And a specially trained and qualified physician-in-charge to interpret the radionuclide examinations is needed for the best benefit of the liver transplanted patient.

References

1. Blumgart HL, Weiss S: Studies on the velocity of blood flow. J Clin Invest 4:389–398, 1927.
2. Vetter H, Falkner R, Neumayr R: The disappearance rate of colloidal radiogold from the circulation and its application to the estimation of liver blood flow in normal and cirrhotic subjects. J Clin Invest 33:1594–1599, 1954.
3. Stirrett LA, Yuhl ET, Cassen B: Clinical applications of hepatic radioactivity survey. Am J Gastroenterol 21:310–314, 1954.
4. Silverstein SC, Steinmamm RM, Chon ZA: Endocytosis. Am Rev Biochem 46:669–772, 1977.
5. Reske SN, Vyska K, Feinendegene LE: In vivo assessment of phagocytic properties of kupffer cells. J Nucl Med 22:405–410, 1981.
6. George EA, Hendershott LR, Klos DJ, Donati RM: Mechanism of hepatic extraction of gelatinized 99m Technetium sulphur colloid. Eur J Nucl Med 5:241–245, 1980.
7. Lebrec D, Blanchet L, Lacroix S: Measurement of hepatic blood flow in the rat using fractional clearance of indocyanine green and colloidal radiogold. Pflugers Arch 391:353–354, 1981.
8. Pirttiaho H, Pitkänen U, Rajasalmi M, Ahonen A: Comparison of three methods of measuring liver blood flow. Acta Radiol Diagn 21:535–539, 1980.
9. Dobson EL, Jones HB: The behaviour of intravenously injected particulate material: its disappearance from blood stream as a measure of liver blood flow. Acta Med Scan 144 (Suppl.) 273, 1952.
10. Creutzig H, Brölsch CH, Müller ST, Neuhaus P, Gratz KF: Follow up of liver transplanted patients with radionuclides. In: Imaging Methods in Hepatology. Lutz H (ed). Lancaster MIT, 1984.
11. Biersack HJ, Thelen M, Schulz S: Die sequientielle Hepatosplenoszintigraphie zur quantitativen Beurteilung der Leberdurchblutung. Fortschr Roentgenstr 126:47–53, 1977.
12. Creutzig H, Schober O, Brölsch CH, Pichlmayr R, Hundeshagen H: Der arterielle Anteil an der Lebergesamtperfusion. Nucl Med 20:25–29, 1981.
13. Creutzig H: Nuklearmedizinische Diagnostik. In: Bock HE, Gerock W, Hartmann F (eds). Klinik der Gegenwart. Band VII:E436–E440, 1984.
14. Rypins EB, Fajman W, Sarper R: Radionuclide angiography of the liver and spleen. Am J Surg 142:574–579, 1981.
15. Peschl C, Kroiss A, Funovics J, Neumayr A: Untersuchungen zur Leberdurchblutung bei portosystemischen Shuntpatienten. Z Gastroenterol 17:589, 1979.
16. Calne RY, Williams R: liver transplantation. Cur Prob Surg 16:24–33, 1979.
17. Gratz KF, Creutzig H, Brölsch CH, Pichlmayr R, Hundeshagen H: Szintigraphie des Gallelecks. In: R. Höfer (ed.) Radioaktive Isotope in Klinik und Forschung. Wien, Egermann, 1982.
18. Zeeman RK, Lee CH, Stahl R, Viscomi GN: Strategy for the use of biliary scintigraphy in non-

iatrogenic biliary trauma. Radiology 151:771–777, 1984.

19. Pistolesi M, Fazio F. Marini G, Giunti C: Lung uptake of 1231-HIPDN in man: an index in lung metabolic function. J Nucl Med All Sci 27:180–182, 1983.

20. Creutzig H, Sturm JA, Schober O, Nerlich ML, Kant CJ: Diagnostik des pulmonary capillary protein leakage. Nuklearmedizin (in press).

21. Creutzig H, Brölsch CH, Neuhaus P. Gonda S, Pichlmayr S, Hundeshagen H: Five years experience in the follow-up of liver transplanted patients with radionuclides. J Nucl Med 23:P16, 1982.

22. Creutzig H, Brölsch CH, Müller ST, Neuhaus P. Gratz KF, Schober O, Pichlmayr R, Hundeshagen H: Nuklearmedizinische Diagnostik des Gallelecks. Dtsch Med Wschr (in press).

Section 5

SELECTION. PEDIATRIC LIVER TRANSPLANTATION

18. Selection of patients for liver transplantation and results

R. WILLIAMS, J. NEUBERGER, B. PORTMANN and R.Y. CALNE

In this chapter I am going to discuss the type of patient who should be considered for liver transplantation and the results that can be obtained in the different disease categories. The likelihood and significance of disease recurrence is also considered.

Indications

Liver transplantation is indicated in any patient who has a progressive and otherwise fatal disease, for whom standard therapy is no longer effective and who is fit enough to withstand the considerable trauma of the surgery involved. In practice, the decisions as to which patients should be offered liver transplantation and when to perform such surgery are often very difficult.

During the course of the joint transplant programme of liver grafting (Addenbrooke's Hospital, Cambridge and King's College Hospital, London), almost every type of liver disease has been included over the past 15 years. The one major area that is not well represented in our series is biliary atresia. Although published results from Starzl's group have always been better in children than in adults [1], in the United Kingdom the extreme difficulty in obtaining suitable donor organs in this age group has resulted in few children being transplanted. Also, until the recent advent of cyclosporin, we have always been worried about the complications associated with the long term use of corticosteroids in children, including retardation of growth.

Overall results and long-term survival

Up to July 1984 166 patients had received liver grafts in our series (Table 1 and Figure 1). These cases can be divided into those with malignant disease and those with non-malignant disease, the latter being the larger category and the group

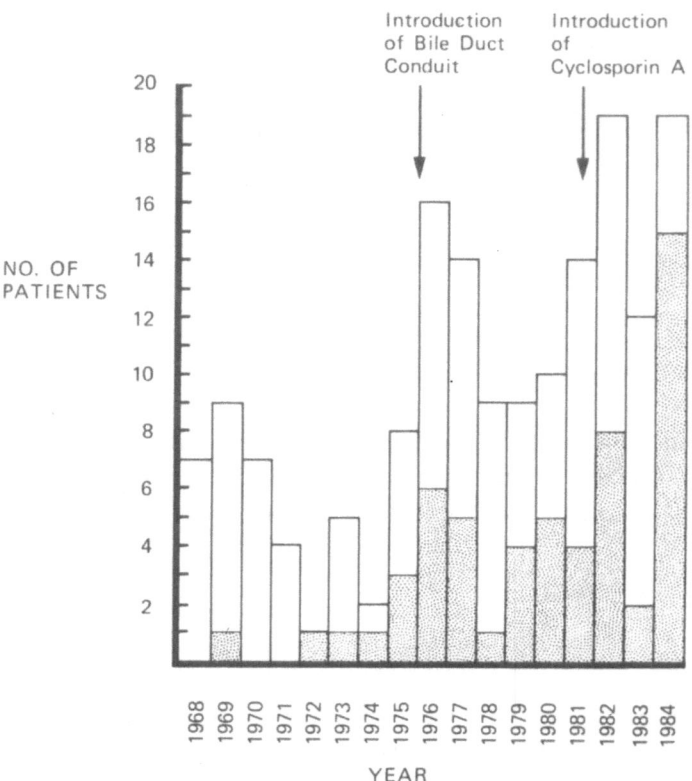

Figure 1. Number of patients receiving liver grafts in the Addenbrooke's/King's College Hospital series. Shaded areas represent those patients surviving for more than 1 year. (Patients grafted as of 1 July 1984: estimated survival.)

from which we are currently grafting the majority of patients. However, our early experience was gained largely from patients with malignant disease.

During the course of the transplant programme there have been many advances in both surgical techniques and methods of organ harvesting and transplantation that have resulted in improved survival and a greater number of patients being able to receive a graft. Before the introduction of the conduit technique for biliary tree anastomosis many patients died from complications associated with fistula formation and sepsis. A further major advance in the maintenance of immunosuppression is the introduction of cyclosporin A, although in our experience intravenous use of the drug in the early peri-operative period is associated with considerable toxicity, including nephrotoxicity, pulmonary oedema and convulsions [2].

In this series, as at 18 July 1984, 39 patients had survived for over 1 year, of whom 22 were currently alive. As can be seen from Table 2, nine patients have

Table 1. Orthotopic liver transplantation: Addenbrooke's/King's College Hospital series (May 1968–July 1984).

Malignant disease		Non-malignant disease		
Primary liver tumours	47	Cirrhosis		89
Hepatocellular carcinoma	34	Primary biliary cirrhosis	35	
Intrahepatic cholangiocarcinoma	9	Chronic active hepatitis	20	
Sarcoma	4	Cryptogenic cirrhosis	13	
		Alcohol	6	
Carcinoma of the hepatic ducts	8	Sclerosing cholangitis	6	
Hepatic metastases	6	Secondary biliary cirrhosis	3	
		Galactosaemia	1	
		α_1 Antitrypsin deficiency	3	
		Wilson's disease	1	
		Oxaluria	1	
		Budd-Chiari syndrome		8
		Subacute hepatic necrosis		2
		Biliary atresia		6
Total 166 patients	61			105

survived for periods of 4 or more years after grafting, can lead a normal life and may succumb to diseases unrelated to the primary disease or the liver graft, as described elsewhere. One patient (OL5) was grafted for a primary liver carcinoma and led a normal life for over five years. She died after a short illness from biliary sepsis secondary to sludging in the biliary tract. Other causes of late deaths included myocardial infarction and colonic carcinoma. A tragic development in one patient (OL34) was cirrhosis. This was in a woman who had presented with a primary hepatocellular carcinoma arising in a non-cirrhotic liver. She had been taking the oral contraceptive pill and this was considered to be the cause of the tumour [3]. She was first treated by partial resection but when the tumour recurred in the remaining liver transplantation was carried out and she made an excellent recovery. However, following a termination of pregnancy she received a blood transfusion, following which she developed a non A non B hepatitis. This

Table 2. Prolonged survival (>1 year) in patients in the Addenbrooke's/King's College Hospital series of liver transplantation (as of 1 July 1984).

Period (years)	Alive	Dead
1–2	3	9
2–4	10	4
4–6	4	4
>6	5	0
Total	22	17

progressed to a cirrhosis and she died in 1979, nearly six years after grafting, from bleeding oesophageal varices.

Our longest survivor had a hepatocellular carcinoma in association with a chronic hepatitis B viral infection (OL43). He had a positive family history with a younger brother dying from a hepatoma and a brother having already died from a hepatoma (Figure 2). During the anhepatic phase of the operation (carried out in 1975) he was given high titre anti-HBs immunoglobulin. He remains well over seven years later and is currently working as a mechanic. In our experience the use of high titre immunoglobulin was effective in clearing the circulation of HBsAg in four patients and we have not found any evidence of re-infection of the donor liver. These results contrast with the findings from the Denver group [1] who have reported late deaths occurring from re-infection of the donor liver with the HB-virus. Part of the explanation for the difference may lie in the e antigen status since all our patients were e antigen negative and it is therefore unlikely that active viral replication was occurring. In future it will be possible to investigate more fully the evidence for viral replication by testing for HBV and DNA genome using nucleic acid hybridisation techniques as well as for DNA polymerase and staining for HBV core antigen in the liver. There is now increasing evidence that the virus replicates also in extrahepatic tissues, notably the pancreas and bone marrow, and these sites will provide a reservoir for the virus.

Currently the risks of recurrence of disease in the patients who are e antigen positive are too great to consider them suitable candidates for transplantation, although it may be possible to consider these patients for grafting if e antigen/antibody conversion occurs after therapy with suitable anti-viral agents such as interferon, arabinoside, arabinoside monophosphate or acyclovir.

One type of case that may figure more frequently in the future series is the patient who has developed a hepatoma in a long-standing cirrhotic liver. With the more widespread use of ultrasound or radionucleide scanning and regular testing of the serum for alpha fetoprotein, these tumours may be detected at an early stage and before extrahepatic spread has occurred. One such case, OL131, is now well over 13 months after grafting. He had been followed at King's College Hospital for 4 years for management of his cryptogenic cirrhosis. In 1982 serum alpha fetoprotein was found to be elevated and subsequent investigation confirmed a small hepatocellular carcinoma.

Current position with transplantation for malignant disease

There are two major types of malignant disease which are no longer considered as suitable for grafting. The first is carcinoma of the hepatic duct, the Klatskin tumour [4]. This tumour often presents early with biliary obstruction on account of its site at the porta hepatis and it rarely metastasises. However, in eight patients grafted for this condition local recurrence has occurred in all, although

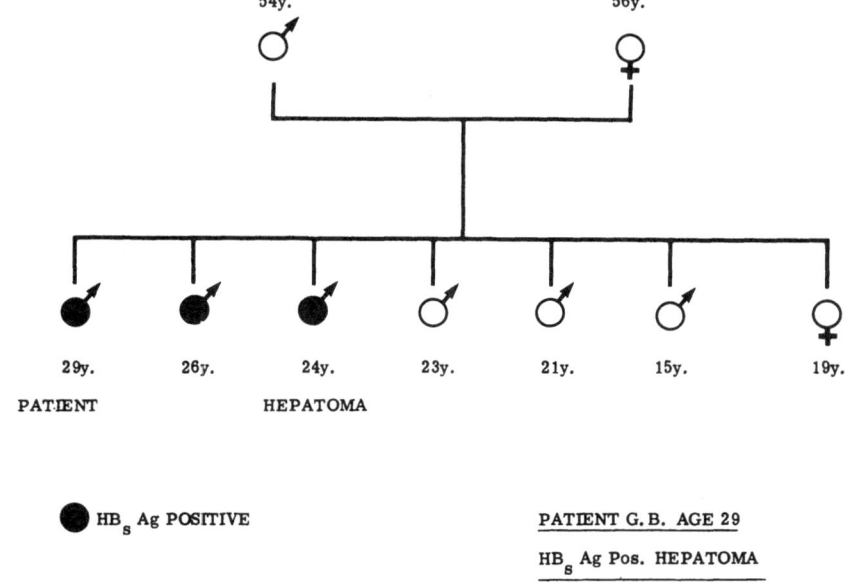

Figure 2. Family tree of patient OL43 with familial HBsAg positive hepatoma: ● = HBsAg positive.

the longest survivor lived for 11 months. It is of interest that all patients had undergone some form of intubation of the tumour for either diagnostic or therapeutic reasons and it is probable that the mechanical intervention resulted in an accelerated dissemination of the disease.

The second group is the isolated hepatic metastasis. Early in the series five patients received liver grafts for a solitary hepatic metastasis developing some time after resection of the primary tumour. These secondaries have arisen from primaries in the colon, pancreas and kidney, as well as a duodenal leiomyosarcoma and meningioma. In each instance, except the leiomyosarcoma, the tumour had been resected at least three years before grafting and all techniques then available had precluded other sites of spread. In all cases extrahepatic spread occurred. In none of the published series have there been recorded cases of a long-term cure for secondary hepatic metastases.

The current view with respect to transplantation for malignant disease is illustrated by the case with an apparently slow growing tumour which is not resectable occurring in a young person who has no underlying liver disease, or if the tumour arises on the basis of well-compensated cirrhosis. In our experience the degree of elevation and rate of rise of serum alpha fetoprotein are useful indications of the rate of growth of the tumour. One of the more recently recognised subgroups of alpha fetoprotein negative liver tumours is the fibrolamellar hepato cellular carcinoma variant, which is slow growing and tends to metastasise late. With adherence to such criteria and with better methods for detecting extrahepatic spread it is likely that the recurrence rate will become more acceptable. Indeed, an analysis of the first 40 patients with intrahepatic hepatocellular carcinoma and cholangiocarcinoma showed that 60% (24) of these patients were 'cured' of the tumour and six were alive and well over one year after grafting. Of the 16 patients in whom recurrence occurred 13 have survived for periods over one year. However, even with the use of all available methods for screening for extrahepatic spread, including ultrasound, CT scanning of the abdomen and lung fields and skeletal surveys, small metastases in the lymph nodes or porta hepatis can be missed.

Indications in cirrhosis and other non-malignant disease

In contrast to those with malignancies, those with end-stage parenchymal disease present a much greater surgical problem to the surgeon, particularly with removal of the diseased liver where the presence of portal hypertension and abdominal collaterals add considerably to the difficulties involved. There is usually associated disease and other organ failure, such as renal failure, and pulmonary disease with arterio-venous shunting. In addition cirrhotic patients are often malnourished and this leads to impaired healing and decreased resistance to infection.

Only a small proportion of those patients with alcoholic cirrhosis are likely to be considered as suitable candidates for surgery since not only is there the risk that they may return to their previous habit but heavy alcohol ingestion is associated with cardiac and cerebral impairment and malnutrition greatly increasing the hazards of transplantation. Nevertheless if the patient is assessed carefully excellent results can be achieved as evidenced by one patient, OL117, who, although he had drunk heavily in the past was able to abstain from alcohol completely once liver disease had been diagnosed. Although his clinical state improved temporarily the severity of the cirrhosis was such that despite increasing doses of diuretics his ascites became increasingly difficult to control and he developed chronic encephalopathy and the appearance of oesophageal varices. Despite a very stormy post-operative course, as illustrated in Figure 3, he made an excellent recovery and is now extremely well, with virtually normal liver function tests.

Patients with chronic encephalopathy who are only poorly controlled by standard therapy present a further group of patients who show dramatic improvement following a successful transplant. One such example is OL22, a 49-year-old woman admitted to King's College Hospital five times in 4 months for recurrent encephalopathy due to an underlying cirrhosis. Post-operatively she remained well for 6 months, but died from an infection with pneumocystis. At post-mortem examination she was found to have a reticulum cell sarcoma which, on nuclear chromatin staining, was found to arise from the host [5] since the donor was a male.

R.C. MALE AGE 47

JUNE 1980	- ASCITES, JAUNDICE, GRADE I ENCEPHALOPATHY
SEPTEMBER 1981 ONWARDS	- PROGRESSIVE DETERIORATION ALBUMEN 2.2 GRMS/L PROTHROMBIN TIME 22 SECS SMA 1/80 VARICES ⋔ SIZE
3.1.82.	- TRANSPLANTATION AT CAMBRIDGE
4.1.82.	- INTRA-ABDOMINAL HAEMORRHAGE - RE-EXPLORED
13.1.82.	- BILIARY PERITONITIS - RE-EXPLORED RENAL FAILURE
21.1.82.	- TRANSFERRED BACK RESPIRATORY FAILURE STEROID PSYCHOSIS
8.2.82.	- ↑ JAUNDICE/BILIARY FISTULA/SEPTICAEMIA TRANSHEPATIC PERCUTANEOUS DRAINAGE REVERSAL OF JAUNDICE
6.3.82.	- WEIGHT 50 → 65 KG / ENTERAL NUTRITION

Figure 3. Post-operative course of patient OL117.

Transplantation has a useful place in those patients where recurrent bleeding from varices cannot be controlled. The benefits that can be obtained are exemplified by the case of OL61, a 34-year-old man with cryptogenic cirrhosis. He first bled from oesophageal varices in December 1970 (Figure 4). Because of continued bleeding he was treated by mesocaval shunting but, because of thrombosis of the shunt and repeated bleeding, he underwent oesophageal transection and then sclerotherapy. The patient himself demanded a transplant having been stimulated by the presence of a recent transplant patient on the ward attending for routine follow-up. Since the time of transplantation he has remained extremely well, working full-time as a mechanic and running daily. Liver function tests are normal.

Primary biliary cirrhosis

This is in many ways at present the most suitable variety of cirrhosis for transplantation once a certain stage of the disease has been reached. Indeed, it constitutes

182

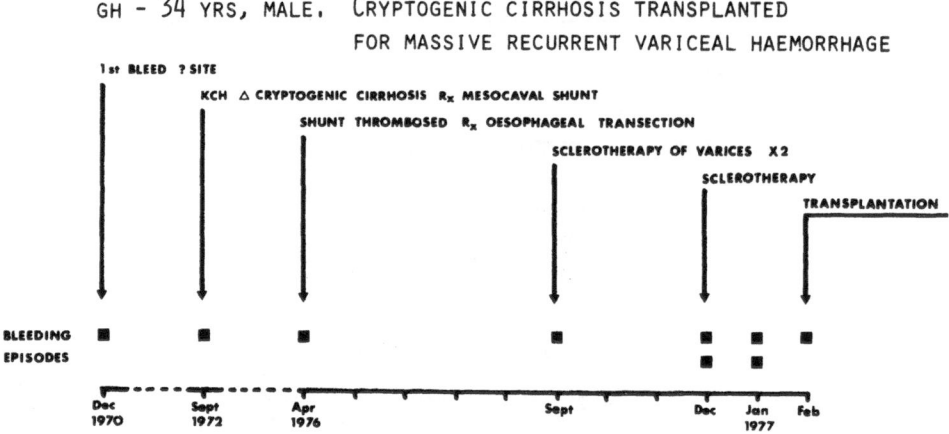

GH - 34 YRS, MALE. CRYPTOGENIC CIRRHOSIS TRANSPLANTED
FOR MASSIVE RECURRENT VARICEAL HAEMORRHAGE

Figure 4. Clinical course of patient OL61 prior to liver transplantation.

the largest group of patients transplanted in our series. The synthetic aspects of liver function tend to be well preserved until a late stage of the disease and patients seem to withstand surgery better than those with other types of chronic liver disease. In the later stages of the disease patients tend to have a striking disability from their disease, with deepening jaundice, pigmentation, pruritus that is intractable and diarrhoea. In selecting the optimum time for grafting the decision is usually made on clinical criteria, such as chronic encephalopathy, resistant ascites or intractable pruritus, or the inability to carry out housework without recording changes in laboratory tests. The serum bilirubin is currently the most useful guide and once this has exceeded 150 μmol/l the prognosis is limited to less than 1 year in the average case [6].

In 1982 we described the possibility of recurrence of the disease in the donor liver following our experience with three patients who developed histological features of the disease in the donor liver three or more years after grafting (Figure 5). The histological features observed indicated granuloma formation and bile duct destruction with lymphoid follicles. Disease recurrence was suggested not only by the persistence of antimitochondrial antibodies (Figure 6) and elevated IgM levels and increasing levels of serum bilirubin (Figure 7), but also by the development of the sicca syndrome in two patients and mild hypothyroidism and sclerodactyly in one [7]. However, examination of the material available from Starzl's series raised the suggestion that the histological features seen in these patients may be due to rejection [8]. In our experience the lesions of chronic rejection and those described in patients with recurrence of PBC are quite distinct. It is of interest that the three patients we originally described had been maintained on low doses of azathioprine and corticosteroids. The former agent is of limited value in controlling PBC and the benefit of the latter remains to be proven. In the last two years the immunosuppression has been altered to cyclo-

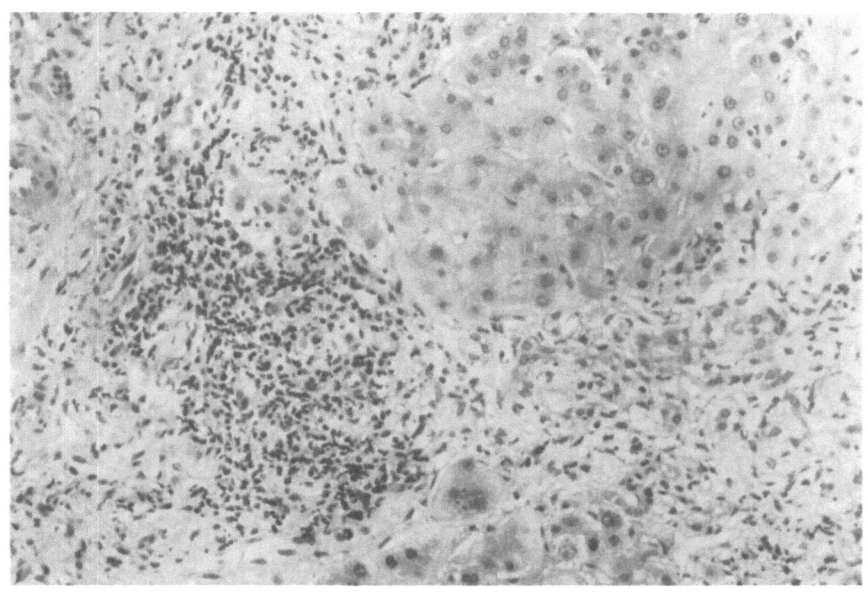

Figure 5. Liver biopsy of patient OL64 4 years after grafting, showing features of PBC (H&E ×350) (by permission of the Editor, New England Journal of Medicine).

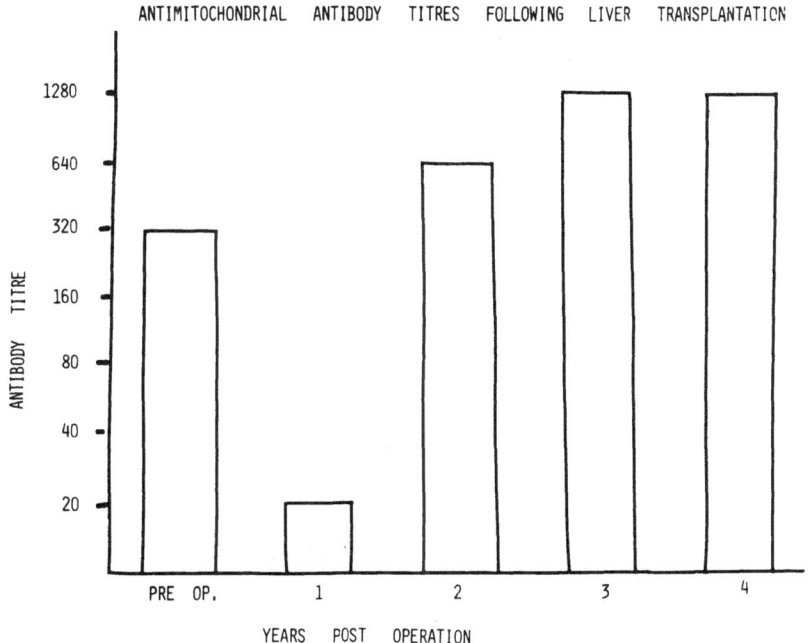

Figure 6. Antimitochondrial antibody titres of patient OL74 following liver transplantation for PBC.

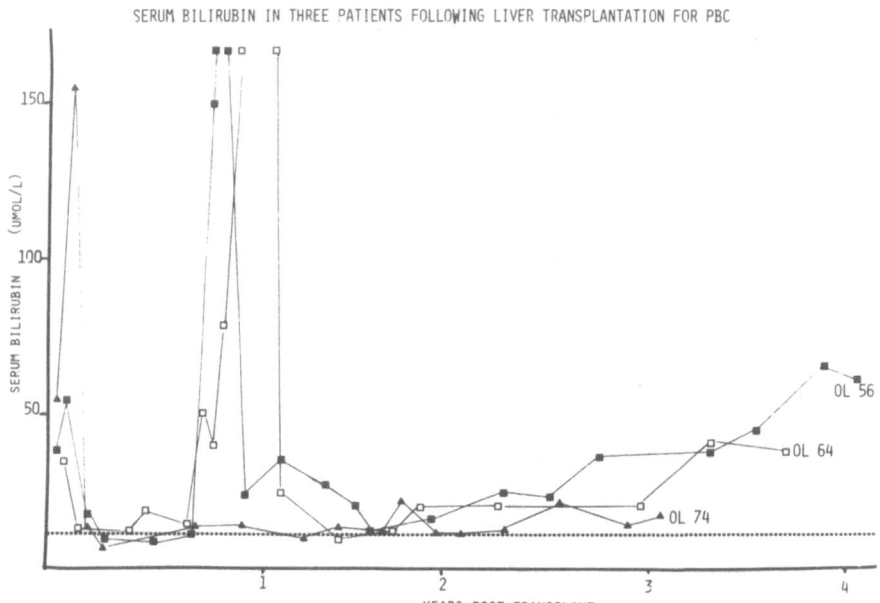

SERUM BILIRUBIN IN THREE PATIENTS FOLLOWING LIVER TRANSPLANTATION FOR PBC

Figure 7. Serum bilirubin in three patients grafted for PBC and maintained on prednisolone and azathioprine. Dotted line represents upper limit of normal.

sporin A. There is preliminary evidence that this drug is of benefit in the treatment of PBC [9], and no further histological evidence of progression has been observed in those transferred to cyclosporin A. It is to be emphasised also that in these three patients the disease is still at an early stage and all patients have been able to return to their previous occupations. Thus in all cases transplantation has resulted in a remarkable improvement in the quality of their lives.

Chronic active hepatitis

Chronic active hepatitis is like PBC, in which the pathogenetic mechanisms are thought to include an immune mediated attack against normal liver antigens, and it might be anticipated that recurrence of the disease may also occur. Evidence of such recurrence has been seen recently in a 21-year-old woman, OL99, with autoimmune chronic active hepatitis [10], who underwent liver grafting in 1980. Immediately following surgery the spider naevi resolved and the serum immunoglobulins and autoantibodies fell to normal levels. She was maintained initially on cyclosporin A and prednisolone (Figure 8). The dose of prednisolone was gradually reduced, but she remained well until 9 months later when she developed a constitutional illness with anorexia and weight loss. Her spider naevi returned together with elevation of serum transaminases, immunoglobulins and

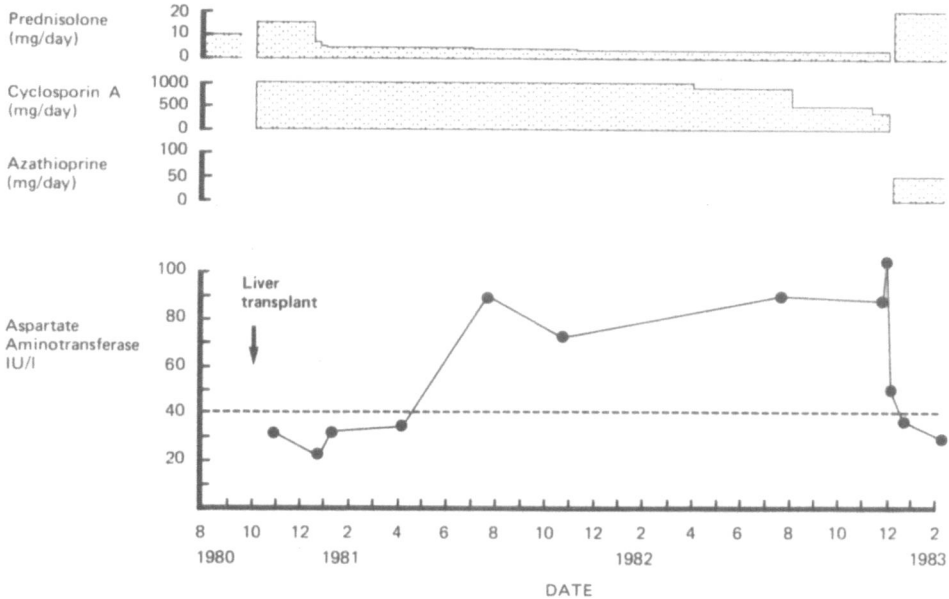

Figure 8. Serum transaminases and immunosuppressive regime in patient OL99 following liver transplantation (by permission of the Editor of Transplantation).

autoantibodies. A liver biopsy at that time showed histological features of chronic active hepatitis (Figure 9), with piecemeal necrosis and a predominantly mono-nuclear cell portal tract infiltrate. The cyclosporin was discontinued, the pred-nisolone dose increased and azathioprine added. All signs and symptoms sub-sequently resolved and a repeat liver biopsy showed features of chronic persistent hepatitis. During her illness all markers for viruses were negative and the pos-sibility of a non A non B hepatitis was considered unlikely on the basis of both negative serology (kindly performed by Dr H. Thomas, London) and elevated levels of antibodies to liver specific lipoprotein (LSP). These antibodies are characteristically absent in non A non B hepatitis. In our experience cyclosporin A is of little value in the therapy of chronic active hepatitis, whereas prednisolone and azathioprine are of proven benefit. In patients with CAH, as in those with PBC, the immunosuppressive regime should be selected according to the nature of the original disease.

Budd-Chiari syndrome

Another important group of patients in which excellent results can be obtained, but where the original disease may recur, is the Budd-Chiari syndrome. Often these patients are referred at a stage too late to be considered for side-to-side

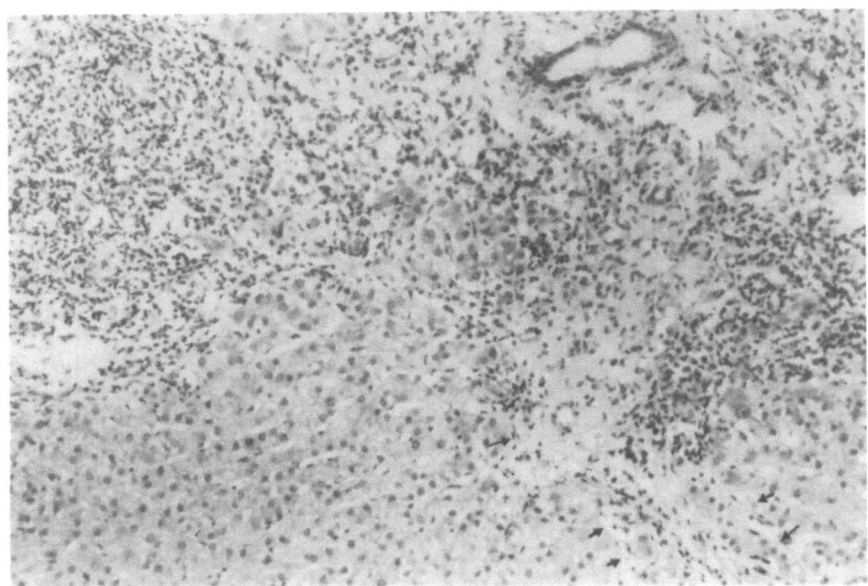

Figure 9. Liver histology of patient OL99 9 months after liver transplantation showing features of chronic active hepatitis (by permission of the Editor of Transplantation).

portocaval shunting. The progressive ill health and emaciation which are often associated with massive ascites, requiring high doses of diuretics, make a normal life no longer tenable. Of the eight patients grafted in this group the last developed thrombosis of the portal and hepatic veins immediately post-operatively at sites away from the anastomotic lines. Since then all such patients have received anti-coagulation post-operatively. Nonetheless, thrombosis of the hepatic veins has occurred in three despite full anti-coagulation and one of these, in addition, has developed a portal vein block. Thus it seems that these patients have an underlying disturbance in blood coagulation, although all tests of coagulation are normal.

Metabolic disorders

In contrast to those diseases which may recur in the donor liver, grafting may be curative in a number of metabolic conditions involving or arising in the liver. These included α_1 antitrypsin deficiency, some glycogen storage disorders and galactosaemia [1]. Another disease cured by grafting is Wilson's disease. Patient OL119, a 20-year-old male, underwent liver transplantation for Wilson's disease because of severe liver failure, recurrent encephalopathy and gross wasting. He made an excellent post-operative recovery and has returned to work as a farmer.

He was not maintained on any chelating agent post-operatively. Studies of copper metabolism were carried out by Dr John Walshe of Addenbrooke's Hospital, Cambridge and these were found to be entirely normal.

Extent of rehabilitation

We have assessed the extent of the rehabilitation of those patients who have survived the major hazards of surgery and the post-operative period. Of 34 1-year survivors, rehabilitation has been considered excellent in 21 cases. Most of these patients have returned to work in full-time jobs, including accounting, mechanics, gardeners and laboratory technicians. The women have been able to return to household duties and look after their families again – perhaps the hardest job of them all. In addition, patients have taken up full physical activities, including running, fell walking and rafting. In four cases only was rehabilitation considered to be poor because of chronic rejection (OL92), partial extrahepatic biliary obstruction (OL63, 76) and chronic encephalopathy (OL107).

On this basis, and with increasing availability of suitable donor organs and a better understanding of the post-operative problems, liver transplantation will be a more widely used and acceptable form of treatment for the patient with end-stage liver disease in whom no other therapy is effective.

Acknowledgements

The generous time and experience given by all those involved in the transplant programme in the Liver Unit, King's College Hospital and the Surgical Department at Addenbrooke's Hospital, Cambridge, can never be adequately acknowledged.

References

1. Starzl T, Iwatsuki S, Van Thiel DA, *et al.*: Evolution of liver transplantation. Hepatology 2:614–636, 1982.
2. Rolles K, Williams R, Neuberger J, Calne R: The Cambridge and King's College Hospital experience of liver transplantation 1968–1983. Hepatology 4:50S–55S, 1984.
3. Neuberger J, Portmann B, Nunnerley H, *et al.*: Oral contraceptive associated liver tumours: occurrence of malignancy and difficulty in diagnosis. Lancet 1:247–276, 1980.
4. Klatskin G: Adenocarcinoma of the hepatic duct at its bifurcation within the porta hepatis. Am J Med 38:241–256, 1965.
5. Portmann B, Schindler AM, Murray-Lyon IM, Williams R: Histological sexing of a reticulum cell sarcoma arising after liver transplantation. Gastroenterology 70:82–84, 1976.
6. Shapiro JM, Smith H, Schaffner F: Serum bilirubin: a prognostic factor in primary biliary cirrhosis. Gut 20:137–140, 1979.

7. Neuberger J, Portmann B, Macdougall B, *et al.*: Recurrence of primary biliary cirrhosis after liver grafting. N Engl J Med 306:1–4, 1982.
8. Fennel RH, Shikes RH, Vierling JN: Relationship of pre-transplant hepatobiliary disease to bile duct damage occurring in the liver allograft. Hepatology 3:841–849, 1983.
9. Routhier G, Epstein O, Janossy G, *et al.*: Effects of cyclosporin A on suppressive and inducer T lymphocytes in primary biliary cirrhosis. Lancet 2:1223–1226, 1980.
10. Neuberger J, Portmann B, Calne RY, Williams R: Recurrence of autoimmune chronic active hepatitis after liver transplantation. Transplantation 37:363–365, 1984.

19. Liver transplantation for hepatic tumors

C.E. BRÖLSCH, P. NEUHAUS, K. WONIGEIT and R. PICHLMAYR

The incidence of hepatocellular carcinoma is increasing within the population of Western Europe and North America. Improved diagnostic means and improved general medical care account for the more frequent detection of hepatic malignomas rather than the incidence of hepatic cirrhosis and chronic active hepatitis [2]. Surgical treatment regularly precedes any alternative therapy. Early detection of the hepatic lesion has frequently resulted in a successful hepatic resection when the tumor was found to be confined to an anatomical lobe of the liver. In addition, in cases of irresectability, intraarterial or systemic infusion of chemotherapy or embolization could be started by the same laparotomy, inserting a pump infusion system selectively into the hepatic artery [1]. Trials on the effect of tumor treatment by local application are still to be performed. However, it will become an increasingly more important approach since reports on the ultimate mode of treatment for irresectable hepatic malignancies by liver replacement have been discouraging in the long-term prognosis (Aigner *et al.* 1984, personal communication). Various types of hepatic malignomas have been transplanted in the past, all of which spontaneously have a different prognosis which makes comparison of survival rates and determination of prognosis very difficult (Table 1).

Cholangiocellular carcinoma, hepatic sarcoma and rare types of hemangio-endotheliosarcoma are known to grow rapidly and mostly have already spread metastases at the time of their recognition. However, long-term survivors have been observed after liver transplantation with our oldest patient surviving more than 9 years, and other series have reported similar individual successes [4, 8, 12]. The following report of the Hannover experience evaluates the experiences of liver transplantation with particular respect to tumor patients and the current approach to treat patients with hepatic tumors.

The number of patients referred for hepatic surgery has increased drastically since hepatic transplantation opened an alternative to otherwise irresectable malignancies in the past. The first case in Germany was performed on a tumor patient [7] with the ultimate hope of long-term treatment. The risk of the operation and the uncertain outlook was justified by the lack of alternative treatments [11].

Even at the price of considerable risk, hepatic resection should be carried out since its operative mortality is relatively low and long-term prognosis is better in almost any case compared with the outcome of transplantation [9, 14].

Among the first fifty (50) cases of liver transplantation in our series there was a relatively high number of tumor patients who characterized the approach in the past. Any center to start with a liver transplant program can circumvent a number of difficulties related to the procedure itself and the postoperative management if they choose to operate on tumor patients. Even in patients with an underlying cirrhosis and chronic active hepatitis who developed a tumor almost two-thirds of these patients had no signs of portal hypertension and secondary organ involvement, such as hepatorenal syndrome or encephalopathy.

Generally, tumor patients are physically healthier, although some patients with hepatomegalia due to the gigantic size of the tumor and advanced cancer disease showed pulmonary complications preoperatively which affected the course postoperatively. In addition, some patients presented with severe jaundice due to an intrahepatic biliary duct tumor and reduced general condition and were likely to develop secondary organ complications. It is still impossible to determine the significance of preoperative secondary organ involvement and its relation to the development of consequent organ failure while the trauma of liver replacement is added to an already impaired organ system.

Among the risk factors most important to determine the postoperative outcome are age and preexisting infectious complications. Age accounts for a variety of factors involving cardiac and respiratory function and physical reserve. Preexisting infections mostly occur in the biliary tract system due to outflow obstruction or in bacterial pneumonia due to ineffective ventilation. Despite these factors which present prior to the operation, liver transplantations have been successfully performed but the majority of patients succumbed. It is concluded therefore that these general factors should be taken into consideration more thoroughly.

Preoperative assessments have therefore to aim in two directions simultaneously: (1) evaluating risk factors thoroughly and (2) evaluating the proper diag-

Table 1. Indications for liver transplantation in 50 tumor patients.

Primary Liver Tumors	
1. Irresectable hepatocellular carcinoma	17
2. Cirrhosis with hepatocellular carcinoma	15
3. Cholangiocellular carcinoma	5
Adenocarcinoma of the biliary tract	9
Metastatic liver tumors	4

Med. Hochschule, Hannover 8/84.

nosis. Viewing the diagnostic workup, many risk factors will be determined by the patient's history, the time of tumor growth, intermittent complications, therapeutical load and psychological expectations which all together influence the indication. In particular, psychological expectations provoked by information regarding the possibility of liver transplantation sometimes predetermine the patient's desire to undergo a liver transplantation in an otherwise slowly progressive deleterious course.

Determination of the tumor diagnosis proved to be the most important factor as to prognosis after liver transplantation. The diagnosis should focus on the site, the size, the intrahepatic infiltration of the tumor, histological features and differentiation of the tumor cells and on the possibility of extrahepatic tumor growth. The latter can sometimes only be identified by laparotomy, which is either performed prior to transplantation or at the same time, while another patient is already alerted in case extrahepatic tumor growth proves to be present. However, this approach is sometimes cruel to the patient awakening from anesthesia and still carrying the same tumor-containing liver. In any case, when there is suspicion of lymph node enlargement within the porta hepatis and around the aorta, and in cases when the tumor indicates irresectability, laparotomy should be performed by the same surgeon who eventually carries out the liver transplantation. Specimens should be taken from the tumor as well as from periportal lymph nodes and periaortal lymph nodes (Table 2). If the tumor proves to be irresectable while the lymph nodes are free of microcellular infiltration, and while there is no other organ system involved, the prognosis of this patient after liver transplantation becomes significantly better. In addition, better hepatic tumor specimens can be obtained and more precise determinations can be made regarding the grade of malignancy of the tumor itself. It has been clearly shown that well-differentiated hepatocellular carcinomas carrying parts of fibrous tissue have a favorable prognosis following liver transplantation [14]. If they are solid, unilocular and irresectable, a liver transplantation should be carried out. The same indication applies for hepatoblastomas in children which cannot be resected, although a laparotomy is mandatory in children to establish irresectability. Chil-

Table 2. Results of liver transplantation in tumor patients (38 transplants in 37 patients) (Medizinische Hochschule, Hannover) (1983).

Tumor spread at time of operation	Number of patients	Survival time (months)[a]				Alive	Longest survivor
		<1	1–6	6–12	>12		
Extrahepatic growth	20	8	7 (4)	4 (–)	1 (–)	4	2 years
No extrahepatic growth	17	5	2 (1)	6 (2)	4 (4)	7	6³/₄ years

[a] Number of living patients in brackets.

dren tolerate extended resections very well so that the diagnosis of irresectability should be established by an experienced liver surgeon. Transplantation in pediatric tumor patients, however, is limited due to the lack of suitable donor organs which, when they eventually become available, should be used for a child with a benign disease such as atresia.

Cholangiocellular carcinoma, hemangiosarcomas or metastatic diseases should no longer be considered to be an indication for liver transplantation. In all series it has been shown that there is early tumor recurrence when the patient survives the first 6 months after operation. Metastatic diseases will occur despite the time of long tumor-free interval. As to whether immunosuppression therapy is of support in promoting recurrence of the disease remains an empirical observation, but it is likely [3, 4, 8, 12, 14].

At the time when metastases are detected, it is definitely foreseeable that the tumor disease is generally recurring (Table 3). For these patients, a different approach has to be obtained, such as total body irradiation and bone marrow transplantation and additional chemotherapy (Huber *et al.* 1984, personal communication). The patients transplanted in our institution for metastatic disease have been individuals with primary colorectal cancer removed up to 5 years prior to transplantation and patients with the diagnosis of a primary hepatic tumor which turned out to be a metastasis of a melanoma of the retina.

As far as indications are concerned, it is certainly not settled that liver transplantation is not an adequate procedure for primary or secondary hepatic tumors but, thus far, its indication has to be restricted to certain types of hepatocellular tumors with a well-defined location in the absence of extrahepatic tumor growth. Other indications will eventually become possible but they lack a biological basis and are aimed to meet the patient's desire in a critical situation. On the basis of the research approach, other management protocols related to the use of monoclonal antibodies, chemotherapy, total body irradiation and bone marrow transplantation and, just recently, liver transplantation may very well be carried out in the future.

The *acute and chronic complications* with patients transplanted for hepatic

Table 3. Results of liver transplantations depending on tumor diagnosis (38 transplantations in 37 patients).

Type of tumor	Survival time			Alive
	>3 months	>6 months	>12 months	
Hepatocellular carcinoma n = 23	13	10	3(12%)	7
Cholangiocellular carcinoma n = 6	1	1	1(16%)	3
Biliary tract carcinomas and rare others n = 4	3	3	1(25%)	1
Metastases n = 4	1	1	–	–

cancer reflex the overall complication rate except that the perioperative mortality is lower compared to surgery in cirrhotic patients. Major complications in those patients concern the recurrence of the disease which is, more precisely, a general metastatic spread of the removed primary tumor. It affects primarily the lungs, the transplanted liver and secondarily, bone and brain [8]. From the observations of early pulmonary metastases, it is probable that micrometastases have already been present at the time of operation without documentation.

The performance of a CT scan of the lung, as well as a bonescintigraphy, is, therefore, recommended [4]. The earliest detection in our series was in an 18-year-old boy who was transplanted because of uncontrollable bleeding after blunt liver injury. His liver presented as a hemangiomatosis, ruptured following blunt injury. Suspicion of a malformation or a cancerous lesion of the liver as frozen section of liver tissue. When the diagnosis of cancer of the tissue was confirmed without specification of the tumor, the liver was removed. Six weeks after transplantation, metastases were detected in the lungs as well as in the transplanted liver, followed by rapid metastatic spread due to an unknown teratoid sarcoma which was thought to be the original tumor and finally found at autopsy.

However, more than 2/3rd of the patients left the hospital and returned to a somewhat limited but useful life until they finally succumbed.

Specific complications arise from *damage of the graft* in the postoperative period. Either acute vascular thrombosis of the hepatic artery or of the portal vein can occur in the graft, or the graft itself turns out to be nonviable due to irreversible damage in the agonal phase in the donor in combination with subsequent perfusion damage. Both complications can only be treated by immediate retransplantation. Thus far, no reliable determination of graft function is available to predict reliability following harvesting and perfusion. The incidence of portal vein thrombosis or hepatic entry thrombosis occurred in three patients

Table 4. Main causes of death in 33 tumor patients after liver transplantation.

	n
Tumor recurrence	15
Ischemic liver necrosis	3
Non-viable graft	2
Chronic rejection	3
Acute, irreversible rejection	2
Sepsis due to	
bowel perforation	1
biliary leakage	1
Pulmonary embolism	1
Multiorgan failure	5

with no chance of successful management, although arterialization of the liver was attempted in one case.

Graft rejection is an equally important complication which could be treated more successfully once Cyclosporine A became available [4, 12]. With the previous application of Azathioprine and steroids, and initially antilymphocyte globulin, two acute, uncontrollable rejections were observed in our institution while our experience with Cyclosporine A has been that acute uncontrollable rejection becomes a rare entity although it is still observed. With Cyclosporine A uncontrollable rejection presents in a more progressive manner leaving more time for the exact diagnosis to establish and leaving more time to search for a second transplant. In the early postoperative period, it is still a matter of controversy to distinguish rejection from prolonged perfusion damage, acute cholangitis, and toxic and secondary secretory damage. Repeated biopsies may provide the final differentiation in combination with a broad spectrum of functional screening of the liver.

A variety of *surgical complications* has to be considered since major abdominal surgery causes regular problems such as intestinal obstruction, peritonitis or intraabdominal hemorrhage. Previously, the most deleterious complications such as biliary leakage were managed by improved surgical choledochocholedochostomy and early detection of leakage by radionuclide scintigraphy. However, under immunosuppressive therapy, diagnosis is sometimes difficult to establish and was over looked in one patient who finally died from septic peritonitis.

A number of patients were lost due to a final multiorgan failure. All these patients were initially categorized as high-risk patients with pre-existing secondary organ damages. Two of them have been transplanted at a very late stage of their cancerous disease with gigantic tumor masses, extrahepatic tumor spread and removal of adjacent organs to the stomach, duodenum and the pancreas. Preexisting pulmonary infections and impaired renal function, perioperatively determined a chain of subsequent complications which finally ended up as a multiorgan failure.

We conclude from our experiences with transplantation for primary and secondary hepatic tumors that the indication for transplantation has to be done on a very selective basis. Whenever the decision comes up, it is an urgent indication because of the uncontrollable growth of the tumor. The indication should favor unilocular and solid liver tumors, with a high cellular differentiation or a high grade of fibrolamellar tissue [6]. The operative mortality of these patients is low with few pre-existing organic lesions. They are identified, and, after operation, many patients regain a high quality of life. The individual survival time is somewhat unpredictable, and extended survival of a few patients is possible. Liver transplantation for hepatic tumors is indicated in the future on a more selective basis and will eventually continue in combination with adjuvant chemotherapy.

References

1. Blumgart LH, Allison DJ: Resection and embolization in the management of secondary hepatic tumors. Wld J Surg 6(1):32–45, 1982.
2. Bengmark S, Hafstrom L, Jeppson B, Sundquist K: Primary carcinoma of the liver: improvement in sight? Wld J Surg 6(1):54–60, 1982.
3. Broelsch CE, Neuhaus P, Wonigeit K, Pichlmayr R: Ergebnisse der Lebertransplantation. Chirurgie der Leber, Edit. Medizin Hrsg. R. Häring, Berlin, 1983.
4. Calne RY: Liver transplantation for liver cancer. Wld J Surg 6(1):76–80, 1982.
5. Calne RY, MacMaster P, Portmann B, Wall WJ, Williams R: Observation on preservation, bile drainage and rejection in 64 human orthotopic liver allografts. Ann Surg 186:282–289, 1977.
6. Craig JR, Peters RC, Edmondson HH et al.: Fibrolamellar carcinoma of the liver. Cancer 46:372–379, 1980.
7. Guetgemann A, Lie TS, Esser G, Schriefers KH: Operative Aspekte bei der Orthotopen humanen Lebertransplantation. Chirurg 42:167–172, 1971.
8. Iwatsuki S, Klintmalm GBG, Starzl TE: Total hepatectomy and liver replacement (orthotopic liver transplantation) for primary hepatic malignancy. Wld J Surg 6(1):81–85, 1982.
9. Lee NW, Wong J, Ong GB: The surgical management of primary carcinoma of the liver. Wld J Surg 6(1):66–75, 1982.
10. MacDougall BRD, Williams R: Indications and assessment for orthotopic liver transplantation. In: Calne RY (ed.). Liver transplantation. Grune and Stratton, pp 59–66, 1983.
11. Neuhaus P, Broelsch CE, Ringe B, Gratz KF, et al.: Diagnostik und Therapie von Lebertumoren. Therapiewoche 34:4018–4032, 1984.
12. Pichlmayr R, Broelsch CE, Neuhaus P, Lauchart W, et al.: Report on 68 human orthotopic liver transplantations with special reference to rejection phenomena. Transplant Proc XV(1):1279–1283, 1983.
13. Rosen BT, Kamada N, Zimmermann F, Davies HS: Immunosuppressive effect of experimental liver allografts. In: Calne RY (ed.). Liver transplantation. Grune and Stratton, pp 35-54, 1983.
14. Starzl TE: Experience in hepatic transplantation. WB Saunders, Philadelphia, pp 1–553, 1969.

20. Pediatric liver transplantation

S. IWATSUKI, T.E. STARZL, B.W. SHAW, JR., J.C. GARTNER,
B.E. ZITELLI and J.J. MALATACK

Introduction

The value of cadaveric organ transplantation in infants and children has been often questioned because of the unsatisfactory survival and high morbidity associated with the conventional immunosuppressive regimen which includes azathioprine and prednisone, with or without antilymphocyte globulin. Even after so-called 'successful' transplantation the quality of life has been degraded too often by the side effects of high-dose steroid therapy, such as Cushingoid changes, growth retardation and osteoporosis.

Despite the continued efforts over the last 20 years to improve the survival and the quality of life after organ transplantation, real progress had to await the discovery [1, 2] and clinical use [3–6] of cyclosporine, a potent immunosuppressive agent derived from the fungi Cyclidrocarpon lucidum and Trichoderm polysporum.

We are reporting here the progress of liver transplantation in infants and children comparing the results obtained by using a regimen of cyclosporine and low dose steroids to those obtained in the past with the use of conventional immunosuppressive therapy.

Case materials and methods

Since the first human orthotopic liver transplantation on March 1, 1963, 296 patients with various diseases have received liver homografts as of April 30 1983 at the University of Colorado and the University of Pittsburgh. Of those 296 recipients, 170 were treated before March, 1980 with conventional double or triple drug therapy, including azathioprine (or cyclophosphamide), prednisone and antilymphocyte globulin. The remaining 126 were transplanted since March, 1980, and were treated with cyclosporine and low dose prednisone. Among the 170 patients given conventional immunosuppression therapy, 86 were pediatric recipients under age 18. Of 100 consecutive liver graft recipients under cyclo-sporine-low dose steroid therapy since March, 1980, there were 40 pediatric recipients under age 18. The experiences obtained from the total of these 126 pediatric liver recipients form the basis of this report.

Age distribution

The age distribution of the 86 pediatric recipients under conventional therapy and the 40 patients under cyclosporine therapy is shown in Figure 1. Seventy-four recipients were younger than 6 years; 29 were between 6 and 12 years; and 23 were older than 12 years.

Indications for liver transplantation

The main indications for liver transplantation in 126 pediatric orthotopic liver recipients are shown in Table 1. Biliary atresia or hypoplasia accounted for over one half of the total pediatric liver transplantations and was the most common diagnosis. The second most common indication was an inborn error of metabo-lism, such as alpha-1-antitrypsin deficiency disease, Wilson's disease, tyrosine-mia, glycogen storage disease, and sea blue histiocyte syndrome.

Primary liver malignancy which could not be treated by partial hepatic resec-tion once was thought to be an ideal indication for orthotopic liver transplanta-tion. However, previous experiences [7–12] indicated that malignant tumor recur-red in most cases if the malignancy was diagnosed before transplantation and was the major indication for transplantation. On the other hand, if the malignancy was an incidental finding, whether known in advance or found only after exami-nation of the removed specimen, or the malignancy is confined wholly to the liver, cure could be achieved by an orthotopic hepatic transplantation. Ten pediatric patients with primary hepatic malignancy (9 hepatomas and 1 hepato-blastoma) have received liver grafts. In three of them a malignant tumor was the main indication for transplantation but it was an incidental finding in the remain-ing seven. Of the seven patients with incidental malignancies, three were among 71 recipients with biliary atresia, two were patients with tyrosinemia, one a patient with alpha-1-antitrypsin deficiency disease and one patient with sea-blue histiocyte syndrome (Table 1).

Immunosuppressive therapy

The conventional method of immunosuppression, involving the combination of azathioprine and prednisone with or without antilymphocyte globulin [7–9,

13–15] or the substitution of cyclophosphamide [16] for azathioprine, has been reported extensively and in detail elsewhere.

Since March, 1980, combination immunosuppressive therapy with cyclosporine and low-dose prednisone has been used in all liver transplantations [12, 17, 18]. Cyclosporine is administered before liver grafting in an oral dose of 17.5 mg/kg or an intravenous dose of 5–6 mg/kg. Soon after the operation cyclosporine is given intravenously as a dose of 5–6 mg/kg/day in 2–3 divided doses. When the patient can resume oral intake, 17.5 mg/kg/day of cyclosporine in two divided doses is given and intravenous doses are gradually withdrawn, depending upon the renal function, graft function and blood level of cyclosporine. Maintenance doses of cyclosporine are adjusted mainly on the nephrotoxicity of the drug. Usually the

Table 1. Indications for transplantation in pediatric patients (<18 years).

	Pre-cyclosporine era (before 1980) number	Cyclosporine era (after 1980) number	Total number
Biliary atresia and hypoplasia	51	20	71
Inborn metabolic errors	13[a]	10[d]	23
Chronic aggressive hepatitis	13	3	16
Hepatoma	3[b]	0[e]	3
Neonatal hepatitis	2	1	3
Congenital hepatic fibrosis	2	0	2
Secondary biliary cirrhosis	2[c]	1[f]	3
Byler's disease	0	3[g]	3
Budd-Chiari syndrome	0	1	1
Cellular inflammatory pseudotumor	0	1	1
Total	86	40	126

[a] Inborn errors: Alpha-1-antitrypsin deficiency 9
    Wilson's disease 2
    Tyrosinemia 1
    Type IV glycogen storage disease 1
[b] Five other patients had incidental malignancies (4 hepatomas and 1 hepatoblastoma) in their excised liver. The principal diagnoses in these 5 cases were biliary atresia (3 examples), alpha-1-antitrypsin deficiency (1 example), and congenital tyrosinemia (1 example). The diagnosis of the neoplastic change was known in advance only in 2 of the 5 cases.
[c] Secondary to trauma or choledochal cyst (one each).
[d] Inborn errors: Alpha-1-antitrypsin deficiency 6
    Wilson's disease 1
    Tyrosinemia 1
    Type I glycogen storage disease 1
    Sea-blue histiocyte syndrome 1
[e] Two patients had incidental hepatomas: one with tyrosinemia, another with sea-blue histiocyte syndrome.
[f] Secondary to choledochal cyst.
[g] Diagnosis equivocal in one case.

dose is in the 12 mg/kg/day range at 1 month and 10 mg/kg/day at 6 months in pediatric recipients.Infants and younger children seem to tolerate the drug better than older children and adults.

Steroids are a necessary addition to cyclosporine to achieve adequate immunosuppression, but the doses used are much less than those required in combination with azathioprine. Soon after revascularization of the liver, graft recipients receive 250 or 500 mg of intravenous methylprednisolone succinate, with those recipients weighing more than 20–30 kg usually receiving the higher dose.

Postoperatively, the daily dose of methylprednisolone or prednisone is tapered by 20 mg daily, from 100 mg daily on the first day down to a maintenance dose of 10 mg on the sixth day. Further reduction of the steroid dose depends upon graft function. Usually the children are discharged with a maintenance dose of prednisone of 5 mg/day one to two months after transplantation. Initial and maintenance doses of steroids are reduced in infants and smaller children, and are increased in larger children.

If rejection occurs despite the above outlined immunosuppressive therapy, boluses of intravenous steroid therapy and/or a recycle of the original 5-day burst of prednisone therapy are given immediately. Although cyclosporine does not permit much dose maneuverability, it is often possible in infants and children to increase the dose with little risk of nephrotoxicity.

If severe nephrotoxicity was suspected, cyclosporine doses were reduced or the drug was substituted by azathioprine, often with rapid reversal of acute renal failure. The dose of cyclosporine was also reduced in the face of severe infectious complications.

Donor operation

The liver, heart and kidneys can be procured from a single donor without compromising the anatomy and function of any of the organs. The technique of multiple organ procurement and the early functions of each organ graft have been reported [19, 20]. The incidence of first week dialysis in patients receiving renal allografts procured in combination with livers and hearts or both is less than 15%. In addition satisfactory livers and hearts usually can be obtained unless there has been faulty donor selection.

The techniques of donor hepatectomy in children are essentially the same as those in adults [7, 19]. However, it is advisable in pediatric liver donors to obtain the celiac axis in continuity with the upper abdominal and thoracic aorta and use the latter for anastomosis with the recipients lower abdominal aorta if it is necessary. If the hepatic graft receives an additional blood supply from the superior mesenteric artery, both the celiac axis and the superior mesenteric artery can be obtained in continuity with the upper abdominal and thoracic aorta, particularly in an infant or small child donor [20].

Recipient operation

The techniques of orthotopic liver transplantation had been established more than 15 years ago [7] and several minor modifications have been reported [8, 21–24].

In children a bilateral subcostal incision or upper abdominal transverse incision using a previous incision almost always gives an adequate exposure. Recipient hepatectomy in children is usually easier than that in adults.

The most important area wherein pediatric hepatic transplants require particular attention to detail is in the performance of the vascular anastomosis. We employ a continuous suture using monofilament polypropylene for all vascular anastomoses. To avoid the purse stringing which can easily occur with this technique, care is taken to prevent undue traction upon the sutures. Nevertheless, a 'growth factor' technique, described elsewhere in detail [24] is left in all vascular suture lines, particularly the arterial and portal vein anastomoses. Every effort should be directed toward eliminating strictures in these suture lines so that turbulent flow and pressure gradients are minimized across the anastomoses.

The order of anastomoses can vary following completion of the suprahepatic vena cava connection. Most commonly the infrahepatic vena cava anastomosis is made next followed by the portal vein, followed by release of the flow through the latter, the lower and the upper vena cava channels. The arterial anastomosis is then completed while the liver is perfused by portal vein flow.

In the face of cardiodynamic instability caused by vena caval interruption, or if portal vein clamping appears to be causing undue damage to the intestine the portal vein anastomosis can be done following the upper vena cava and flow through the liver restored with the infrahepatic vena caval ends clamped. The latter can then be reconnected as the third anastomosis.

In addition, one may wish to complete the arterial anastomosis before the portal vein if portal vein flow appears to be inadequate, as may be the case, for example, in some biliary atresia patients with small, sclerotic native portal veins. Finally, all four vascular anastomoses often can be completed in less than 60–70 min and arterial and portal vein flow restored to the hepatic graft simultaneously.

Bile duct reconstruction methods in pediatric cases are similar to those in adults [7, 25, 26]. End-to-end choledochocholedochostomy with a T-tube stent is used whenever recipient anatomy and size permit. In-dwelling internal stents are often necessary for very small bile ducts. In cases of biliary atresia and other bile duct disorders a satisfactory native bile duct is not available and end-to-side anastomosis of graft common duct to a Roux-en-Y loop of jejunum is employed. These also are stented internally.

Cholecystojejunostomy or other methods which depend entirely upon drainage via the cystic duct are now avoided entirely because of the high incidence of obstruction of the cystic duct by sludge in transplanted livers which undergo even minor rejection episodes [25, 27]. Operative cholangiograms through either a T-tube or the graft cystic duct stump are performed to document duct anatomy, patency and competency.

Results

Causes of death

Fifty-three of the 86 pediatric liver recipients between 1963 and 1980 (pre-cyclosporine era) and 14 of the 40 between 1980 and 1982 (cyclosporine era) died within a year after transplantation. Detailed clinical-pathologic analyses of almost all of these deaths has been reported, using OT code numbers [7–9, 12, 28]. Although the causes of deaths in these patients were usually multiple, they were categorized to the best of our knowledge as shown in Table 2.

During the precyclosporine era bacterial, fungal and viral infections were the main cause of deaths within a year after transplantation (20 of 53 deaths), see also Chapter 11. There were 9 deaths from abdominal sepsis, 5 deaths from viral infection (adenovirus, chickenpox and herpes), 4 deaths from systemic bacterial and fungal sepsis and 2 deaths from pulmonary infection. Although infectious complications continue to be a major threat to life after transplantation none of the 14 deaths under cyclosporine therapy was categorized death from infection.

Significant numbers of deaths were caused by surgical technical complications of arterial, venous or biliary anastomoses. In the precyclosporine era there were

Table 2. Main causes of death within a year after liver transplantation among 86 children in precyclosporine era and 40 children in cyclosporine era.

	Pre-cyclosporine era (86 children)	Cyclosporine era (40 children)
Intra- & peri-operative death	3	1
Surgical technical complication	15	7
Unsatisfactory liver graft	3	1
Graft rejection	9	4
Infection	20	0
Recurrent malignancy	1	0
Other	2[a]	1[b]
Total	53	14

[a] One died from pulmonary emboli at 52 days and another from respiratory insufficiency due to an over-sized graft.
[b] One died from graft hypoxia due to marked pulmonary arteriovenous shunt.

15 deaths in this category. Eight of the 15 were failures in biliary duct reconstruction, 4 in hepatic artery anastomosis, 2 in portal venous anastomosis and 1 in suprahepatic inferior vena caval anastomosis. In the cyclosporine era surgical technical complications were the direct cause of death in 7 of the 14 children. There were three failures in hepatic artery anastomoses, and one each in both the hepatic artery and portal vein anastomosis, portal venous anastomosis, suprahepatic vena caval anastomosis, and biliary duct reconstruction.

Acute and chronic graft rejection were the third main cause of death in the precyclosporine era and the second in the cyclosporine era. Despite the better immunosuppression therapy and the improved survival with cyclosporine approximately 10% of the recipients died from graft rejection both in the precyclosporine era and in the cyclosporine era.

Survival

One-year survival
Actual survival of 86 pediatric liver recipients in the precyclosporine era and actuarial survival of 40 pediatric recipients in the cyclosporine era are shown in Figure 1. After the introduction of cyclosporine the 1-year survival after liver transplantation improved from 40% to 62%.

Age and survival
Because the majority of deaths within the first year occurred within three months after liver transplantation the three month survival of each age group is compared in Figure 2. In the precyclosporine era 28 of 53 (53%) infants and preschool children (less than 6 years old), 8 of 16 (50%) school age children (between 6 and

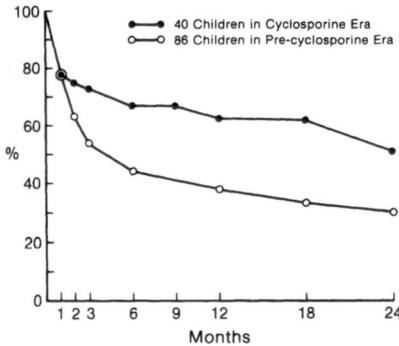

Figure 1. A comparison of survival after liver transplantation between 86 pediatric liver recipients under conventional immunosuppression therapy (azathioprine, prednisone and ALG) and 40 pediatric recipients under cyclosporine-prednisone therapy.

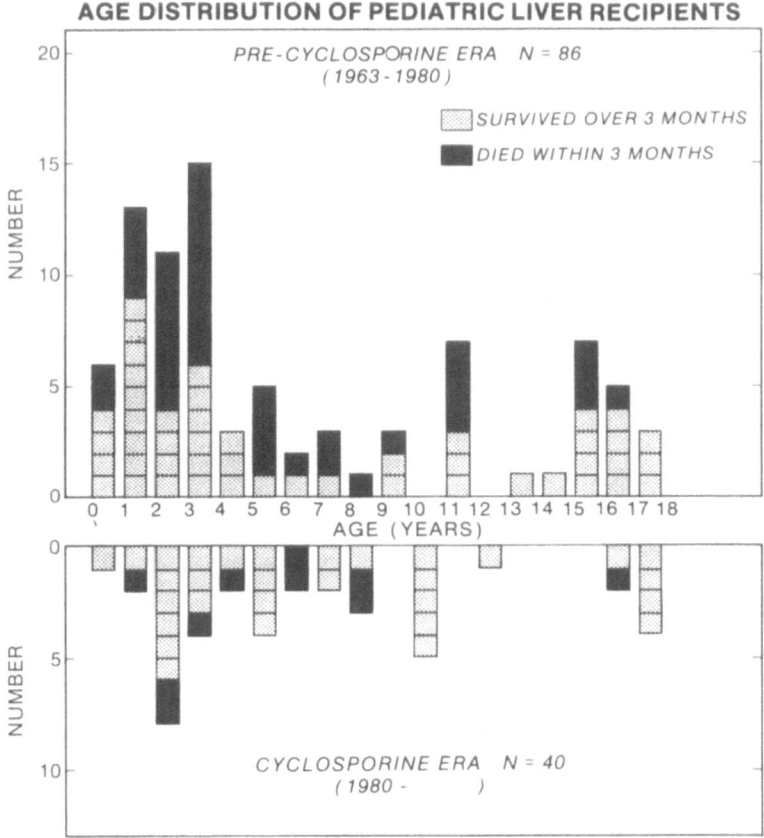

Figure 2. Age distribution of 126 pediatric liver recipients. A shaded square represents a child who survived more than 3 months, and a black square represents a child who died within 3 months.

12 years old), and 13 of 17 (76%) adolescents lived more than 3 months. In the cyclosporine era 16 of 21 (76%) infants and preschool children, 8 of 12 (67%) school children and 6 of 7 (86%) adolescents lived more than three months. Both in the precyclosporine era and in the cyclosporine era 3-month survival of infants and preschool children was statistically not different from those of school children. Three-month survival of the adolescents was slightly better than those of younger children in both eras.

It is worthwhile to note that 5 of 7 (71%) infants (less than a year old) lived more than three months. The technical difficulties in infant surgery have been fairly well overcome in liver transplantation as well. The age of children should not be a consideration in accepting them as candidates for liver transplantation. Our youngest recipients have been 3 and 6 months.

Liver disease and survival
The influence of original liver disease upon survival was analyzed in the two most common indications (biliary atresia and inborn metabolic errors) of pediatric liver transplantation, and shown in Figures 3 and 4. Both in the precyclosporine era and the cyclosporine era survival of children with inborn metabolic errors was significantly better than those of children with biliary atresia. The survival of children with biliary atresia was lower than overall survival in the precyclosporine era, but it was similar to the overall survival in the cyclosporine era. This improvement in survival of children with biliary atresia may well reflect the better surgical techniques, management and immunosuppression with cyclosporine.

Five-year survival
Seventy-five pediatric patients received liver transplantation more than 5 years ago (precyclosporine era). Sixteen of the 75 (21%) lived more than 5 years, and 15 are still alive between 5 and 14 years after transplantation as of April, 1983. All but two have normal liver function and attend school or work full time. Two patients with abnormal liver function lost their jobs recently.

Long-term survival data in the cyclosporine era is not available yet, but 13 children are alive and in good health between one and three years after transplantation.

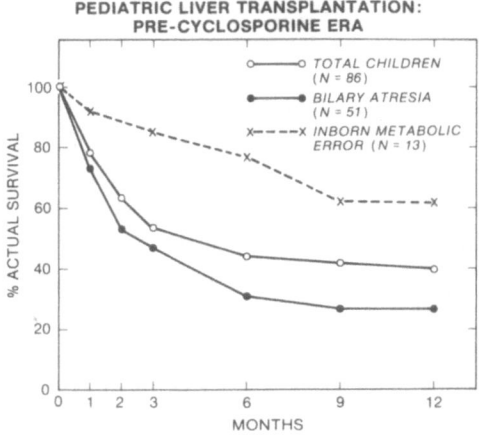

Figure 3. Influence of original liver disease upon one year survival under conventional immunosuppression therapy.

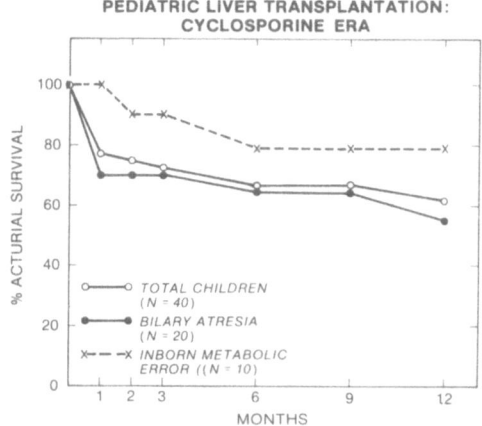

Figure 4. Influence of original liver disease upon one year survival under cyclosporine-steroid therapy.

Discussion

Since the introduction of cyclosporine, the results of organ transplantation such as kidney [5, 6, 29], liver [12, 17, 18], and heart [30], have improved significantly.

In combination with a low dose steroid, cyclosporine provides more effective and safer immunosuppression than conventional double or triple drug immunosuppression therapy (azathioprine and prednisone with or without antilymphocyte globulin). In pediatric liver transplantation the one year survival improved from 40% to 62% with cyclosporine and low dose steroid therapy. Infectious complications, which had been the most frequent direct cause of death after liver transplantation with conventional immunosuppression therapy, became less frequent and more treatable under this new immunosuppression therapy. Children can grow at a normal or better rate after transplantation and complications of high dose steroids such as Cushingoid feature and osteopathy have been virtually eliminated.

The opinion that infants and small children may not be good candidates for liver transplantation because of age and size has been proved incorrect. Survivals of infants and smaller children have been as good as larger children, and survivals of pediatric recipients have been better than those of adults both in the precyclosporine and the cyclosporine era.

The original liver disease has had some influence upon the outcome of transplantation. Children with liver-based inborn metabolic errors have done better than those with biliary atresia or hypoplasia. This is partly due to the fact that previous major surgeries such as Kasai operation (for biliary atresia) make the transplantation operation more difficult; anatomic anomalies have been an additional factor. However, in the cyclosporine era the results of liver transplantation for biliary atresia has raised to the level of overall survivals of pediatric cases, but it is still inferior to that after treatment of inborn metabolic errors.

Survival and quality of life after liver transplantation have improved significantly since the introduction of cyclosporine, and it has become a reliable method of therapy for otherwise untreatable liver diseases. As the experience in pediatric liver transplantation expands and deepens, further improvement of outcomes and better understanding of various liver disease can be expected.

Acknowledgements

This research was supported by grants from the Veterans Administration, National Institutes of Health, Bethesda, grant no. AM29961.

References

1. Borel JF, Feurer C, Gubler HU, Stahelin H: Biological effects of cyclosporin A; a new anti-lymphocytic agent. Agents Act 6:468–475, 1976.
2. Borel JF, Feurer C, Magnee C, Stahelin H: Effects of the new antilymphocytic peptide cyclosporin A in animals. Immunology 32:1017–1025, 1977.
3. Calne R, White DJG, Thiru S, Evans DB, McMaster P, Dunn DC: Cyclosporin A in patients receiving renal allografts from cadaver donors. Lancet 2:1323–1327, 1978.
4. Calne RY, Rolles K, White DJG, Thiru S, Evans DB, McMaster P, Dun DC, Craddock GN, Henderson RG, Aziz S, Lewis P: Cyclosporin A initially as the only immunosuppressant in 34 recipients of cadaveric organs; 32 kidneys, 2 pancreases, 2 livers. Lancet 2:1033–1036, 1979.
5. Starzl TE, Wel R III, Iwatsuki S, Klintmalm GBG, Schröter GP, Koep LJ, Iwaki Y, Teraskai PI, Porter KA: The use of cyclosporin A and prednisone in cadaveric kidney transplantation. Surg Gynecol Obset 151:17–26, 1980.
6. Starzl TE, Klintmalm GBG, Weil R III, Porter KA, Iwatsuki S, Schröter GP, Fernandez-Bueno C, MacHugh N: Cyclosporin A and steroid therapy in 66 cadaver kidney recipients. Surg Gynecol Obstet 153:486–494, 1981.
7. Starzl TE, (With the assistance of CW Putnam): Experience in hepatic transplantation. Philadelphia, WB Saunders, 1969.
8. Starzl TE, Porter KA, Putnam CW, Schröter GPJ, Halgrimson CG, Weil R III, Hoelscher M, Reid HAS: Orthotopic liver transplantation in 93 patients. Surg Gynecol Obstet 142:487–505, 1976.
9. Starzl TE, Koep LJ, Halgrimson CG, Hood J, Schröter GPJ, Porter KA, Weil R III: Fifteen years of clinical liver transplantation. Gastroenterology 77:375–388, 1979.
10. Iwatsuki S, Klintmalm GBG, Starzl TE: Total hepatectomy and liver replacement (Orthotopic liver transplantation) for primary hepatic malignancy. World J Surg 6:81–85, 1982.
11. Calne RY: Liver transplantation for liver cancer. World J Surg 6:76–80, 1982.
12. Starzl TE, Iwatsuki S, Van Thiel DH, Gartner JC, Zitelli BJ, Malatack JJ, Schade RR, Shaw BW Jr, Hakala TR, Rosenthal JT, Porter KA: Evolution of liver transplantation. Hepatology 2:614–636, 1982.
13. Starzl TE, Marchioro TL. Huntley RT, Rifkind D, Rowlands DT Jr, Dickinson TC, Waddell WR: Experimental and clinical homotransplantation of the liver. Ann NY Acad Sci 120:739–765, 1964.

14. Starzl TE, Marchioro TL, Faris TD, McCardle RJ, Iwasaki Y: Avenues of future research in homotransplantation of the liver: With particular reference to hepatic supportive procedures, antilymphocyte serum, and tissue typing. Am J Surg 112:391–400, 1966.

15. Starzl TE: Experience in renal transplantation. Philadelphia, WB Saunders, 1964.

16. Starzl TE, Putnam CW, Halgrimson CG, Schröter GP, Martineau G, Launois B, Corman JL, Penn I, Booth AS Jr, Porter KA, Groth CG: Cyclophosphamide and whole organ transplantation in humans. Surg Gynecol Obstet 133:981–999, 1971.

17. Starzl TE, Iwatsuki S, Klintmalm GBG, Schröter GPJ, Weil R III, Koep LJ, Porter KA: Liver transplantation, 1980, with particular reference to Cyclosporin A. Transplant Proc 13:281–285, 1981.

18. Starzl TE, Klintmalm GBG, Porter KA, Iwatsuki S, Schröter GP: Liver transplantation with use of Cyclosporin A and prednisone. N Engl J Med 305:266–269, 1981.

19. Shaw BW Jr, Hakala T, Rosenthal JT, Iwatsuki S, Broznick B, Starzl TE: Combination donor hepatectomy and nephrectomy and early functional results of allografts. Surg Gynecol Obstet 155:321–325, 1982.

20. Shaw BW Jr, Rosenthal JT, Griffith BF, Hardesty RL, Broznik B, Hakala T, Bahnson HT, Starzl TE: Techniques for combined procurement of hearts and kidneys with satisfactory early function of renal allografts. Surg Gynecol Obstet 157:261–264, 1983.

21. Shaw BW Jr, Iwatsuki S, Starzl TE: Alternative methods of hepatic graft arterialization. Surg Gynecol Obstet 159:491–493, 1984.

22. Starzl TE, Koep LJ, Weil R III, Halgrimson CG: Development of a suprahepatic recipient vena cava cuff for liver transplantation. Surg Gynecol Obstet 149:76–77, 1979.

23. Starzl TE, Groth CG, Brettschneider L: An everting technique for intraluminal vascular suturing. Surg Gynecol Obstet 127:125–126, 1979.

24. Starzl TE, Iwatsuki S, Shaw BW Jr: A 'Growth Factor' in fine vascular anastomoses. Surg Gynecol Obstet 159:164–166, 1984.

25. Starzl TE, Putnam CW, Hansbrough JF, Porter KA, Reid HAS: Biliary complications after liver transplantation; with special reference to the biliary cast syndrome and techniques of secondary duct repair. Surgery 81:212–221, 1976.

26. Iwatsuki S, Shaw BW Jr, Starzl TE: Biliary tract complications in liver transplantation under cyclosporine-steroid therapy. Transplant Proc 15:1288–1291, 1983.

27. Martineau G, Porter KA, Corman J, Launois B, Schröter G, Palmer W, Putnam CW, Groth CG, Halgrimson CG, Penn I, Starzl TE: Delayed biliary duct obstruction after orthotopic liver transplantation. Surgery 72:604–610, 1972.

28. Starzl TE, Koep LJ, Porter KA, Schröter GPJ, Weil R III, Hartley RB, Halgrimson CG: Decline in survival after liver transplantation. Arch Surg 115:815–819, 1980.

29. Starzl TE, Hakala TR, Rosenthal JT, Iwatsuki S, Shaw BW Jr: Variable convalescence and therapy after cadaveric renal transplantations under cyclosporin A and steroids. Surg Gynecol Obstet 154:819–825, 1982.

30. Shumway NE: Recent advances in cardiac transplantation. Transplant Proc 15:1221–1224, 1983.

21. Child and Turcotte's classification of hepatic functional reserve and its modifications by Campbell and by Pugh in predicting blood loss during liver transplantation

E.B. HAAGSMA, C.H. GIPS, H. WESENHAGEN, G.M.TH. DE JONG, G.W. VAN IMHOFF and R.A.F. KROM

Introduction

In orthotopic liver transplantation (OLT) the function of the diseased recipient liver to a great extent determines the effectiveness of hemostasis during the operation. Patients with seriously compromised function of the liver show an increased blood loss already early in the operation and we found in a prospective study that this was correlated with large blood loss in the last phase of the operation – although the donor liver was in situ – and also that it took longer in these patients to end the operation because of the defective hemostasis [1]. The strongest preoperative parameters indicating large blood loss were found to be those of the hepatorenal syndrome, followed by tests indicating defective protein synthesis in the liver. The stage of disease rather than the type was shown to influence blood loss during OLT.

The problems of defective hemostasis during operation and subsequent decreased survival in abdominal surgery for chronic liver disease have been well known for many years and it is not amazing that parameters have been looked for to assess the risk of major surgery in cirrhotic patients [2–6]. Child and Turcotte classified in 1964 three types of patients with chronic liver disease with regard to their aptness to survive porta-systemic shunt surgery [4]. Serum bilirubin and serum-albumin, ascites, neurological disorder and nutritional state were the elements they used in composing their class A, B and C patients, where A had minimal disturbance of hepatic functional reserve and C advanced. The class C patients had an about 50% mortality following shunt surgery, a figure that has not improved with time [7].

It proved difficult for subsequent investigators to place every patient in one of the Child classes, as a patient has to meet all the elements of that particular class [8]. Campbell et al. [5], using the Child and Turcotte elements, designed a scoring system. For all patients a total score is calculated and a classification A, B or C is made on predefined total score ranges per class. Another scoring system, using other total score ranges per class, is that of Pugh et al. [6]. They eliminated nutrition and included prothrombin time in their investigations on patients who were to undergo transection of the oesophagus for variceal bleeding and made some other, minor, changes. As every patient necessarily fits in such scoring systems they are essentially different from Child and Turcotte's. Crucial for every scoring system is the scientific basis of the definition of the boundaries of the total score of the classes.

As part of the prospective investigation mentioned above, we have been able to include the elements of the Child-Turcotte classification and the two scoring systems. We have related the classes and the elements from which their classifications are made up to blood loss in the first and last phase of OLT and we have compared the results with our own findings.

Methods and patients

Child and Turcotte's classification of hepatic functional reserve and the modifications of Campbell et al. and of Pugh et al. (Table 1)

Child and Turcotte's classification is presented in Table 1. To be graded, the patient has to conform to all elements of a class. In Campbell *et al.*'s modification

Table 1. Child and Turcotte's 'clinical and laboratory classification of patients with cirrhosis in terms of hepatic functional reserve' and modifications by Campbell *et al.* (scoring using the classification as such) and Pugh *et al.* (scoring using an altered classification). Child and Turcotte stated that serum bilirubin was 'equivocal in biliary cirrhosis'. PTT: prothrombin time; Pbc: primary biliary cirrhosis.

	minimal A	moderate B	advanced C	Campbell A 5–8	B 9–11	C 12–15	Pugh A 5–6	B 7–9	C 10–15
bilirubin, μmol/l	<34	34–51	>51	1	2	3	1	2	3
albumin, g/l	>35	30–35	<30	1	2	3	1		
ascites	–	easily controlled	poorly controlled	1	2	3	1	2	3
neurological disorder	–	minimal	advanced, coma	1	2	3	1	2	3
nutrition	excellent	good	poor, wasting	1	2	3			
Pugh's alterations									
bilirubin (in pbc)	17–68	68–171	>171		(in pbc:	1	2	3)	
albumin		28–35	<28					2	3
PTT, + sec.	1–4	4–6	>6				1	2	3

the elements of class A get 1, of class B 2 and of class C 3 points each. Grade A scores 5–8 points and this implies that of the five elements two only need be A (three then will be B) and also that $3A + 1B + 1C$ still are graded A. Grade B scores 9–11 points and this makes combinations like $2A + 2B + 1C, 1A + 2B + 2C$ or $3A + 2C$ possible. For grade C (12–15 points) at least $2C$ elements are needed. Combinations that conform to this grade are for example $3B + 2C$ and $1A + 1B + 3C$. Using this scoring system Child-Turcotte class A would obtain 5, B 10 and C 15 points.

Pugh *et al.* also score 1, 2 and 3 points for increasing abnormality. They have excluded nutritional state and included prothrombin time, there still being five elements per class. Serum albumin is graded differently from Child in classes B and C and a correction is made for bilirubin in primary biliary cirrhosis patients. Ascites, 'easily' or 'poorly controlled' (Child's B and C) is 'slight' or 'moderate' in Pugh's 2 and 3 grading, while Child's neurological disorder, 'minimal' in B and 'advanced, coma' in C, has its equivalent in Pugh's scoring, where encephalopathy grades 1 and 2 according to Trey *et al.* [9] get 2 points and encephalopathy grades 3 and 4 three points. Pugh's class A scores 5–6 points, i.e. one B element can be included. Class B (7–9 points) includes $3A + 2B$ or $3A + 2C$. Class C scores 10–15 points and thus the 5 B's together score C.

Our definition of the clinical elements used in the classifications

Because a strict definition for the clinical elements in the classifications is lacking, we mention our definition of these elements:

Ascites: Presence of ascites means that it is manifest on clinical examination. Many patients show some ascites under laparoscopy but these were not classified as such. Easily controlled (slight) ascites, class B, disappears on absolute bedrest and sodium and water restriction and does not recur on mobilization when at most a thiazide diuretic (hydrochlorothiazide 50 mg daily) is added. Poorly controlled (moderate) ascites, class C, does or does not disappear or recurs already during bedrest, water- and extreme (17 mmol daily) sodium restriction, diuretics and if needed paracenthesis. Upon mobilization recurrence can be avoided or not, often a combination of diuretics and sometimes a LeVeen shunt is needed.

Neurological disorder: No clinical encephalopathy in class A. In class B episodes of encephalopathy elicited by gastrointestinal bleeding or other events, no treatment needed outside these episodes. Class C: chronic porta-systemic encephalopathy, needing continuous treatment.

Nutritional state: In class A no weight loss, no muscle wasting, 'excellent' condition. Class B, 'good': some weight loss, some muscle atrophy on examination. Class C, 'poor, wasting': considerable weight loss, easily visible wasting.

Patients, clinical and laboratory data

These are described in full in our earlier report [1]. The investigation comprised 25 adult consecutive OLT patients, 19 women and 6 men, median age 47 (17–58) years. Thirteen had chronic active or inactive cirrhosis (cac/ic), 10 primary biliary cirrhosis (pbc), 1 hepatocellular carcinoma without cirrhosis and 1 Budd Chiari's syndrome. None had evidence of preexistent renal disease, none had used cyclosporin A. Of the 25, 14 were alive 1 year after OLT.

Twelve patients had a history of ascites, all these were salt and fluid restricted and 11 were on diuretics. The ascites was grade B in 5 and C in 7 patients. Porta-systemic encephalopathy was B in 2 and C in 3 patients. Nutritional state was A in 6, B in 9 and C in 10 patients. Urinary sodium and creatinine clearance (ml/min/1.73 m^2) were determined in the pretransplant assessment period and blood tests were done at donor organ announcement, about six hours before the operation. Urinary sodium was determined in 22 patients during a 3–5-day test period, without diuretics, on a fixed fluid and sodium intake. The laboratory methods are found in our earlier report.

Blood loss was measured in the three phases of the operation in 23 patients and for the whole operation in 25. In phase 1 the diseased liver is dissected, phase 2 is the anhepatic phase and phase 3 starts when the portal and caval circulations have been restored. Blood loss was considered to be 'medical' when it could be related to hemostasis problems and 'surgical' when surgical events were primarily responsible. Five of the deaths, 3 under and 2 after the operation, 15 and 36 days, were due to complications of major 'medical' blood loss and one, 43 days after the operation, to complications of major 'surgical' blood loss. Hemostasis problems arising from the degree of liver disease would be expected to emerge in phase 1, while in phase 3 hemostasis ultimately depends on the viability of the donor liver. The amount of blood transfused was used to express blood loss. The median blood losses in the phases 1, 2, 3 and in the total operation were 1.5, 2.2, 3.2 and 9.2 l respectively and the median durations 2$^1/_4$, 1$^1/_4$. 2$^1/_2$ and 6 h. Total blood loss was under 6 l in 11 patients, 6–10 l in 4 and over 10 l in 10.

The one patient with major 'surgical' blood loss had losses of 1.5 l and 2.8 l in phases 1 and 3 respectively. In phase 2 the loss was 8.5 l due to rupture of the spleen, which made total blood loss 12.7 l. For the purpose of this work total blood loss in this patient was graded to be in the 6–10 l group, as medical blood loss was moderate.

Our classification in 'better' and 'worse' patients

In our previous study we have demonstrated a correlation between blood loss and several preoperative parameters. Table 2 shows them for the five patients with the lowest and the highest blood loss. Considering the most significant para-

Table 2. Preoperative parameters associated with 'medical' blood loss during OLT in the five patients with lowest and highest blood loss respectively (medians and ranges) and grading according to Campbell's and Pugh's modifications of Child and Turcotte's classification. APTT: activated partial thromboplastin time.

Blood loss	lowest	highest
n	5	5
liver disease	cac/ic 1, pbc 3, hcc 1	cac/ic 4, pbc 1
blood transfused, 1	3.0 (1.6–3.2)	39.0 (34.0–47.2)
ascites, past or present, no. of patients	0	5
serum Na (137–145 mmol/l)	140(137–146)	134(130–139)
24 h urinary Na, mmol	111 (81–166)	5(0–10)
creatinine clearance (90–130 ml/min/1.73 m²)	102 (76–117)	78 (64–85)
albumin (37–47 g/l)	41 (26–43)	35 (21–37)
cholinesterase (1600–4400 U/l)	2400 (1300–3600)	1113 (820–1452)
antithrombin III, (80–120%)	134 (66–177)	50 (22–67)
prothrombin time ($-1- +1$ s)	+0.2 (−0.8– +2.1)	+2.4 (+2.0– +4.6)
APTT ($-5- +5$ s)	+0.5 (−12– +9)	+9 (+7– +16)
platelets (150–300 · 10⁹/1)	217 (36–362)	40 (27–135)
gastrointestinal varices, no. of patients	1	5

	A	B	C	A	B	C
Campbell, no. of pts.	4	1	0	2	0	3
Pugh, no. of pts.	3	2	0	0	2	3

meters the following values were found to discriminate for a total blood loss of more or less than 10 liters: urinary sodium 10 mmol/24 h, negative/positive history of ascites, creatinine clearance 90 ml/min/1.73 m², serum Na 135 mmol/l, antithrombin 3 (AT 3) 60% and cholinesterase 1250 U/l.

Using these results we can classify our patients as 'better' or 'worse' patients with regard to peroperative hemostasis. In this investigation we will study besides the Child-Turcotte, Campbell and Pugh classifications the value of our classification in the prediction of blood loss in phase 1 and 3 of the operation.

Statistical analysis

Wilcoxon's two sample test and the sign test were used. A difference was regarded to be significant with a p-value ≤0.05, while 0.1 ≥p >0.05 was designated as a trend and shown in brackets. Where not stated medians and ranges were used to indicate group results.

Results

Child-Turcotte classification

Four patients out of 25 could be classified. Three fell into class A, 1 in C. The results using the separate elements are mentioned under Campbell's and Pugh's classifications.

Campbell's and Pugh's classifications (Tables 3 and 4)

In the classifications of Campbell and Pugh blood loss did not differ between classes A and B. With Campbell's classification blood loss was higher in group C than in B, B + A and A in phases 1, 3 and total operation. Blood loss was not different in A from B + C in phases 1 and 3, while total blood loss was lower. In Pugh's classification blood loss was higher in C than in B + A in phases 1, 3 and total operation and than in A in phase 3 and total operation. There were trends for higher blood loss in C than A in phase 1 and than B in phase 3 and total operation.

The elements of the Child-Turcotte (Campbell) and the Pugh classification (Tables 3 and 4)

Blood loss did not differ in the bilirubin classes A, B and C in phases 1, 3 or total operation in the two classifications. In albumin class C blood loss was in phase 1 higher than in B + A, B or A (trend only in Campbell's classification) and for total blood loss there were trends between C and A and (Pugh only) C and B + A. Between classes A and B or B + C there were no differences. Severity of ascites was in phase 3 highly significant correlated with higher blood loss in C or C + B than B, B + A or A; in the total operation blood loss was higher in C and C + B than in B + A or A. In phase 3 and total operation there was a trend between blood loss in B and A. In phase 1 blood loss was higher in C or C + B than in B + A or A.

Neurological disorder was associated only with a trend towards higher blood loss in class B than in class A in phases 1 and 3. Nutritional state class A had a lower blood loss in phase 1 than B + C or C and there was a trend towards lower blood loss in A + B than in C. In phase 3 there was a trend towards lower blood loss in A than in B + C. Total blood loss was lower in A than in B, B + C and (trend) C.

Table 3. Blood loss during OLT in the Child-Turcotte-Campbell and Child-Turcotte-Pugh classes and separate components. Bilirubin and neurological disorder are not included in the Table (see Table 5). Phases 1 and 3: n = 23, total operation n = 25.

Classes Blood loss, 1 No. of patients	A n	median, range	B n	median, range	C n	median, range
Campbell, over all						
phase 1	12	1.2 (0.1–6.0)	5	0.7 (0.3–1.0)	6	3.3 (2.2–7.2)
phase 3	12	2.6 (0.6–28.0)	5	1.5 (0.1–6.1)	6	14.8 (5.8–39.7)
total operation	13	5.8 (1.6–39.0)	5	4.3 (3.0–11.6)	7	32.0 (9.5–47.2)
Pugh, over all						
phase 1	9	1.0 (0.1–2.8)	7	0.8 (0.1–6.0)	7	3.0 (0.7–7.2)
phase 3	9	2.4 (0.6–5.1)	7	1.5 (0.1–28.0)	7	12.4 (5.8–39.7)
total operation	10	5.7 (2.8–10)	7	4.3 (1.6–39.0)	8	28.0 (9.5–47.2)
Campbell, albumin						
phase 1	10	1.2 (0.1–6.0)	6	0.7 (0.1–5.0)	7	3.0 (0.8–7.2)
phase 3	10	2.6 (0.6–28.0)	6	3.8 (1.1–39.7)	7	11.0 (0.1–17.9)
total operation	10	5.7 (2.8–39.0)	7	10.0 (1.6–47.2)	8	20.6 (3.0–40.5)
Pugh, albumin (class A identical to Campbell)						
phase 1	10	1.2 (0.1–6.0)	8	0.9 (0.1–5.0)	5	3.5 (0.8–7.2)
phase 3	10	2.6 (0.6–28.0)	8	4.4 (1.1–39.7)	5	12.4 (0.1–17.9)
total operation	10	5.7 (2.8–39.0)	9	9.5 (1.6–47.2)	6	28.0 (3.0–40.5)
Campbell/Pugh, severity of ascites						
phase 1	12	0.9 (0.1–2.8)	4	1.4 (0.3–5.0)	7	3.5 (0.7–7.2)
phase 3	12	2.0 (0.1–5.1)	4	5.1 (1.5–14.3)	7	17.1 (6.1–39.7)
total operation	13	4.5 (1.6–10.0¹)	5	9.5 (4.3–40.5)	7	32.0 (11.6–47.2)
Campbell, nutritional state						
phase 1	6	0.3 (0.1–2.8)	7	1.0 (0.3–6.0)	10	2.4 (0.6–7.2)
phase 3	6	2.2 (0.6–5.1)	7	3.2 (1.5–28.0)	10	8.4 (0.1–39.7)
total operation	6	3.9 (1.6–9.2)	9	10.0 (4.3–40.5)	10	15.0 (2.8–47.2)
Pugh, prothrombin time						
phase 1	22	1.2 (0.1–7.2)	1	3.0	0	
phase 3	22	3.1 (0.1–39.7)	1	12.4	0	
total operation	23	6.4 (1.6–47.2)	2	28,9 (17.2–40.5)	0	

Blood loss in 'better' and 'worse' patients (Table 5)

There was a highly significant larger blood loss in phase 3 and total operation for urinary sodium ≤10 mmol/day and presence of ascites, followed by AT 3 ≤60% in the phases 1, 3 and total operation, serum sodium ≤135 mmol/l and creatinine clearance ≤90 ml/min/1.73 m² in total operation, urinary sodium ≤10 mmol/day in phase 1, serum sodium ≤135 mmol/l in phase 3 and cholinesterase in phase 3. Differences were also present in all other instances. Blood loss was not higher

Table 4. Differences in blood loss (p-values) between the Child-Turcotte-Campbell and the Child-Turcotte-Pugh classes, with analysis of separate components. Blood loss did not correlate with bilirubin in either classification and with neurological disorder A vs B p = 0.1 and 0.08 in phases 1 and 3 only. Prothrombin time was A (Pugh) in 23 patients and B in 2 (n = 25). N.s.: not significant. Trends in brackets.

Classes	A vs B	B vs C	A vs C	A + B vs C	A vs B + C
Campbell, over all					
phase 1	n.s.	0.008	0.05	0.005	n.s.
phase 3	n.s.	0.01	0.02	0.004	n.s.
total operation	n.s.	0.009	0.009	0.003	0.05
Pugh, over all					
phase 1	n.s.	n.s.	(0.1)	0.01	(0.1)
phase 3	n.s.	(0.07)	0.001	0.003	(0.09)
total operation	n.s	(0.07)	0.001	0.002	(0.07)
Campbell, albumin					
phase 1	n.s.	0.05	(0.06)	0.03	n.s.
phase 3	n.s.	n.s	n.s.	n.s.	n.s.
total operation	n.s.	n.s.	(0.1)	n.s.	n.s.
Pugh, albumin (A vs B + C identical to Campbell)					
phase 1	n.s.	0.05	0.04	0.02	n.s
phase 3	n.s.	n.s.	n.s.	n.s.	n.s.
total operation	n.s.	n.s.	(0.07)	(0.09)	n.s.
Campbell/Pugh, severity of ascites					
phase 1	n.s.	n.s.	0.005	0.006	0.02
phase 3	(0.1)	0.05	0.0005	0.0005	0.0007
total operation	(0.08)	n.s.	0.0005	0.002	0.0005
Campbell, nutritional state					
phase 1	n.s.	n.s.	0.03	(0.1)	0.04
phase 3	n.s.	n.s.	n.s.	n.s.	(0.1)
total operation	0.02	n.s.	(0.07)	n.s.	0.02

than 2.8 l in phase 1 when urinary sodium was over 10 mmol/day or when the history of ascites was negative or the creatinine clearance over 90 ml/min/1.73 m². During phase 3 these maximal losses were 5.8, 5.1 and 6.1 l respectively and for the total operation they were 10, 10 and 11.6 l.

Blood loss in patients with preoperative antithrombin 3 levels between 40 and 70% (Table 6)

The five patients with AT three levels between 40 and 70% who had an urinary sodium over 10 mmol/day had a total blood loss ranging from 1.6 to 10 l. All five belonged to the 'better' ascites and serum sodium classes and 4 and 3 respectively to the 'better' creatinine clearance and cholinesterase classes. The four patients with an AT 3 level between 40 and 70% who had an urinary sodium ≤10 mmol/

Table 5. Blood loss during OLT in 'better' and 'worse' patients. Creatinine clearance: ml/min/1.73 m^2.

liver function blood loss, 1 no. of patients	n	better median, range	n	worse median, range	difference, p
urinary Na, mmol/24 h		>10		≤10	
phase 1	14	0.9 (0.1–2.8)	7	3.5 (0.7–7.2)	0.004
phase 3	14	2.2 (0.1–5.8)	7	17.1 (6.1–39.7)	0.0005
total operation	15	4.7 (1.6–10.0)	7	32.0 (11.7–47.2)	0.0003
history of ascites		negative		positive	
phase 1	12	0.9 (0.1–2.8)	11	3.0 (0.3–7.2)	0.02
phase 3	12	2.0 (0.1–5.1)	11	12.4 (1.5–39.7)	0.0007
total operation	13	4.5 (1.6–10.0)	12	28.0 (4.3–47.2)	0.0007
creatinine clearance		>90		≤90	
phase 1	12	0.9 (0.1–2.8)	10	3.3 (0.3–7.2)	0.02
phase 3	12	2.2 (0.1–6.1)	10	13.4 (1.5–39.7)	0.01
total operation	12	4.6 (1.6–11.6)	11	24.0 (2.8–47.2)	0.004
serum Na, mmol/l		>135		≤135	
phase 1	14	0.9 (0.1–5.0)	9	3.0 (0.3–7.2)	0.03
phase 3	14	2.2 (0.1–14.3)	9	12.4 (1.5–39.7)	0.005
total operation	15	4.7 (1.6–34.3)	10	28.0 (4.3–47.2)	0.003
antithrombin 3, %		>60		≤60	
phase 1	13	0.6 (0.1–3.5)	10	2.7 (0.7–7.2)	0.003
phase 3	13	2.0 (0.1–17.9)	10	11.7 (2.4–39.7)	0.003
total operation	14	5.0 (1.6–34.0)	11	24.0 (4.5–47.2)	0.003
cholinesterase, U/l		>1250		≤1250	
phase 1	14	0.9 (0.1–3.5)	9	3.0 (0.3–7.2)	0.03
phase 3	14	2.0 (0.1–39.7)	9	11.0 (2.9–28.0)	0.007
total operation	14	4.4 (1.6–47.2)	10	14.4 (4.7–39.0)	0.02

day had total blood losses ranging from 11.6 to 47.2 l. All four were of the 'worse' category as to ascites and serum sodium and all but one as to creatinine clearance and cholinesterase.

Grading of total blood loss during OLT and preoperative classification (Table 7), sign test

C patients in Campbell's and Pugh's classifications had more chance of blood loss over 6 l (p<0.02) and A + B patients more chance of a blood loss of 10 l or less (Campbell p = 0.05, Pugh p = 0.01). Blood loss in patients with poorly controlled ascites (class C) was over 10 l (p<0.02) and in patients without ascites (A) 10 l or less (p<0.01). Blood loss in easily controlled ascites (B) was variable. Patients with urinary sodium ≤10 mmol/24 h all had a blood loss over 10 l, and all with a larger sodium excretion had a smaller blood loss (p<0.02).

Table 6. Total blood loss during OLT in the patients with preoperative antithrombin 3 levels between 40 and 70%, related to the other most important preoperative parameters (Table 7). Ascites was in all four patients poorly controlled (class C).

AT 3, 80–120%	history of ascites	creat. cl. 90–130 ml/ min/173 m^2	serum Na, 137–145 mmol/l	CHE 1600– 4400 U/l	Total blood loss, l
Urinary Na >10 mmol/24 h					
46	–	115	140	1476	9.2
47	–	148	136	970	4.7
51	–	121	141	1384	4.5
66	–	117	146	1300	1.6
70	–	58	137	420	10.0
Urinary Na ≤10 mmol/24 h					
46	+	104	127	1099	11.6
50	+	73	134	820	39.0
60	+	64	135	1452	47.2
67	+	85	130	1150	34.0

Table 7. Grading of total blood loss during OLT and preoperative indexing of patients with the two variants of Child and Turcotte's classification, with ascites classes alone and using the urinary sodium element of the better/worse classification. Percentages of patients in the different classes. N = 25, for urinary sodium 22.

n	Total blood loss, l	Campbell			Pugh			Ascites			Urinary sodium	
		A	B	C	A	B	C	A	B	C	B	W
11	<6	7	4	0	6	5	0	9	2	0	11	0
5	6–10	4	0	1	4	0	1	4	1	0	5	0
9	>10	2	1	6	0	2	7	0	2	7	0	7
% of total		50	20	30	40	30	30	50	20	30	70	30

Discussion

We were unable to grade more than 15% of the patients when using the Child-Turcotte classification. By definition, the two modifications allowed all the patients to be graded and here problems became visible already after classifying the patients with minimal and maximal blood loss: they were not clear-cut A's or C's. In the patients with maximal defective hemostasis during OLT there were A's (Campbell) and B's (Pugh).

That bilirubin classes were of no value in the definition of blood loss during OLT can easily be understood. Cholestasis per se is not associated with a serious increase in surgical mortality [10, 11]. Serum bilirubin can be predictive as to survival in particular diseases, such as primary biliary cirrhosis or acute alcoholic hepatitis, but then serves as a marker of disasters to come, which may be life threatening but need not in the first place be related to liver function as such. Also Linton found bilirubin less important [2]. Serum albumin classes showed blood loss differences in phase 1 of the operation only. Although albumin is synthesized exclusively in the liver, serum albumin is influenced by several variables and therefore is not so strong an indicator of hepatic synthesis function [8]. We found antithrombin 3 and cholinesterase more useful [1]. Ascites separated both A from B + C and C from A + B, in phases 1 and 3, but most strongly in phase 3, which by and large is responsible for high blood loss during OLT. There were no differences in the porta-systemic encephalopathy classes. Campbell *et al.* made blood ammonia classes and did not find these relevant either [5]. It might be that differences would come out when using refined tests including subclinical porta-systemic encephalopathy. Nutritional state classes appear to be important, as blood loss in class A has narrow ranges in both phases 1 and 3. Unlike what was found for the overall classifications and for albumin where the separation was between C and A + B but in accordance with ascites nutritional state separated A from B + C.

An excellent nutritional state is associated with moderate blood loss during OLT. More or less outspoken defects in nutritional state may or may not be associated with increased blood loss depending on the pathogenesis (under or malnutrition, malabsorption biliary steatorrhoea, decreased ability to synthesize proteins and fat or combinations). Apart from more or less expressing functional hepatic reserve, nutritional state is one of the components telling us something about the condition of the patient. Severe muscle wasting may imply longer postoperative artificial respiration because the intercostal muscles are not able to do their work properly and the preoperatively bedridden patient may not be able to come out of bed shortly after the operation because of over all lack of muscle. A more sophisticated definition of nutritional state could prove to be useful in further defining B and C patients especially with regard to the postoperative state.

Prothrombin time classes perhaps have been defined too arbitrarily by Pugh *et al.* We earlier [1] found the division line for severely defective hemostasis to be at a prolongation of 2 s and we did not find prothrombin time a strong indicator or peroperative hemostasis problems.

The better/worse parameters were derived from our calculation of chances of total blood loss to be over 10 l or less than 10 l [1]. We now have done the reverse and we also have applied them to phases 1 and 3 of the operation. The differences were significant for all the parameters used in both phases 1 and 3 and total operation. The best separation between less and more blood loss was found with urinary sodium in phase 3 and total operation and in fact, others [12, 13] have found this parameter to correlate most closely with survival without operation, when compared with routine parameters in liver disease. An urinary sodium

>10 mmol/24 h, a negative history of ascites and a creatinine clearance >90 ml/min/1.73 m² were all associated with moderate blood loss with well defined ranges. Although the differences between the groups were (highly) significant, the separation of moderate and high blood loss was less good with serum Na, antithrombin 3 and cholinesterase. After urinary sodium and ascites the strongest significance was with antithrombin 3. In the abnormal 40–70% range there was an overlap of patients with or without urinary sodium of 10 mmol/24 h or less – and for the same patients – with or without ascites. Urinary sodium rather than antithrombin 3 determined whether blood loss was high or not. It should be noted that there were no ascites class B patients in this group.

When we compared the Campbell classification, the Pugh classification the element ascites and the parameter urinary sodium, we found that about 30% of the patients were C or 'worse' in any of the classifications, with blood loss of 6 l or more; 'ascites' and 'urinary sodium' predicted a blood loss over 10 l. Absence of ascites and Pugh's A were best able to predict a blood loss less than 10 l, leaving this uncertain for ascites class B and over all Pugh class B. Urinary sodium >10 mmol/24 h was the sharpest predictor of low or moderate blood loss.

The problem with the two scoring systems presumably is with the scientific basis of the definition of the total scores. Campbell et al. state it's absence by mentioning that they arbitrarily defined the total scores for classes A, B and C. With Pugh's classification an other difficulty is with the prothrombin time as outlined above. A further aspect concerns the relative importance of the separate items. Linton is the only author known to us who has dealt with this subject [2]. The relative importance of the hepatorenal syndrome is high because it in chronic liver disease always implies end stage and problems ahead.

It has to be stated that we define hepatorenal syndrome as a disturbance in renal function in the presence of liver disease and in the absence of other diseases. This disturbance of renal function consists of a decreased sodium- and water clearance which is sooner or later combined with a decreased glomerular filtration rate.

Measurement of urinary sodium is discriminating because under the test conditions only right sided cardiac failure [14], toxemia of pregnancy and salt depletion will give the low sodium values, possibly through the same mechanisms, while primary renal disease will have other characteristics.

Conclusion

When we assume that the originators have laid most weight on class C and class A and that in their mind ascites, poorly controlled, was of paramount importance in class C and excellent nutrition in class A with the other parameters relatively less important, then the Child-Turcotte classification is better than any modification.

Nutritional state should be included as item to be charted in the general routine for potential OLT candidates after some form of standardization has been made.

Patients with an excellent nutritional state and/or absence of a history of ascites, an urinary sodium >10 mmol/l under test conditions, a creatinine clearance >90 ml/min/1.73 m² (preexistent renal disease excluded) will have the best chances of low or moderate blood loss during OLT. Those with poorly controlled ascites will have great chances of high blood loss as will all patients with an urinary sodium of 10 mmol/24 h or less. The presence of ascites, anyway class C, overrules an otherwise acceptable antithrombin 3.

Addendum

While this manuscript was made ready to go to press, an analysis of the Child-Turcotte criteria in patients with medically treated cirrhosis was published [15]. Survival decreased significantly with increasing degree of abnormality (A → B → C) of albumin, ascites, bilirubin and nutritional state. The criteria were found to be inferior to a prognostic index based on multivariate analysis of prognostic factors.

References

1. Haagsma EB, Gips CH, Wesenhagen H, van Imhoff GW, Krom RAF: Liver disease and its effect on hemostasis during liver transplantation. Liver, 1985, in press.
2. Linton RR: The selection of patients for portacaval shunts. Ann Surg 134:433–443, 1951.
3. Wantz GE, Payne MA: Experience with portacaval shunt for portal hypertension. N Eng J Med 265:721–728, 1961.
4. Child CG, Turcotte JG: Surgery and portal hypertension. In: Child CG (ed.). The liver and portal hypertension. Philadelphia, WB Saunders, p 50, 1964.
5. Campbell DP, Parker DE, Anagnostopoulos CE: Survival prediction in portacaval shunts: a computerized statistical analysis. Am J Surg 126:748–751, 1973.
6. Pugh RNH, Murray-Lyon IM, Dawson JL, Pietroni MC, Williams R: Transection of the oesophagus for bleeding oesophageal varices. Brit J Surg 60:646–649, 1973.
7. Turcotte JG, Lambert MJ: Variceal hemorrhage, hepatic cirrhosis and portacaval shunts. Surgery 73:810–817, 1973.
8. Conn HO: A peek at the Child-Turcotte classification. Hepatology 1:673–676, 1981.
9. Trey C, Burns DG, Saunders SJ: Treatment of hepatic coma by exchange blood transfusions. N Eng J Med 274:473–481, 1966.
10. Harville DD, Summerskill WHJ: Surgery in acute hepatitis. JAMA 184:257–261, 1963.
11. Hatfield ARW, Tobias R, Terblanche J et al.: Preoperative external biliary drainage in obstructive jaundice. Lancet ii:896–899, 1982.
12. Arroyo V, Rodés J: A rational approach to the treatment of ascites. Postgrad Med J 51:558–562, 1975.
13. Arroyo V, Bosch J, Gaya-Beltrán J et al.: Plasma renin activity and urinary sodium excretion as prognostic indicators in nonazotemic cirrhosis with ascites. Ann Intern Med 94:198–201, 1981.
14. Hollander W, Judson WE: The relationship of cardiovascular and renal hemodynamic function to sodium excretion in patients with severe heart disease but without edema. J Clin Invest 35:970–979, 1956.
15. Christensen E, Schlichting P, Fauerholdt F, Gluud C, Andersen PK, Juhl E et al.: Prognostic value of Child-Turcotte criteria in medically treated cirrhosis. Hepatology 4:430–435, 1984.

22. Hepatic transplantation in a child using a reduced-sized orthotopic liver graft

H. BISMUTH and D. HOUSSIN

Introduction

In some cases, transplantation of the liver is difficult to achieve due to the large size of the graft. This is particularly the case for heterotopic liver transplantation when there is not enough room in the abdomen for a normal sized liver graft or for orthotopic liver transplantation in children when the liver graft comes from an older donor.

In these conditions, the volume of the graft makes abdominal closure difficult [6] and may lead to early death [11]. To avoid these difficulties, the use of liver grafts from child donors has been widely adopted by Starzl *et al.* for orthotopic liver transplantation in children [10]. However, in most countries, it appears that obtainment of liver grafts from child donors is exceedingly rare. For these reasons, we adopted, in these last years, the principle of a reduced-sized adult liver graft anytime when there was no sufficient room in the abdominal cavity to place the graft either orthotopically or heterotopically. We report here the case of an orthotopic transplantation of a reduced-sized adult liver in a 10-year-old child with Byler's disease.

Case report

In September 1981, a 10-year-old male child with Byler's disease was admitted to our department for liver transplantation. Physical examination revealed an underdeveloped child (26 kg for 1,21 meter) with intense jaundice, severe pruritus and deep asthenia. The liver was enlarged and hard and the spleen was enlarged. There were several spider angiomas and moderate ascites. Biology revealed: Total bilirubin: 460 µml/l; Alkaline phosphatase: 220 mu/ml; ASAT: 171 mu/ml; ALAT: 138 mu/ml; Albuminemia: 30 g/l. HBsAg was negative; α-fetoprotein level was normal; α-1-antitrypsin level was normal; platelets count was: 118,000/mm^3; RBC were 3,600,000/mm^3 and WBC: 3000/mm^3; the Quick test was 35% of control; factors II, V and VII + X were 40, 40 and 35% of control, respectively. Endoscopy revealed the presence of esophageal varices.

On October 25, 1981, an ABO compatible, cross-match negative, three haplotype mismatched adult donor was found. Because of the large discrepancy in weight between donor (75 kg) and recipient, orthotopic transplantation of the whole donor liver was not possible: only the left lobe of the donor liver was implanted in the recipient.

The whole liver graft was cooled in the donor. An extended right hepatectomy [1], which removed segments IV, V, VI, VII and VIII (according to the nomenclature of Couinaud [4] of the liver graft was performed ex situ. The hepatectomy was performed using our standard technique: the vessels of the quadrate lobe, the right hepatic artery, portal branch and right hepatic duct were dissected free, ligated and divided; the liver parenchyma was transected along the insertion of the falciform ligament towards the right side of the vena cava and to prevent diffuse bleeding at the level of the transected surface of the graft at the time of revascularization, this surface was dried and immediately covered with a gelatin-resorcin-formaldehyde glue. When the glue was polymerized the absence of vascular leakage was verified by injecting Collins' solution into the portal vein, hepatic artery and left supra-hepatic vein.

Then, the recipient's liver was removed, and the graft, consisting of the left lobe (segments II and III) and Spiegel lobe (segment I) of the donor liver, was implanted in the recipient according to the usual orthotopic technique (Figure 1). Despite some discrepancy in caliber between donor and recipient's vessels, end-to-end suprahepatic vena cava, portal vein, hepatic artery and infra-hepatic vena cava anastomoses were performed (Figure 1). Revascularization of the graft was satisfying. Total ischemia time of the graft was 4 h. The bile duct of the graft was anastomosed end-to-side to the jejunum of the recipient using a Roux-en-Y loop. The amount of blood transfusion to the recipient during operation was 1200 ml.

Post operatively, the patient was given prednisolone and cyclophosphamide. Immediate evolution was good with normal consciousness, decrease in bilirubin, alkaline phosphatases, and return of coagulation factors to normal. Five days after operation, a severe acute rejection crisis occurred, marked by a sharp increase of ASAT and ALAT levels and, histologically, by signs of hepatocellular necrosis with intense congestion. Within a few days, signs of acute rejection disappeared. During the following weeks a progressively increasing cholestasis was observed, with normal intra and extra hepatic bile ducts, and characterized histologically by a progressive disappearance of the interlobular bile ducts with signs of interlobular bile duct necrosis in some places. More than two years after transplantation, the physical status of the patient is good but there is a persisting jaundice with moderate pruritus. Immunosuppression consists of prednisone (10 mg, every two days) and cyclosporin A (15 mg/kg/day).

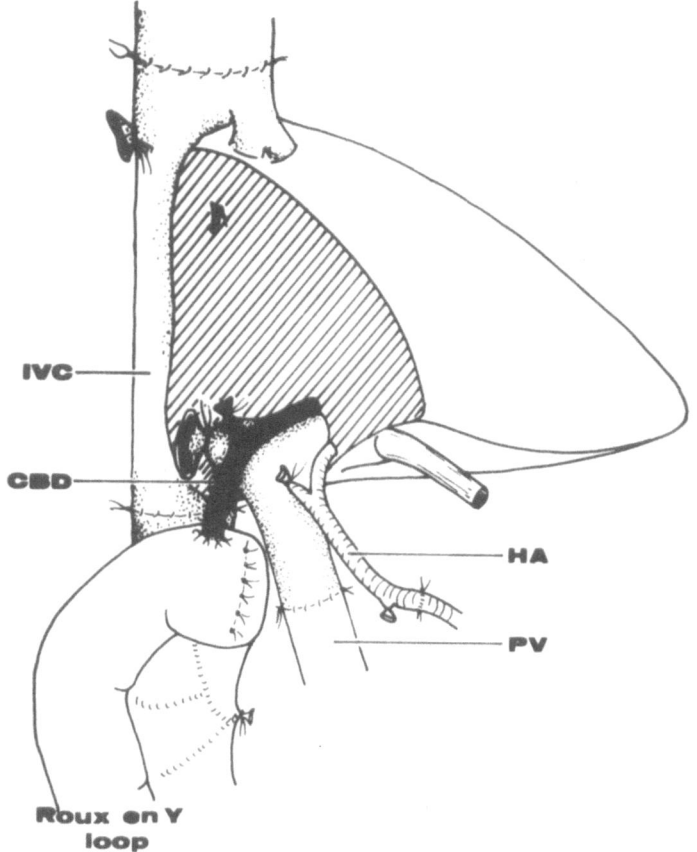

Figure 1. Reduced-sized orthotopic liver graft. IVC: inferior vena cava; CBD: common bile duct; HA: hepatic artery; PV: portal vein.

Discussion

This observation shows that orthotopic transplantation of a liver graft reduced to the left lobe can be satisfactorily achieved in man. A few unsuccessful attempts to transplant heterotopically a part of the liver have already been reported: Shumakov and co-workers [9] used a left anatomical liver lobe grafted retroperitoneally in the iliac fossa, Fortner *et al.* conducted a left lobectomy on a liver graft heterotopically transplanted in a child in order to facilitate abdominal closure. However, in these cases, the technique used was different from ours since, in our patient, the graft was an hepatectomized liver transplanted orthotopically with all its normal vascular connections. As a matter of fact, the large size of an adult liver graft creates a difficult technical obstacle to orthotopic liver transplantation in children and to heterotopic liver transplantation, due to the absence of sufficient room in the abdomen of the recipient. In three patients with end-stage hepatic failure, in one case sub-acute hepatitis due to sodium valproate [8], in a second case primary biliary cirrhosis and in the third case chronic graft rejection after orthotopic liver transplantation, we used an adult liver graft which was reduced to the left lobe and transplanted heterotopically. This procedure aims to achieve an equivalent of the heterotopic auxiliary transplantation that we had done previously with success by using a child liver graft in an adult recipient [7]. Survival times in these three patients were 24, 10 and 21 days, respectively. Causes of death were liver failure in two patients and medullar aplasia with septicemia in one patient. The present observation reports the use of a similar procedure of graft reduction for an orthotopic liver transplantation in a child.

Technically, the procedure of graft reduction exposes to two hypothetical risks. The first one is related to the prolongation of the ischemic time (about 1 h) which is necessary to perform an ex-situ hepatectomy. This risk can be minimized if donor and recipient are operated on simultaneously in the same operative theatre and if rewarming of the graft is prevented during its partial resection. In our observation, post-operative function of the graft was good and it may be advanced that ischemic damage to the graft was minimal. The second risk is that of an intraperitoneal hemorrhage, due to the presence of a raw liver surface. This risk has been prevented by applicating a rapidly polymerizing glue to this raw surface prior to revascularizing the graft: in this patient, as well as in the three heterotopically liver transplanted patients, intra-operative bleeding was moderate and no bleeding was observed post-operatively. It is most improbable that, in our patient, the intrahepatic cholestasis observed later on had any connection with the technique used: a similar complication has been reported [4] in patients who underwent a standard orthotopic liver transplantation.

Since child donors are very rarely found, the main advantage of this technique is that it allows to perform orthotopic liver transplantation in children using an adult liver graft. The liver graft can be reduced to 30 or 50% of its volume using a right hepatectomy, a right lobectomy, or a left lobectomy combined to a right lateral sectoriectomy. In children younger than our patient, the graft should be submitted to a larger hepatectomy: the segmental anatomy of the liver allows to perform the reduction of liver parenchyma which is the most suitable in each circumstance [2].

It appears from recent reports that results of liver transplantation have improved in these last years, particularly in children transplanted for biliary atresia [10] and that a further improvement is foreseeable with the use of cyclosporin A as an immunosuppressive drug [12]. In this rather favorable context concerning liver transplantation in children, it may be advanced that the procedure of a reduced-sized orthotopic liver graft transplanted from an adult donor to a child could facilitate the performance of liver transplantation in this category of patients.

References

1. Bismuth H: Surgical anatomy and anatomical surgery of the liver. Wrld J Surg 6:3–9, 1982.
2. Bismuth H, Houssin D, Castaing D: Major and minor segmentectomies 'réglées' in liver surgery. Wrld J Surg 6:10–24, 1982.
3. Couinaud C: Le foie. Etudes anatomiques et chirurgicales. Paris, Masson, 1957.
4. Fennel RH: Ductular damage in liver transplant rejection. Pathol Ann 16(2):289–294, 1981.
5. Fortner JG, Kim DK, Shin MH, Yeh SDJ, Howland WS, Beattie EJ: Heterotopic (auxiliary) liver transplantation in man. Transplant Proc 9:217, 1977.
6. Fortner JG, Yeh SDJ, Kim DK, Shin MH, Kinne DW: The case for and technique of heterotopic liver grafting. Transplant Proc 11:269–275, 1979.
7. Houssin D, Franco D, Berthelot P, Bismuth H: Heterotopic liver transplantation in HBsAg-positive end-stage cirrhosis. Lancet 5:990–994, 1980.
8. Lebihan G, Coquerel A, Houssin D, Bourreille J, Szekely AM, Bismuth H, Hemet J, Samson M: Insuffisance hépatique aiguë mortelle au cours d'un traitement par le valproate de sodium. Gastroenterol Clin Biol 6:477–481, 1982.
9. Shumakov VI, Galperin EI: Transplantation of the left liver lobe. Transplant Proc 11(2):1489, 1979.
10. Starzl TE, Koep LJ, Halgrimson CG, Hood J, Schröter GP, Porter KA, Weil R: Fifteen years of clinical liver transplantation. Gastroenterology 77:375–388, 1979.
11. Starzl TE, Klintmalm GB, Porter KA, Iwatsuki S, Schröter GP: Liver transplantation with use of cyclosporin A and prednisone. N Engl J Med 305:266–269, 1981.
12. Starzl TE, Iwatsuki S, Van Thiel DH, Carlton Gartner J, Zitelli BJ, Malatack JJ, Shaw BW, Hakala TR, Rosenthal JT, Porter KA: Evolution of liver transplantation. Hepatology 2:614–636, 1982.

Section 6

MANAGEMENT AND OVERALL RESULTS

23. Organisation of liver transplantation

C.H. GIPS, M.J.H. SLOOFF, H. WESENHAGEN, H. VAN GOOR,
C.M.A. BIJLEVELD and R.A.F. KROM

Introduction

Although results are improving, even in the best centres liver transplantation carries a considerable mortality when compared to other therapeutic modalities in medicine. Since the procedure is complex, the liver transplant team must be well organised. The patient must be provided with the best multidisciplinary skills available. Unnecessary risks (risk-free liver transplantations do not exist) should not be taken. Provisions for data analysis should be made to enable improvement of results and, where possible, simplification of procedures.

In Groningen, the divisions of hepatology and paediatric gastroenterology work as integrated units with the department of general surgery. These three disciplines unite with anaesthetics to make up the clinical core of the multi-disciplinary liver transplant team. The organisation of liver transplantation is described starting with the patient's course through all the stages. The development of the liver transplant team including the management of politics and the skills and resources needed for liver transplantation have been reported on elsewhere [1, 2].

The patient

Entrance to the system

The patient enters the system (flow chart) via a telephone referral from his internist/paediatrician. The internist/paediatrician in charge completes a form and often requests further documentation consisting of a referral letter, all available scans and x-rays, an ECG and sometimes histological slices. Rarely is a case refused at first glance. During weekly rounds the internists, paediatricians, radiologists and surgeons belonging to the transplant team assess the medical file received and prepare a consult letter. Thereafter a team member telephones the referring physician, who may be asked to proceed with more investigations depending on his hospital facilities, or be advised that the patient is unsuitable for liver transplantation and be given an alternative treatment plan, or the patient may be admitted to the division of paediatric gastroenterology or hepatology for further evaluation. Patients who seem to be good candidates or about whom some doubt exists are admitted. A patient is never accepted for transplantation on verbal or written documentation alone.

Admission

Selection stages

After admission the diagnostic protocol is put into motion. When, after screening, the patient seems to be a good candidate the Possible Candidate stage (a selection stage from the view-point of the transplantation team) is entered and specific diagnostic procedures which are connected in part to the post-transplantation phase are performed. Because of the integration of hepatology, paediatric gastroenterology and general surgery, the surgeons see the patient throughout all the admission stages whereas the anaesthesist sees the patient in the Possible Candidate stage.

A patient becomes a Candidate for liver transplantation when according to

Flow chart. Course of the liver transplant patient.

1. telephone referral or letter to internist/paediatrician of liver transplant team.
   a. (further) documentation requested and multidisciplinary assessment of file → b, c or a repeated.
   b. admission to hepatology/paediatric gastroenterology.
   c. refused by team.
2. admission.
   a. refused after screening.
   b. Possible Candidate → c or refused.
   c. Candidate: requirements have been met.
3. final discussion and decision. Discharge.
   a. transplantation offer accepted. Timing. Appointment with previous transplant patients.
   b. refusal by team or patient.
4. preparation for transplantation.
   T⁻, T. Amber, green, red light. semidefinitive donor announcement.
5. orthotopic liver transplantation.
   intensive treatment, medium care.
6. discharge to half-way house of the Netherlands Liver Foundation.
7. final discharge to home, check ups in local hospital,
   immunological monitoring by internist/paediatricians of liver transplant team.
8. protocolled admissions in Groningen once a year.
   Other admissions in local hospital or in Groningen.

current knowledge all the requirements for a successful liver transplantation have been met. Occasionally consultations from other specialties are necessary to reach this stage. There is a danger that a specialist not wishing to bear the responsibility for refusal of the patient may tend to express too optimistic a view. Older patients especially may have a number of relative contraindications. These have to be weighed and a decision made.

Final discussion and decision: Discharge
Representatives of the team: the internists/paediatricians, surgeon, anaesthesist, attending physician and nurse discuss with the patient and relatives the outcome of the investigations and the medical opinion with regard to liver transplantation. Parents accompany their sick child and an adult patient is asked to be accompanied by his partner and children. If the team considers that the risks of liver transplantation are too great, i.e. the procedure would shorten the lifespan, other therapeutic measures are discussed. Liver transplantation, however important, is only one treatment modality. If a liver transplantation is thought feasible, it is offered to the patient with an explanation of the current known risks. Relative contraindications are also discussed. If the patient and his relatives accept a liver transplantation, timing the transplantation is the next step. The timing for patients who have hepatocellar carcinoma and who are offered a diagnostic laparotomy with donor liver standby status is easy, as quickly as possible. For some patients with cirrhosis early transplantation may be the only solution. Nowadays, most of the patients who enter our system have more time because they are evaluated in a relatively early stage of the disease. The patient is told that a series of liver transplants is planned half a year ahead and he is asked when he thinks the optimal time for his transplant would be. The patient is also asked whether he thinks it would be safe to wait another two years or one year before having a transplant. The discussion results in a decision as to timing. A few patients are told that there is an indication for liver transplantation but that a complicating disease (or diseases) poses potential problems that are beyond the ability of current knowledge, which presumably with increased experience can be solved; thus, some of them remain Possible Candidates. Possible Candidates or not, all patients are followed up.

Candidates who accept the offer made by the transplant team are transferred to the transplantation phase. Candidates and their family are asked to contact previous liver transplant recipients to clarify for themselves the implications of liver transplantation. The liver transplantation secretary provides the Candidate with a brochure on liver transplantation in Groningen and its costs.

Transplantation phases

T minus
In this phase all the requirements of the protocol except HLA typing are completed. Pre-transplant blood transfusions are given at the local hospital according to the liver transplant protocol.

T
In the T phase the patient is ready for a transplantation. Check-ups are done at the referring hospital. Incidental examinations, e.g. once yearly, are done in the liver transplant centre. If either the patient or the referring physician thinks there is a deterioration, they are to report this immediately to the liver transplant team. If necessary, the individual transplantation plan is revised according to a more pessimistic or optimistic view. In the T phase, a patient may be given the Red Light (see appropriate section) because of concomitant diseases.

Amber Light
The Amber Light is given when all the administrative preparations for the actual transplantation have been done. This includes transportation from home to the transplant centre, post-transplant housing near the transplant centre, HLA typing, availability of immediate pre-transplant medication etc. The patient is informed that he and several other patients will have the Amber Light at the same time.

Green Light
The Green Light indicates that the search for a suitable donor liver for this recipient-to-be has begun. Because of this country's small size, travelling distances are short, thus with a few exceptions, a patient carrying a portable paging device can stay at home. Children and adults, different blood groups, the cytomegalovirus seronegativity requirements of the donor, size of the liver and distance between the donor and recipient make it desirable to have several recipients to choose from, in order to make optimal use of the donor livers available. The patient is informed that for various reasons several patients have the Green Light simultaneously. The search is made by the donor organ transplant coordinator in regional hospitals and in collaboration with Eurotransplant. In the Green Light period, the adults are seen every week by an internist at the hospital closest to the patient (not necessarily the referring hospital), and there, investigations are performed according to the transplant team's requirements. Every four weeks, all patients are seen at the transplant centre.

Red Light
The Red Light can be declared in any of the transplantation phases if there are patient-related circumstances (concomitant disease, social reasons) or team-

related factors (incomplete team, insufficient facilities, e.g. no bed available in the intensive care unit).

Semidefinitive donor announcement
When an appropriate donor liver becomes available a timetable is drawn up starting from the recipient-to-be, i.e. travelling time, preparation in hospital, start of anaesthesia, start of recipient operation and expected return of the donor and home teams. The donor team's departure from Groningen is determined by a reverse timetable, counting down from the moment of the team's expected reunion. This way the recipient's interests and the shortest possible liver preservation time are secured. The patient is informed that a donor liver is available and is requested to swallow the pre-transplant medication while still on the telephone. The semidefinitive nature is explained again, i.e. the quality of the donor liver on macroscopic appearance may be unsatisfactory or there may be other reasons including problems with the team's return, thus preventing transplantation.

It is also reiterated to the patient that the operation never goes beyond the point of no return before the donor and home teams are reunited. When the patient arrives at the transplant centre, the internist/paediatrician takes a history and does a physical examination. The findings are reported to a second internist and a decision is made jointly with anaesthetists and surgical team as to the patient's suitability for the operation.

Transplantation and post transplantation phase

These phases proceed according to the diagnostic and therapeutic protocols. The phases are: intensive treatment (department of surgery), medium care (department of medicine or paediatrics), discharge to the Netherlands Liver Foundation halfway house (this accommodation is close to the University of Groningen's Academic Hospital and thus the hospital's facilities are readily available to the patient) and final discharge.

Home
Once home, the patient is seen once a month for the first year by an internist/ paediatrician at the hospital closest to the patient. Laboratory investigations are done at the shorter intervals than the monthly visits. Some are done at the local hospital, others are sent to Groningen. The liver transplant team monitors the immunosuppressive regimen. A telex system has been developed for patients living abroad thus making it possible to receive the results and to give treatment advice the same day the samples are taken.

The patient is seen once a year in Groningen. Intermittent admissions are to the patient's local hospital except when special expertise is needed. Ailments occurring outside the upper abdomen can be treated (operations included) in other hospitals. When the patient's condition is uncertain as far as the liver is concerned the local hospital is also the best treatment centre. In the event of a hospital admission, the transplant team can, if needed, offer advice on a daily basis.

Organisational aspects

Organisation of the surgical team

Liver procurement and the recipient's operation

The surgical team has two main responsibilities: organ procurement and the transplant operation including treatment of any post-surgical complications.

The transplant coordinator (a staff doctor from the surgical department) organises the organ procurement; the logistics of which include collecting information on liver quality and donor-recipient compatibility. Then the coordinator, the transplant team's surgeons, anaesthetists, internists and/or paediatricians discuss this information and decide jointly to accept the donor; after which the transplant coordinator notifies the donor hospital as the team's expected time of arrival, checks the surgical equipment and arranges the transport.

The donor team consists of a transplant surgeon and a transplant surgeon in training or senior resident, an anaesthetist and the transplant coordinator. Two surgeons are necessary because after the liver has been removed, the kidneys must be retrieved.

When the donor team arrives, the donor is taken to the operating room. Prior to operating, the surgeon makes a careful physical examination while the anaesthetist checks the data and the donor's condition. The sequence and the technical aspects of the surgical procedures are discussed with the other team and O.R. assistants. During the first part of the operation the transplant coordinator collects blood and liver samples according to the diagnostic protocol. In the meantime, the transplant coordinator contacts the home team, informs them about the course of the operation and the appearance of the liver. If necessary, the timetable is adjusted.

Before harvesting the organs, perfusion systems are carefully prepared. The organs are perfused simultaneously, then the heart, liver and kidneys are removed, in that order. This procedure also allows for a segmental pancreatectomy.

The home team is telephoned, given details of the quality and condition of the perfused liver, and the donor team's arrival time is set. The team is provided with rapid transportation to Groningen, to minimise liver ischaemia. Meanwhile the home team starts to prepare for the recipient's operation. This team consists of a transplant surgeon and a transplant surgeon in training or a senior resident. When the donor team returns, it joins the home team to make up the recipient's team; thus, the recipient's operation is continued by one of the two transplant surgeons assisted by one of the training transplant surgeons plus two residents, a total of four. This recipient's team may seem a bit large; however, the first part of the recipient's operation is a hepatectomy. This part is difficult because portal hypertension, coagulation disturbances and multiple adhesions are often present from previous operations. To minimise blood loss and operating time, the exposure must be excellent and the operation must be performed by a surgeon experienced with this type of surgery.

The other team members are temporarily relieved for other duties and are to be available for the next transplantation.

Organisation of the anaesthesia team

Orthotopic liver transplantation is a complex surgical procedure which causes extensive alterations to the vital body functions; thus, in view of this procedure's complexity it requires one of the most difficult kinds of anaesthesias currently known. There are many aspects to the anaesthetist's job during a liver transplantation, including: correction of biochemical and coagulation disturbances, compensation for the massive blood loss, management of the interrupted central venous circulation and extensive intravascular monitoring.

General aspects
For everyone to become as experienced as possible, it is vital that the anaesthetic team consists of fixed members. Furthermore, the anaesthetists must have prior experience in intensive care treatment and major surgery other than transplantations. To guarantee that a complete, fully qualified team is available at all times, reserve team members cover during holidays, illnesses and days off, and they always carry portable paging devices. Although the 12 liver transplantations performed each year do not require continuous participation from the anaesthetists, the department was, nevertheless, enlarged by one staff position to fulfill the requirements of the actual transplantations and to accommodate the additional demands these entail (such as round-the-clock availability) which do tax the department as a whole.

Anaesthesia team: Composition and division of work
The team consists of seven anaesthetists. There is one coordinating anaesthetist who preoperatively evaluates and decides on a particular candidate's suitability for a liver transplantation. His expertise covers a vast area: he must foresee the possibility of any complicating factors affecting the vital body functions that may both have a bearing on the feasibility of the transplantation and that may arise in the postoperative intensive care phase. He is also expected to predict the recipient's chances of survival and the immediate postoperative morbidity.

During the operation, he coordinates and oversees all the minutiae of the anaesthesia itself and maintains contact with other transplantation team members, i.e. hepatologist, paediatrician, surgeon, blood bank officer and laboratory personnel. During the operation, there are two anaesthetists; one administers the anaesthesia and medication, and maintains the biochemical condition while the second monitors the patient, including the vital signs and the haematological and biochemical condition. Since the functions of these two anaesthetists overlap, one team member can perform all these functions in instances where a transplantation can be predicted to run smoothly, e.g. in children. The fourth anaesthetist travels with the donor team and sees to the donor's condition in order to provide optimal liver and other organ (heart, kidneys) preservation.

Postoperatively the patient is transferred tot the intensive care unit's team member.

In the intensive care phase, two anaesthetists, specially trained to handle postoperative liver transplant patients, maintain the fluid balance, correct the coagulation mechanism, determine the type and duration of ventilation, and detect and treat infections; all important aspects ensuring a succesful outcome to a liver transplantation. There is one reserve anaesthetist.

Additional personnel include an anaesthesia nurse who maintains adequate supplies, prepares the medication and anaesthetic equipment, takes blood samples and keeps the anaesthetic records. There is also a perfusionist, i.e. a biotechnician who maintains, assembles and operates the pumps required for blood transfusions, autologous transfusions and veno-venous bypass.

Additional comments
Anaesthesia techniques, perioperative medication schemes, monitoring methods, transfusion and bypass systems etc. have been included in a protocol to avoid omissions and mistakes that could easily occur under complex circumstances. To improve the anaesthetic and intensive care of liver transplant patients it is essential to maintain contact with foreign liver transplantation centres and to regularly exchange knowledge between various specialists.

Internal medicine/paediatrics and other disciplines

Internists/paediatricians
Internists or paediatricians trained in hepatology fill special appointments that come under the jurisdiction of the hepatology and paediatric gastroenterology divisions. These two divisions provide the liver transplant patient continuity of care starting at the entrance to the system, continuing to the final discharge, and including home aftercare. An internist or paediatrician is always present during the recipient's operation to speak with the relatives. During the intensive treatment phase, these internists or paediatricians also participate in the patient's management. At any time during the peri- and postoperative period, there are always two internists available.

Nursing, social work and chaplaincy/counselling service
There is one primary-care nurse who coordinates all the specific nursing aspects
of liver transplantation. She is the patient's main thread through all the phases
and at home. Occasionally, the social worker gets involved before admission and
if necessary continues his involvement after discharge whether or not there has
been a transplantation. The hospital chaplain (or counsellor) contacts the patient
after admission and is also available during the halfway house period. When the
patient and his family live a considerable distance from the transplant centre (as
many do), the social worker and chaplain/counsellor often play an important
role, whether a transplant is offered or not because there is always a change and
sometimes even a disruption in family life.

Other disciplines (in alphabetical order)
Blood bank, blood grouping, clinical chemistry, clinical immunology, dentistry,
dietetics, haematology and coagulation, hepatochemistry, medical microbiology
and infection control, nuclear medicine, pathology, radiology, rehabilitation and
other disciplines are linked to the clinical core by protocols and by the weekly
transplantation meetings in which they can participate.

Administration and communication

Administration and laboratory coordination
The liver transplant secretary coordinates the administrative work including the
organisation of protocolled medicine and communication within and without the
group. Two laboratory technicians coordinate the protocolled laboratory investigations. One is responsible for clinical chemistry and haematology and for
communicating laboratory matters to the local hospital and the patient. The other
files the sera and coordinates any special investigations done in other laborato-
ries.

Communication and information
A multidisciplinary team of more than a hundred members requires a communication system which allows for both an increase and exchange of knowledge,
plus a means of maintaining the group's coherence. Weekly liver transplant
meetings and weekly assessments of new patients, a monthly newsletter and the
protocols achieve these ends.

Along with the four clinical core disciplines participating in the liver transplant
meeting, there is also the nurse, social worker, secretary, medical microbiologist,
laboratory coordinators, and any other team member wishing to be present. The
newsletter is edited by the liver transplant secretary. Protocols are made for a
period covering a cohort of liver transplantations (currently 15). Changes in the
protocols are reported in the newsletter which all disciplines can contribute to and

238

profit by. The communication with the referring hospital is described in part in the 'Patient' section. Form letters, which ensure rapid availability of information, are sent to all those involved during each phase the patient has to pass.

Netherlands Liver Foundation

A volunteer representative from the Netherlands Liver Foundation working in collaboration with the social worker and hospital chaplain/counsellor contacts the patient after admission and solves any problems beyond the scope of the liver transplant group. The hospital provides the patient's family with accommodation in the perioperative period and the Netherlands Liver Foundation organises half-way housing before discharge home.

Conclusion

The organisation of liver transplantation needs careful planning. Key attributes for a succesful liver transplant team are: sufficient resources, skill, discipline and cohesion.

Acknowledgments

Mrs. M. de Bruijn-Beeching edited in the English and Ms. M.T. Bouritius provided secretarial assistance.

References

1. Krom RAF, Gips CH: Skills and resources needed for liver transplantation. Hepatology (4):72S-75S, 1984.
2. Gips CH, Krom RAF: The development of the liver transplantation team in Groningen. In: Smit Sibinga CT, Das PC, Opelz G (eds). Transplantation and blood transfusion. Boston, Martinus Nijhoff Publishers 1984, pp 3–8.

24. Principles of multiple organ procurement with special reference to the liver

H. VAN GOOR and M.J.H. SLOOFF

Introduction

With the acceptance of liver and cardiac transplantation as a therapeutic modality for end stage liver and cardiac disease and the recent improvements in immunosuppression, the demand for extrarenal grafts has increased enormously. Currently, potential transplant recipients still far outnumber the available donor organs; however, based on health authorities' reports, there are more than enough brain death patients, to provide a surplus of donor organs. Lack of donor identification, no consent from next of kin and a poor condition of the donor are the most important reasons why a sufficient number of transplantable organs is never reached. In addition, suitable organs can be wasted because of logistical and organisational problems. To redress these problems it is not only imperative to intensify donor recruitment programmes but also to make optimal use of every available donor; therefore, it is necessary to consider every brain death donor as a multiple organ donor in order to realise multiple organ harvests.

The measures mentioned above can be taken locally to expand the donor pool. Apart from these local measures, national and even international organisations were founded to offer facilities to solve the logistical and organisational problems of long-distance organ procurement. UK Transplant, Scandia Transplant and Eurotransplant are representative of such national and international efforts. Calne [1] and Starzl [2] pioneered the field of multiple organ procurement. They were the first to describe the technique of combined donor hepatectomy and nephrectomy. Several other authors reported excellent functional results and usual survival after transplantation of organs harvested from a multiple organ donor [3–5]. However, these results can only be obtained by a highly trained team, with an efficient organisation, a stable donor, and a meticulous and flexible operative procedure. These components are considered basic requirements for a successful transplant programme [6].

Composition of the donor team

The donor team consists of an experienced transplant surgeon, a transplant surgeon in training, an anaesthetist and a transplant coordinator. Two O.R. assistants from the donor hospital complete the operating team. The surgeons remove the abdominal organs and assist the cardiac surgeon in dissecting the heart and lungs. The senior surgeon prepares the abdominal organs for removal and perfusion. He himself takes care of the liver perfusion. The transplant coordinator perfuses the pancreas and kidneys. An anaesthetist dealing regularly with multiple organ procurement is essential for the donor team. The management of the donor can benefit from his experience and may thus contribute to the quality of the organs. The transplant coordinator is responsible for the logistical and organisational aspects of procurement, perfusion and packaging of the organs harvested.

Principles of organisation

Protocol and coordination are the two main aspects in the organisation of multiple organ procurement. The operation in multiple organ donors is a very complex procedure, and up till now, is performed by at least two teams, a thoracic team for removing the heart and/or lungs and an abdominal team that removes the abdominal organs. Because each individual team can influence the quality of all grafts by injudiciously handling their part of the operation, the donor operation must be strictly protocolled.

The essentials of the whole procedure are outlined below. After the donor team's arrival, the donor is admitted to the operating room where the surgeon and anaesthetist carefully examine the donor and check his condition and data before deciding to operate.

Technical aspects are discussed with the other teams and O.R. assistants. It is decided which team members will flush and inspect the organs after their removal, and who will close the sternal and abdominal wounds.

The abdominal surgeons start the operation with a median sternotomy extended with a median laparotomy. This allows the cardiac team to arrive at the donor hospital several hours later or to wait for the crossmatch results. After inspecting the liver, kidneys and pancreas, the surgeons prepare these organs for removal; at which time the cardiac team joins the operation and prepares the heart and/or lungs for explantation. The abdominal team places cannulas in the aorta and the portal and lower caval vein. Subsequently, the cardiac team induces cardiac arrest by total inflow occlusion and at the same time both the thoracic and abdominal organs are cooled. The heart, liver, pancreas and kidneys are removed, flushed at separate tables, packed and prepared for transport. To supervise such a procedure and to guide the different teams in often unfamiliar operating theatres an experienced transplant coordinator is mandatory. With his expertise he can ensure the quality of the organs. He informs the recipient centres about the quality and anatomy of the grafts and the timing of the return.

Principles of donor treatment

Accurate and appropriate donor support is becoming more important since the interval between brain death and organ recovery has increased owing to the extensive logistical and organisational aspects of multiple organ procurement. Specific knowledge of vascular, respiratory and hormonal changes after brain death and intensive therapy is required to maintain an optimal condition of the donor for a considerable period. However, most donors are unstable due to dehydration induced either deliberately for treatment purposes or as a result of concomitant diabetes insipidus. Dehydration is the main cause of electrolyte disturbances and low blood pressure in spite of extensive vasopressor support. Consequently myocardial dysfunction, inadequate organ perfusion and ischaemia develop and finally, it is possible to lose all the organs.

The principles of donor management are: optimal organ perfusion, optimal oxygenation and prevention of infection. The premises are: sufficient vascular access for infusion of various solutions in a short period, ventilation with 50–60% oxygen, only low dose vasopressors and intravenously administrated antibiotics.

Colloid containing plasma solutions with normal saline and cross matched blood are the ideal replacement fluids for covering blood and urine losses.

Two reliable intravenous lines and monitoring of central venous pressure are necessary for controlled rapid infusion. A low dose dopamine infusion ($<10\,\mu$g kg^{-1}min^{-1}) can maintain adequate blood pressure and increase splanchnic blood flow.

Some authors consider dopamine contraindicated when the heart is considered for transplantation because it promotes catecholamine depletion in the myocardium [7].

The use of adrenaline and noradrenaline is contraindicated because organ perfusion is drastically reduced and their need reflects severe instability of the donor. Vasopressin supplementation (2–$20\,\mu$E kg^{-1}min^{-1}) is required, administrated as a continuous intravenous infusion, to maintain normal intravascular fluid and electrolyte balance.

Broad spectrum antibiotics are given intravenously in relatively high doses prior to and during surgery.

Principles of the donor operation

The operation must be performed without jeopardising the anatomical and functional integrity of each individual organ. This must be a constant concern for every transplant surgeon because every transplantation starts with the donor operation. The execution of the donor operation determines to a great extent the outcome of the transplantation and its eventual complications.

Multiple organ retrieval has several implications for the liver. Hepatotoxic substances, cardio-respiratory instability and impaired portal flow during the donor operation compromise the hepatic parenchyma and may influence early graft function. A lesion of the hepatic artery or anomalous branches to the right or left liver lobe endangers the vascularization of the liver and the common bile duct anastomosis in the recipient. Damage to the caval vein which remains unnoticed, will lead to severe bleeding during the transplantation.

A prolonged extensive operative procedure will evoke contamination of the liver, which can have a deleterious effect in an immunecompromised host after transplantation.

Combined donor hepatectomy and nephrectomy

The formerly used cruciate abdominal incision has been replaced by a complete midline incision from the suprasternal notch to just above the symphysis pubis to provide the best exposure in the upper abdomen and perfect access to the liver. The diaphragm is incised laterally on both sides. After inspection of the abdominal organs the dissection is started.

The extraperitoneal space is entered in the right lower abdomen. The ascending colon and caecum are mobilized and swept over to the left upper abdomen together with the small intestine in a manner such that compression of the portal vein is avoided. The aorta and inferior vena cava are encircled at their bifurcation and dissected upward at the anterior surface. The inferior mesenteric artery and vein are ligated and divided. The renal arteries are identified on both sides and dissected some distance towards the renal hilus.

Superior to the left renal vein, the superior mesenteric artery is encountered, passing anteriorly, and encircled. The superior mesenteric artery is carefully checked for the presence of a right hepatic artery.

The left and right kidney are freed from Gerota's fascia without traction on the vascular structures. The adrenal glands are slipped off. Both ureters are identified near the bladder and freed over their entire length. Next the structures of the portal triad are skeletonized from the right to the left side.

The common bile duct is transsected as close as possible to the duodenum.

The hepatic artery is dissected towards the coeliac axis, cutting off the gastroduodenal and right gastric artery. The splenic artery and left gastric artery are identified, and the coeliac trunk and the left gastric artery are checked for anomalous hepatic branches. The portal vein is mobilized and encircled just superior to the junction of the splenic and superior mesenteric vein, so that division of the neck of the pancreas is not usually necessary.

The upper abdominal aorta is cleaned circumferentially proximal to the coeliac axis and encircled just below the diaphragm. When there is insufficient space to place a clamp on the upper part of the abdominal aorta, the lower thoracic aorta is encircled just above the diaphragm. Attention is then directed to the caval vein. The right triangular and coronary ligaments are cut with gentle retraction of the right hepatic lobe. The retro- and infrahepatic vena cava is exposed; the right adrenal vein is ligated and divided, and the posterior attachments are cut. No effort is made to dissect the suprahepatic vena cava until the liver is totally perfused with cold solution. Next the posterior surface of the aorta and caval vein are dissected; lumbal arteries and veins are clipped and divided. Alpha blocking agents can be given at this time provided the blood pressure is normal.

After cross clamping the aorta above the renal arteries and below the superior mesenteric artery and the caval vein just above the renal veins, the kidneys can be removed *en bloc*, placed on a back table and flushed with one of the Collins'-type solutions. Sometimes, because of the proximity of the renal arteries and superior mesenteric artery, it is necessary to ligate and divide this latter structure in order to obtain a suitable aortic patch for the renal arteries. This may only be done when there is no hepatic artery originating from the superior mesenteric artery; otherwise, this artery must be preserved and the renal arteries must be cut from the aorta without patches.

Now the circulation of the donor is still intact and providing the liver with both hepatic arterial and portal venous blood. Successively, the portal vein is ligated and cannulated, cooling of the liver is immediately started, the superior mesenteric artery is tied, and the aorta is cross clamped just above the coeliac trunk at the indicated sites. By simple removal of the caval clamp, congestion of the liver is avoided.

An alternative method of organ preservation is *in situ* cooling of both the liver and kidneys. The preparatory steps for this procedure are described in the next paragraph.

Combined cardiectomy, hepatectomy and nephrectomy

The main option of this combined procedure is immediate graft cooling of the heart, liver and kidneys after disconnection of the abdominal and thoracic aorta followed by circulatory arrest. The preparation of the intra-abdominal organs is analogous to the description in the previous paragraph. In order to provide optimal circulation for the heart, the aortic and portal vein cannulas are placed when the dissection of the heart is completed, prior to *in situ* cooling.

The pericardial cavity is opened and the ascending aorta, main pulmonary artery and its bifurcation are mobilized and separated from each other. The superior vena cava is ligated and a Brettschneider needle is inserted into the ascending aorta if *in situ* cooling of the heart is preferred.

When all the cannulas are in position and a last check up has been made the inferior vena cava is clamped near the heart, causing a total inflow occlusion; then the aorta is cross clamped at the ascending part and at the diaphragm, causing an arrest of organ perfusion.

Immediately afterwards, an infusion of a cardioplegic solution into the ascending aorta and cooling of the liver and kidneys through the portal and aortic cannulas begins. Decompression of the abdominal caval vein is obtained simply by opening this vein below the renal veins. The heart is removed first followed by the liver and kidneys.

Hepatectomy in combination with pancreatectomy

With the techniques described, excision of the whole pancreas is not possible. Only a segment of the pancreas can be obtained. The pancreas and its vascular structures are dissected first. Just before *in situ* cooling of the heart, liver and kidneys, the segment is removed without patches and perfused with a cold solution at a back table.

Principles of liver preservation and removal

In several centres 'precooling' of the liver is done with lactated Ringer's solution through the splenic vein during the operation [8]. Its main disadvantage is the decrease in body temperature with a danger of ventricular fibrillation compromising arterial blood supply of the liver and foreshortening the procedure including heart procurement.

In situ cooling by infusion of a Collins' solution through the portal vein and hepatic artery immediately after circulatory arrest is a simple and safe method of liver preservation applied in many European centres for several years now. Rapid portal infusion of 1.5 l of Euro Collins' solution (see Table 1), with 15–20 cm H_2O pressure, in about 5–10 min renders the liver cold and bloodless. This pressure

Table 1. Composition of Euro Collins' solution. pH at 4° C: 7.20. Osmolality 355 mOsm/kg H_2O.

maeq/l	Na$^+$	10	Cl$^-$	115
	K$^+$	115	HCO$_3^-$	10
			HPO$_4^{2-}$	85
			H$_2$PO$_4^-$	15
		125		125
mmol/l	glucose	200		

resembles the normal portal blood pressure in humans. The hepatic arterial system is flushed in combination with the kidneys through the aortic cannula with a total of 2 l of solution all the while maintaining a pressure of approximately 100 cm H_2O.

At the back table, the whole liver is submitted to a thorough inspection. Injuries to the vascular and biliary structures are located and repaired.

The vascular structures of the liver are trimmed and the orifices of the dia-phragmatic veins into the caval vein are accurately sutured. The gall bladder and bile ducts are irrigated, to wash out the bile. The hepatic artery is flushed with approximately 100 ml Euro Collins' solution. The liver is placed in a tightly sealed plastic box floating in Euro Collins' solution at 4° C. The box is packed in three sterile bags and transported in a polystyrene container filled with crushed ice.

Conclusion

Successful multiple organ procurement requires an efficient organisation, excellent donor management and a standard operative procedure performed by a selected team. The procedure described is flexible enough to allow removal of the heart, liver, kidneys, pancreas and intestine from one single donor. Immediate organ function after transplantation, especially in heart and liver recipients, must be kept in mind at all times. Avoidance of liver cell ischaemia, vascular and biliary tract lesions and contamination will increase the survival of liver transplants.

Acknowledgments

Mrs. M.F. de Bruijn-Beeching edited the English and Ms. M.T. Bouritius, and Mrs. A.W.H. van der Velde-Palm provided secretarial assistance.

References

1. Calne RY, Williams R: Liver transplantation in man – I. Br Med J (4):535–540, 1968.
2. Starzl TE: Experience in hepatic transplantation. Philadelphia, WB Saunders, 1969.
3. Shaw BW Jr, Hakala T, Rosenthal JT *et al*: Combination donor hepatectomy and nephrectomy and early functional results of allografts. Surg Gynecol Obstet (155):321–325, 1982.
4. Rolles K, Calne RY, McMaster P: Technique of organ removal and fate of kidney grafts from liver donors. Transplantation (28):44–46, 1979.
5. Slooff MJH, Kremer GD, Lichtendahl DHE, Krom RAF: Surgical and functional aspects of combined donor nephrectomy and hepatectomy: Transplant Proc (16):1346–1347, 1984.
6. Krom RAF, Gips CH: Skills and resources needed for liver transplantation. Hepatology (4):72S–75S, 1984.
7. Cooper DKC, de Villiers JC, Smith LS *et al*: Medical, legal and administrative aspects of cadaveric organ donation in the Republic of South Africa. S Afr Med J (62):933, 1982.
8. Starzl TE, Hakala TR, Shaw BW Jr *et al*: A flexible procedure for multiple cadaveric organ procurement. Surg Gynecol Obstet (158):223–230, 1984.

25. Status of liver transplantation in Europe

B. RINGE

Activity in liver transplantation is steadily growing throughout the world. This is reflected by two surveys from last year. According to the situation in Europe, Starzl reported on 424 recipients treated in nine institutions by July 1, 1984 [1]. Scharschmidt analyzed data on 819 total patients 319 of whom had been transplanted in three experienced European centers between May 1968 and August last year [2].

In a recent inquiry overall figures were obtained directly from centers with active liver transplant programs in Western Europe (Table 1). Deadline for these data was January 1, 1985. Up to that moment a total of 639 liver transplants had been performed in 610 patients. This activity is distributed among 25 institutions in 13 different countries. So far there are 12 centers – the majority of them being experienced in this field for many years – with at least ten patients treated. Additional trials have been done among newly-established groups. Compared to the reviews previously mentioned, there has been a remarkable increased progress in hepatic transplantation.

With respect to these crude data several substantial questions arise. Sooner or later the demand to establish the number of liver transplants as well as transplant centers needed per country is obvious. Intensified cooperation between different organ procurement programs may lead to a European network of liver exchange. The establishment of an international liver transplant registry for collection and analysis of all essential data seems to be of great benefit.

Table 1. Frequency of liver transplantation in Europe (January 1, 1985).

Country	Center	Transplants	Patients
Austria	Innsbruck	16	16
	Vienna	34	33
Belgium	Brussels (Louvain)	10	10
	Brussels (Erasme)	3	3
Finland	Helsinki	2	2
France	Montpellier	40	40
	Nice	2	2
	Rennes	6	6
	Villejuif	25	23
Germany	Berlin (Charité)	32	32
	Berlin (Steglitz)	2	2
	Bonn	18	18
	Hamburg	5	4
	Hannover	147	134
	Tübingen	4	4
Great Britain	Birmingham	17	16
	Cambridge/London (King's)	197	191
	London	9	7
Italy	Milan	3	3
	Rome	6	6
Netherlands	Groningen	41	39
Norway	Oslo	3	3
Spain	Barcelona	13	13
Sweden	Stockholm	1	1
Switzerland	Berne	3	2
total:		639	610

References

1. Starzl TE, Iwazuki S, Shaw BW, Gordon RD: Orthotopic liver transplantation in 1984. Transplant Proc 17:250, 1985.
2. Scharschmidt BF: Human liver transplantation: Analysis of 819 patients from four centers (in press).

26. Human liver transplantation: Analysis of data on 540 patients from four centers

B.F. SCHARSCHMIDT

Abstract

The results of liver transplantation in a total of 540 patients from four centers in the United States and Western Europe have been collated. Twenty-five per cent of all transplants were performed for neoplastic disease. One- and 3-year survivals for this group were approximately 26 and 12% overall, and survival differed little for patients transplanted before and after January 1, 1980. Among the 44% of patients transplanted for endstage cirrhosis, 3-year survival was lowest for patients with alcoholic cirrhosis (20%). Three-year survival was greater for patients with nonalcoholic cirrhosis (29% overall), did not differ markedly among the various subtypes, and was greater for patients transplanted after January 1, 1980 (42%), as compared with before (22%). Patients with biliary atresia, sclerosing cholangitis, and metabolic and miscellaneous disorders constituted the remaining 30% of patients; 3-year survival varied from about 20 to 44% overall for the various subgroups, with a consistent trend toward improved survival among patients transplanted after January 1, 1980. The use of cyclosporin may not wholly explain this improved survival among more recently transplanted patients. Quality of life for transplant recipients surviving at least 3 months, as judged by a limited amount of data regarding time-in-hospital and functional status, appears to be good.

Introduction

Liver transplantation in humans has been performed for at least 20 years, and the experience of several centers active in this field has been periodically summarized in published form. However, because of differences in presentation format, the published data are not readily integratable so as to permit an overview of current

(Reprinted with permission from: *Hepatology*, Vol. 4, no. 1, pp. 95S–101S, 1984).

transplantation experience. The purpose of this project was to analyze in a uniform fashion the data from four selected centers.

Materials and methods

Data gathering

Transplantation data were requested from four centers in the United States and Western Europe. The location of these centers as well as the corresponding physician and total number of patients are summarized in Table 1.

The data requested regarding each transplant recipient are summarized in Table 2. As indicated in the table, some data were not provided by all correspondents or were provided in differing fashions so as to hamper collation. In addition, general statements were requested from each center regarding the criteria for acceptance or rejection of individual patients and the average survival of patients accepted but not transplanted.

Data analyses

Over 30 different diagnoses were represented among transplant recipients, and a number of other factors potentially bearing on survival (age, sex, ethnicity, immunosuppressive therapy, date of transplant, and transplant center) were available for analysis. It was, thus, not feasible to characterize survival for each diagnosis separately and, at the same time, to examine the effects of all other variables.

The problem was, therefore, approached by first identifying potentially important differences among centers in patient selection and survival. Then, using the

Table 1. Transplant centers providing data for the present analysis.

No.*	Location	Corresponding surgeon	Total no. of patients
1	University of Pittsburgh Pittsburgh, Pa.	Dr. Thomas E. Starzl	296
2	University Hospital Groningen Groningen, The Netherlands	Dr. Ruud A.F. Krom	26
3	University of Hannover Hannover, West Germany	Dr. Rudolf Pichlmayr	81
4	University of Cambridge Cambridge, England	Dr. Keith Rolles	137

* Designates the identifying number of the center for the purposes of this analysis.

pooled data, survival was characterized for all patients with neoplastic and nonneoplastic disease as well as for patients in each of the major diagnostic categories, and for each level of the other factors believed to be most critical such as date of transplant and immunosuppressive therapy. At the same time, causes of death and certain other pertinent patient characteristics were tabulated.

For these analyses, all data were coded, transferred to punched cards, and analyzed using the BMDP1L program [1]. Estimated survival probabilities were obtained for 1-month time intervals following transplantation using the adjusted life table method. The effect of selected variables on survival was assessed using the log-rank test, and p values <0.05 were taken to be statistically significant [2].

Results and discussion

Diagnoses and epidemiologic data among transplant recipients

A total of 33 different diagnoses were represented among the 540 patients. For these analyses only the primary diagnoses were considered. Most importantly, if a patient was transplanted for a malignancy superimposed on a nonmalignant condition (e.g. hepatocellular carcinoma arising in a cirrhotic liver), only the malignancy was considered for the purposes of analysis. As summarized in Table 3, the frequency of various diagnoses differed among centers. Tumors were disproportionately represented in centers 3 and 4, whereas neonatal cholestatic disorders, sclerosing cholangitis, and metabolic disorders were disproportionately represented at center 1. Nonalcoholic cirrhosis was a frequent diagnosis at all four centers and the most common diagnosis overall, representing 39% of patients. Neoplastic disease constituted 26% of patients overall and was the next most frequent diagnostic category, followed in order by neonatal cholestatic disorders (predominantly biliary atresia), metabolic disorders, alcoholic cirrhosis, sclerosing cholangitis, and miscellaneous.

Table 2. Data requested for all transplant recipients.

Age	Date of last follow-up
Race	Condition at last follow-up
	Alive/dead
Sex	Functional status[a]
Diagnosis	If alive, evidence of rejection?[a]
Date of transplant(s)	If dead, cause of death?[a]
Immunosuppressive therapy	Total hospitalization time from transplantation
	to last follow-up[a]

[a] Indicates data not provided by all correspondents or provided in varying ways so as to hamper collation.

Table 3. Diagnoses of patients undergoing transplantation.

	Center no.				Total
	1	2	3	4	
Tumors (all types)	36	1	44	58	139
	(12.2)	(3.8)	(54.3)	(42.3)	(25.7)
Hepatocellular carcinoma	25	1	30	32	88
	(8.4)	(3.8)	(37.0)	(23.4)	(16.3)
Cholangiocarcinoma	9	0	9	18	36
	(3.0)	(0.)	(11.1)	(13.1)	(6.7)
Other primary tumors (adenoma,	2	0	0	4	7
angiosarcoma, mesenchymoma)	(0.7)	(0.)	(0.)	(3.6)	(1.3)
Metastatic	0	0	5	4	8
	(0.)	(0.)	(6.2)	(2.2)	(1.5)
Cirrhosis (all types)	123	24	26	62	235
	(41.6)	(92.3)	(32.1)	(45.3)	(43.5)
Alcoholic	17	0	3	5	25
	(5.7)	(0.)	(3.7)	(3.6)	(4.6)
Nonalcoholic (all types)	106	24	23	57	210
	(35.8)	(92.3)	(28.4)	(41.6)	(38.9)
Primary biliary	23	10	3	26	62
	(7.8)	(38.5)	(3.7)	(19.0)	(11.5)
Secondary biliary	8	0	1	4	13
	(2.7)	(0.)	(1.2)	(2.9)	(2.4)
Postnecrotic/chronic active	2	14	19	13	48
hepatitis	(0.7)	(53.9)	(23.5)	(9.5)	(8.9)
Cryptogenic/unspecified	73	0	0	14	87
	(24.7)	(0.)	(0.)	(10.2)	(16.1)
Neonatal cholestasis	79	0	9	2	90
	(26.7)	(0.)	(11.1)	(1.5)	(16.7)
Biliary atresia	72	0	9	2	83
	(24.3)	(0.)	(11.1)	(1.5)	(15.4)
Other (Byler's disease, neonatal	7	0	0	0	7
hepatitis)	(2.4)	(0.)	(0.)	(0.)	(1.3)
Sclerosing cholangitis	16	0	0	3	19
	(5.4)	(0.)	(0.)	(0.)	(3.5)
Metabolic disorders	32	0	0	3	35
	(10.8)	(0.)	(0.)	(2.2)	(6.5)
α_1-antitrypsin deficiency	23	0	0	1	24
	(7.8)	(0.)	(0.)	(0.7)	(4.4)
Wilson's disease	4	0	0	1	5
	(1.4)	(0.)	(0.)	(0.7)	(0.9)
Other (glycogen storage disease,	5	0	0	1	6
protoporphyria, galactosemia,	(1.7)	(0.)	(0.)	(0.7)	(1.1)
hemochromatosis, tyrosinemia,					
etc.)					
Miscellaneous	10	1	2	9	22
	(3.4)	(3.8)	(2.5)	(6.6)	(4.1)

Table 3. Continued.

	Center no.				Total
	1	2	3	4	
Budd-Chiari syndrome	5	1	1	7	14
	(1.7)	(3.8)	(1.2)	(5.1)	(2.6)
Acute hepatic failure	2	0	0	0	2
	(0.7)	(0.)	(0.)	(0.)	(0.4)
Other (cystic disorders, congenital	3	0	1	2	6
hepatic fibrosis, nodular	(1.0)	(0.)	(1.2)	(1.5)	(1.1)
transformation)					

* The number without parentheses represents the actual number of patients, while the number in parentheses represents the per cent of the total.

As would be anticipated, patients in the pediatric age group were disproportionately represented among those centers transplanting patients with neonatal cholestatic disorders (Table 4). Overall, males and females were about equally represented, and the transplanted patients were predominantly white (Table 4).

Center-by-center analysis of survival

A center-by-center analysis of survival was undertaken for both malignant and nonmalignant disease, each analyzed separately for patients transplanted before and after January 1, 1980. As summarized in Table 5, center 1, which accounted for most patients, tended to report higher 1-year survival probabilities than the remaining centers. This difference is attributable at least in part to differences in patient selection.

The center-by-center comparisons summarized in Tables 3 to 5 thus revealed clear-cut differences in patient selection and survival. While not considered so

Table 4. Epidemiology of transplant recipients.

	Center no.				Overall
	1	2	3	4	
Age ≤18 (% of total patients)	46.6	7.7	22.2	8.1	31.3
Sex (male/female)	1.08	2.7	0.93	1.21	1.13
Race					
White (%)	88.9	100.	98.8	98.5	93.3
Black (%)	8.8	0.	1.2	0.	5.0
Other/unspecified (%)	2.4	0.	0.	1.5	1.7

Table 5. Center-by-center analysis of survival.

Diagnosis/transplant date	1-year survival/no. of patients[a]			
	Center no.			
	1	2	3	4
Neoplastic disease				
Before January 1, 1980	30.4%	–[b]	16.7%	14.9%
	(23)	(1)	(6)	(47)
After January 1, 1980	59.3%	–	20.5%	45.4%
	(13)	(0)	(38)	(11)
Nonneoplastic disease				
Before January 1, 1980	32.2%	–	11.1%	27.3%
	(146)	(3)	(9)	(44)
After January 1, 1980	54.0%	60.0%	48.2%	34.3%
	(114)	(22)	(28)	(35)

[a] Per cent indicates per cent 1-year survival, while the total number of patients in each group is enclosed in parentheses.
[b] Indicates insufficient data.

great as to preclude meaningful collation, these important differences need to be kept in mind when interpreting the figures for overall survival as summarized below.

Overall analysis of survival: neoplastic disease

The survival of patients transplanted for neoplastic disease, analyzed both in a 'lumped' fashion as well as separately for a number of variables, is summarized in Table 6. For all 139 patients, a median survival of 4.1 months was calculated with the probability of survival being about 50% at 3 months, 26% at 1 year, and 12% at 3 years. In an attempt to assess the impact of improved surgical technique, better supportive care, and newer immunosuppressive therapy, survival was separately analyzed for patients transplanted before and after January 1, 1980, and was found not to be different (Table 6 and Figure 1). Survival was also not different among additional subgroups analyzed separately including cyclosporin vs. no cyclosporin – both for all patients and only those transplanted after 1980.

Overall analysis of survival: nonneoplastic disease

The survival of patients transplanted for nonneoplastic disease, analyzed both in a 'lumped fashion' as well as separately for a number of variables, is summarized in Table 7. For all 401 patients, a median survival of 3.0 months was calculated,

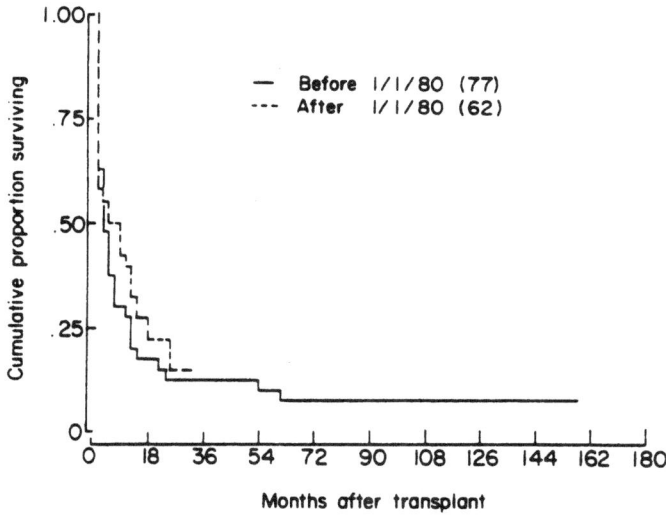

Figure 1. Actuarial survival of 139 patients transplanted for neoplastic disease at all four centers before and after January 1, 1980. In this and subsequent figures, areas in which the two survival plots coincide are represented by a *dashed line.*

with the probability of survival being about 48% at 3 months, 39% at 1 year, and 30% at 3 years. Unlike patients with neoplastic disease, the overall survival was better (p<0.001) for patients transplanted after January 1, 1980, than before (Table 7 and Figure 2). The 1-year survival in these two groups was 50 and 29%, respectively. When patients transplanted after 1980 who received cyclosporin were compared with those transplanted after January 1, 1980 who did not, no

Table 6. Survival of patients transplanted for neoplastic disease at all four centers.

Variable	Median survival (months)	Survival probability at intervals (%)		
		≥3 months	≥1 year	≥3 years
All patients (139)[a]	4.1	50.3	25.8	12.5
All males (71)	3.7	49.1	15.6	7.6
All females (68)	5.0	51.5	34.8	17.1
Transplant before January 1, 1980 (77)	2.9	46.8	20.8	11.7
Transplant after January 1, 1980 (62)	5.9	54.7	32.8	–[b]
Cyclosporin (43)	8.4	58.0	42.7	14.9
No cyclosporin (96)	2.8	46.9	19.8	9.7
Transplant after January 1, 1980 with cyclosporin (42)	8.2	57.0	41.1	–
Transplant after January 1, 1980 without cyclosporin (20)	5.0	50.0	20.0	–

[a] Number in parentheses indicates number of patients in group.

[b] Indicates insufficient data.

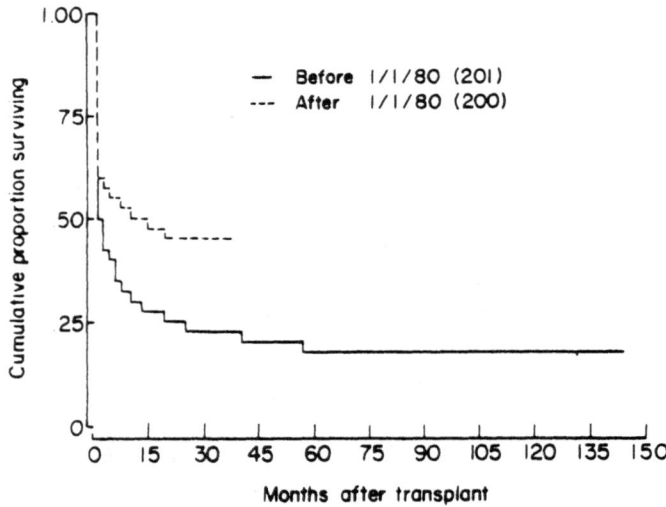

Figure 2. Actuarial survival of 401 patients transplanted for nonneoplastic disease at all four centers before and after January 1, 1980. These two curves were significantly different (p<0.001).

significant difference was observed (p = 0.39) (Table 7 and Figure 3). While this suggests that factors other than cyclosporin contributed most importantly to the improved survival after 1980, this analysis is flawed by a number of factors. For example, all patients transplanted after 1980 at center 1 received cyclosporin, whereas none of the patients transplanted at center 2 received cyclosporin. Thus, the comparison is also, to a certain degree, a comparison among centers. Indeed,

Table 7. Survival of patients transplanted for nonneoplastic disease at all four centers.

Variable	Median survival (months)	Survival probability at intervals (%)		
		≥3 months	≥1 year	≥3 years
All patients (401)[a]	3.0	47.6	38.7	29.9
All males (183)	2.4	42.9	34.4	27.2
All females (218)	4.9	51.4	42.3	32.2
Transplant before January 1, 1980 (201)	2.0	40.3	29.4	21.4
Transplant after January 1, 1980 (200)	14.0	55.8	50.1	45.0
Cyclosporin (170)	19.4	60.3	54.4	49.0
No cyclosporin (231)	1.8	38.9	28.6	20.3
Transplant after January 1, 1980 with cyclosporin (161)	14.5	57.9	51.4	44.8
Transplant after January 1, 1980 without cyclosporin (39)	1.6	47.0	43.8	–[b]

[a] Number in parentheses indicates number of patients in group.

[b] Indicates insufficient data for meaningful analysis.

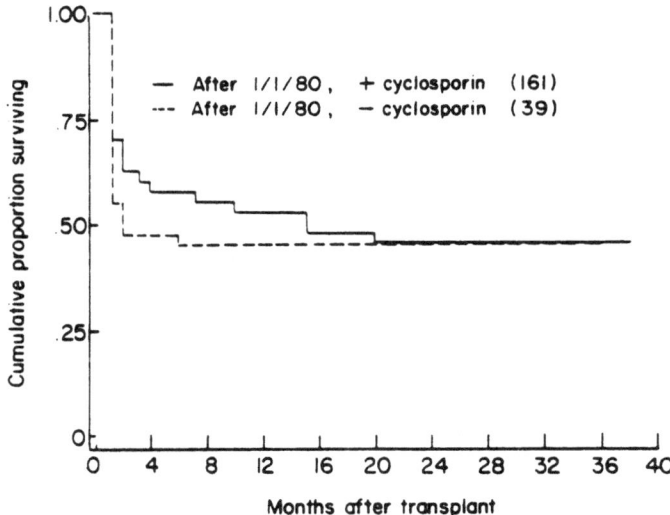

Figure 3. Actuarial survival of 200 patients transplanted for nonneoplastic disease after January 1, 1980 who did or did not receive cyclosporin. These two curves were not significantly different (p = 0.39).

most of the patients transplanted after 1980 who did not receive cyclosporin were from center 2, where stringent selection criteria probably excluded critically ill patients who might have been accepted at the other centers. Moreover, this analysis ignores differences in diagnoses among the cyclosporin and noncyclosporin groups as well as differences in the timing and route of administration of cyclosporin and differences in dosage. Nonetheless, the results do indicate that 1-year survival rates exceeding 50% are achievable without cyclosporin. As for patients with neoplastic disease, a trend toward improved survival for females as compared with males was observed, but it did not reach statistical significance (p = 0.16).

Analysis of survival by disease and date of transplant

The analyses of survival on a disease-by-disease basis stratified by date of transplantation (before and after January 1, 1980) are summarized in Table 8 and Figures 4 to 13. Patients transplanted for neoplastic disease had a lower overall survival than did patients transplanted for nonneoplastic disease, and within the neoplastic disease group, patients with hepatocellular carcinoma tended to have a modestly better survival than patients with cholangiocarcinoma. Among patients transplanted for cirrhosis, survival was greater overall for patients with nonalcoholic cirrhosis as compared with alcoholic cirrhosis. For patients with nonalcoholic cirrhosis, no striking differences were observed among those with primary biliary cirrhosis, postnecrotic cirrhosis/chronic active hepatitis, and cryptogenic or unspecified types (latter group not included in Table 8). Survival

Disease	All patients					Transplant before January 1, 1980					Transplant after January 1, 1980				
	No.	Median survival (months)	Survival probability at intervals (%)			No.	Median survival (months)	Survival probability at intervals (%)			No.	Median survival (months)	Survival probability at intervals (%)		
			≥3 mos	≥1 yr	≥3 yr			≥3 mos	≥1 yr	≥3 yr			≥3 mos	≥1 yr	≥3 yr
Tumors (all types)	139	4.1	50.3	25.8	12.5	77	2.9	46.8	20.8	11.7	62	5.9	54.7	32.8	–
Hepatocellular carcinoma	88	5.4	55.7	32.9	16.7	47	4.8	55.3	29.8	17.0	41	8.1	56.0	37.0	–
Cholangiocarcinoma	36	2.6	47.0	17.4	7.0	22	1.7	31.8	9.1	4.6	14	9.7	71.4	31.8	–
Cirrhosis (all types)	235	2.2	45.9	36.5	28.6	116	1.7	40.5	29.3	21.6	119	5.2	51.6	44.9	40.8
Alcoholic	25	1.1	24.0	20.0	20.0	20	1.3	25.0	20.0	20.0	5	0.6	20.0	20.0	–
Nonalcoholic (all types)	210	2.9	48.6	38.5	29.4	96	1.9	43.8	31.2	21.9	114	5.8	53.0	46.0	41.7
Primary biliary	62	5.3	51.1	41.6	37.6	18	2.0	38.9	33.3	27.8	44	6.4	56.4	45.0	45.0
Postnecrotic/chronic active	48	1.1	43.8	41.2	30.0	13	1.2	38.5	30.8	23.1	35	1.0	46.1	46.1	39.5
Biliary atresia/neonatal cholestasis	90	4.2	50.3	39.1	28.2	52	2.0	38.5	25.0	15.4	38	–	69.2	63.9	–
Sclerosing cholangitis	19	2.0	33.6	20.2	20.2	7	2.5	28.6	14.3	14.3	12	1.8	37.3	24.8	24.8
Metabolic disorders (all types)	35	28.2	55.1	51.8	44.4	16	3.0	43.8	37.8	31.2	19	–	65.5	65.5	65.5
α_1-antitrypsin deficiency	24	28.2	56.5	51.6	41.3	10	4.0	50.0	40.0	30.0	14	–	61.3	61.3	61.3
Wilson's disease	5	–	80.0	80.0	80.0	2	–	100	100	100	3	–	66.6	66.6	–
Miscellaneous															
Budd-Chiari	14	–	71.4	71.4	54.0	5	–	60.0	60.0	60.0	9	19.9	77.8	77.8	47.7
Acute hepatic failure	2	–	0	–	–	1	–	9	–	–	1	–	0	–	–
Caroli's disease	2	–	0	–	–	1	–	0	–	–	1	–	0	–	–
Congenital hepatic fibrosis	2	–	50	50	50	1	–	0	–	–	1	–	100	100	–
Nodular transformation	1	–	100	100	100	1	–	100	100	100	0	–	–	–	–

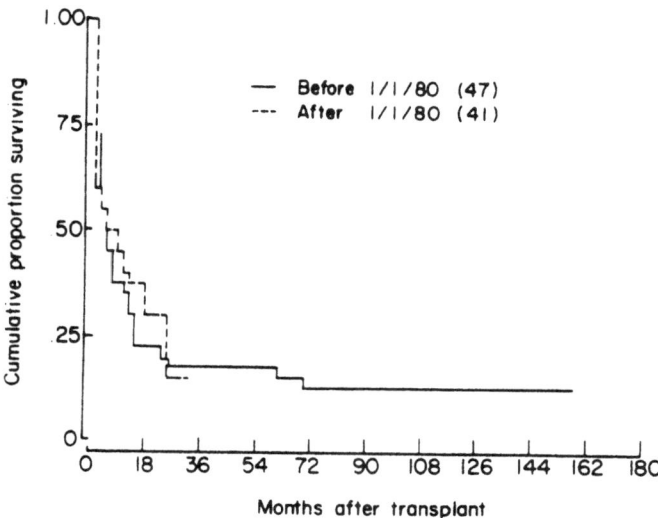

Figure 4. Actuarial survival of 88 patients transplanted for hepatocellular carcinoma before and after January 1, 1980.

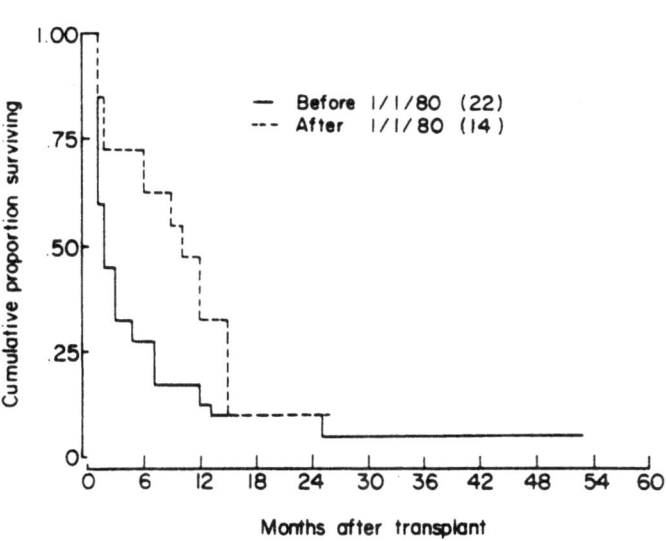

Figure 5. Actuarial survival of 36 patients transplanted for cholangiocarcinoma before and after January 1, 1980.

tended to be greater for patients transplanted after January 1, 1980, as compared with before January 1, 1980 for all groups for which sufficient data was available except for patients with alcoholic cirrhosis and patients with neoplastic disease.

Survival among patients receiving more than one transplant

Fifty-two patients, almost 10% of the total, received a second liver transplant due to failure of the first. The diagnoses among these patients are summarized in Table 9 and included nearly all categories of neoplastic and nonneoplastic disease for which transplants were performed. Not unexpectedly, the survival in this group was less than for patients receiving only one transplant, with the 1-year survival probability being 38% and there being no survivors beyond 3 years.

Survival among patients selected for transplantation but not actually receiving a graft

Detailed information for patients in this category was not provided by any of the four centers. A summary statement from center 1 indicated that the overall 1-year survival of patients who were selected for transplantation but did not actually receive a graft was effectively zero.

Causes of death

Analysis of the causes of death (Table 10) was hampered by the large number of patients for which the precise cause of death was not specified and the difficulty in determining the primary cause, when multiple causes were listed. It is of potential interest that rejection was identified as a cause in less than 10% of cases, and causes of death not necessarily directly liver-related such as infection predominated overall. Recurrent tumor accounted for about 9% of all deaths after 3 months (Table 10).

Quality of life

An attempt was made to assess quality of life by requesting information on the total number of weeks spent in the hospital and functional status. Such data was provided for a minority of patients. Among all patients, living and dead, who survived between 4 and 12 months after transplantation (data base = 23 patients), the mean total number of weeks spent in the hospital after transplantation was 12.6. Among all patients, living and dead, who survived at least 1 year after

Table 9. Diagnoses among patients receiving two or more liver transplants.

Diagnoses	No. of patients	% of total
Hepatocellular carcinoma	3	5.8
Cholangiocarcinoma	1	1.9
Alcoholic cirrhosis	3	5.8
Primary biliary cirrhosis	5	9.6
Secondary biliary cirrhosis	2	3.8
Postnecrotic cirrhosis/chronic active hepatitis	2	3.8
Nonalcoholic cirrhosis (unspecified)	9	17.3
Biliary atresia (all types)	12	23.1
Neonatal hepatitis	1	1.9
Sclerosing cholangitis	5	9.6
α_1-antitrypsin deficiency	6	11.5
Wilson's disease	1	1.9
Glycogen storage disease	1	1.9
Budd-Chiari syndrome	1	1.9
	52	100

Table 10. Causes of death.

Cause	Percentage of patients to which each cause applied[a]	
	Patients dying ≤ 3 months after transplantation (n = 274)	Patients dying >3 months after transplantation (n = 101)
Directly liver-related		
Unspecified	17.8	9.9
Hepatic failure	7.7	21.8
Rejection	8.8	8.9
Recurrent disease (hepatitis, Budd-Chiari, primary biliary cirrhosis)	0	6.9
Not directly liver-related		
Unspecified	25.2	34.6
Operative/technical complications[b]	38.3	17.8
Hemorrhage	11.0	5.0
Infection	26.6	27.7
Recurrent tumor	0.7	8.9[c]

[a] Each number denotes the percentage of patients dying within the specified time to which each cause of death applied. Because certain patients were listed as having more than one cause of death, the total of each column is greater than 100%.

[b] Includes intraoperative deaths as well as late deaths due to biliary tract stricture.

[c] Very likely represents an underestimate inasmuch as causes of death were not specified for many patients transplanted for neoplastic disease.

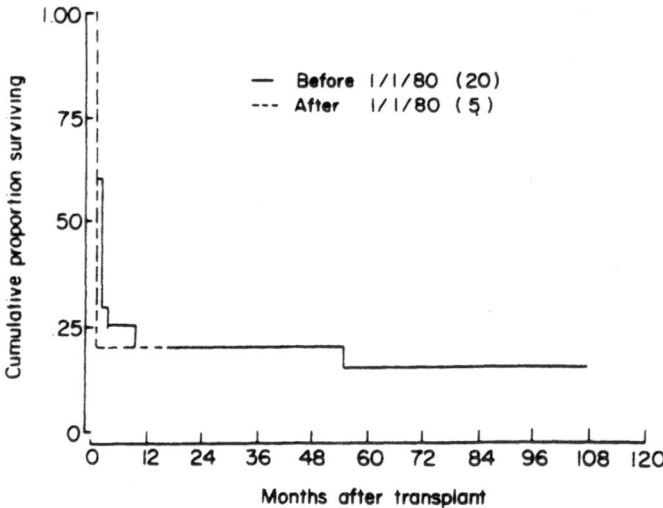

Figure 6. Actuarial survival of 25 patients transplanted for alcoholic cirrhosis before and after January 1, 1980.

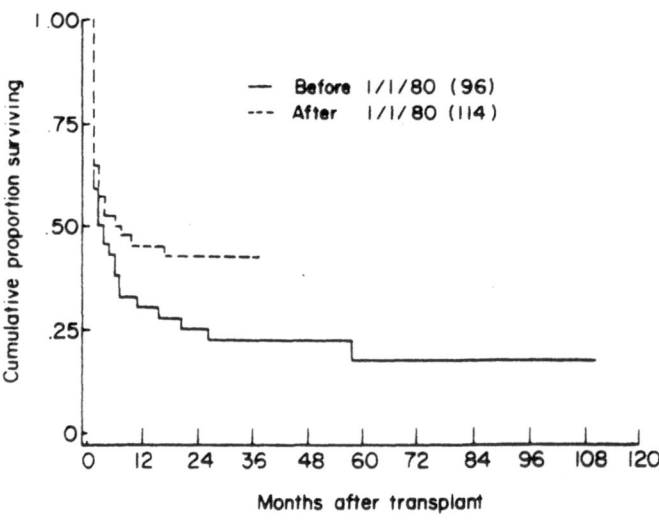

Figure 7. Actuarial survival of 210 patients transplanted for all types of nonalcoholic cirrhosis before and after January 1, 1980. This figure includes data for 100 patients designated as having nonalcoholic cirrhosis (type unspecified) or cryptogenic cirrhosis as well as for the 110 patients included in Figures 8 and 9.

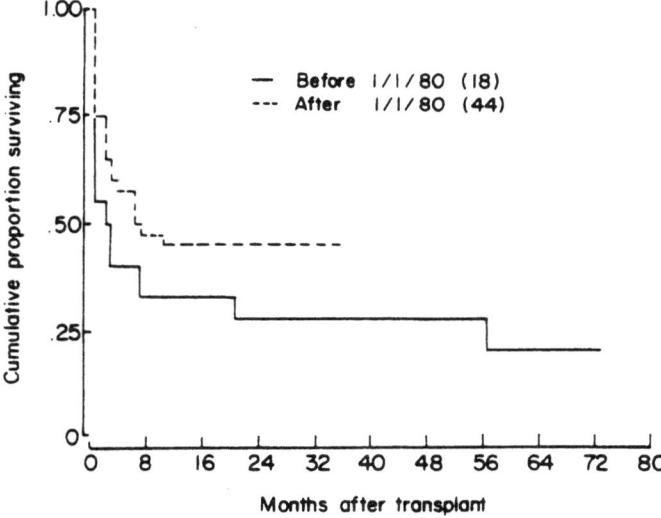

Figure 8. Actuarial survival of 62 patients transplanted for primary biliary cirrhosis before and after January 1, 1980.

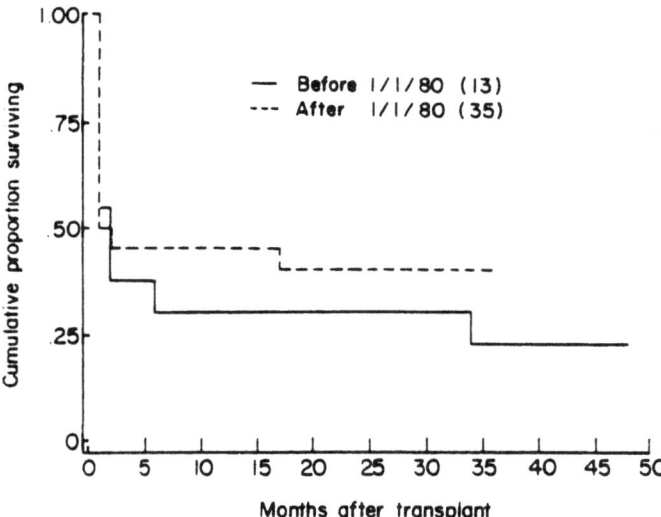

Figure 9. Actuarial survival of 48 patients transplanted for the diagnoses of postnecrotic cirrhosis, chronic active cirrhosis, and chronic active hepatitis before and after January 1, 1980.

264

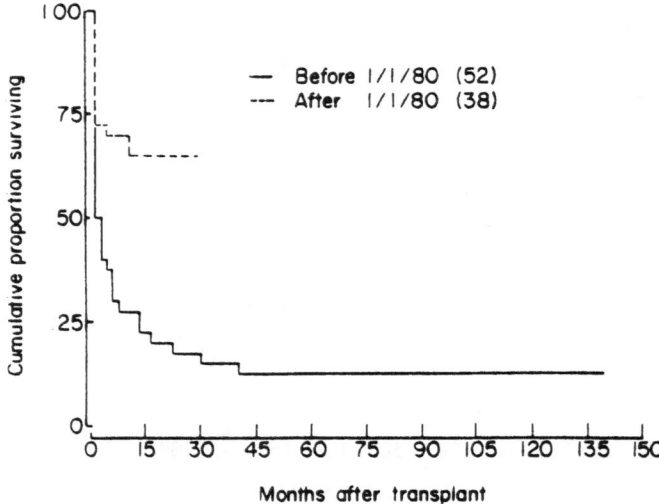

Figure 10. Actuarial survival of 90 patients transplanted for neonatal cholestatic disorders (almost exclusively biliary atresia) before and after January 1, 1980.

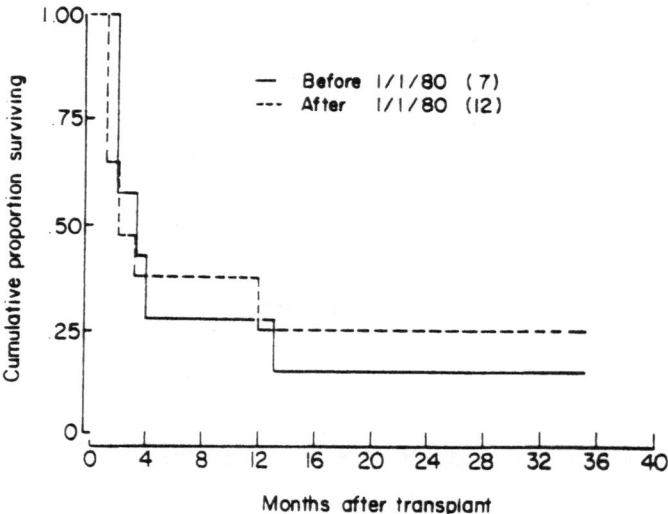

Figure 11. Actuarial survival of 19 patients transplanted for sclerosing cholangitis before and after January 1, 1980.

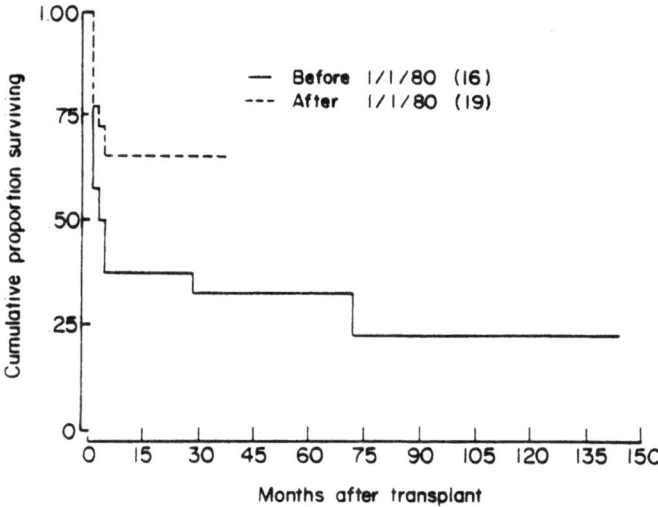

Figure 12. Actuarial survival of 35 patients transplanted for metabolic disorders before and after January 1, 1980.

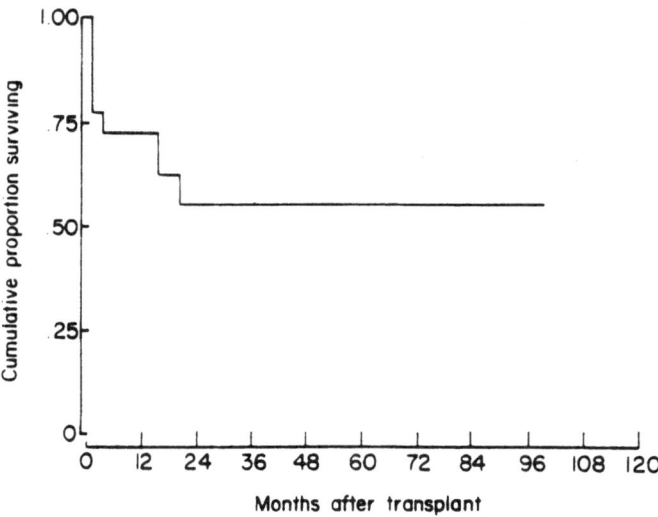

Figure 13. Actuarial survival of 14 patients transplanted for the Budd-Chiari syndrome. The small number of patients precluded meaningful analysis of the pre- and post-January 1, 1980, subgroups.

transplantation (data base = 22 patients), the mean number of weeks spent in the hospital after transplantation was 9.2. When one considers that these average figures reflect the initial hospitalization time for all patients as well as terminal hospitalization time for patients who died after 1 year, it seems reasonable to conclude that patients still living after 1 year spend a very small proportion of their time in the hospital.

Among 184 patients at centers 2 to 4 still living at least 4 months after transplantation for whom data were available, 179 were listed in good condition (fully rehabilitated), while only three were listed in fair condition (able to care for self), and two in poor condition (needs care). A recent survey of transplant recipients at center 1 indicated that greater than 80% of patients surviving longer than 1 year had resumed their former occupation or activities. Thus, as assessed by hospitalization time and functional status, the quality of life for transplant recipients surviving at least four or more months appears to be good.

Conclusions

Based upon an analysis of 540 patients from four centers, the survival of patients transplanted for neoplastic disease is less than that of patients transplanted for nonneoplastic disease. Among patients with nonneoplastic disease, survival is better for patients transplanted after January 1, 1980, as compared with before, and this improvement may not be wholly attributable to the more recent use of cyclosporin. The quality of life for transplant recipients, surviving at least 4 months, as judged by limited data regarding hospitalization time and functional status, appears to be good.

Acknowledgments

The author wishes to acknowledge Drs. David Heilbron and Alan Bostrom of Scientific Computing Services, University of California, San Francisco, for their expert assistance in analysis of the transplantation data, as well as Diana Fedorchak and Michael Karasik for their skillful preparation of the manuscript and continued support throughout this project. Dr. Scharschmidt is supported in part by NIH Research Grants AM-26270 and AM-26743.

References

1. Dixon W-J: BMDP statistical software. Berkeley, CA, University of California Press, 1981.
2. Savage IR: Contributions to theory of rank order statistics – The two sample case. Ann Math Stat 27:590–650, 1956.

27. Liver transplantation: Summary of the National Institutes of Health Consensus Development Conference (Volume 4, Number 7)

Members of the Consensus Development Panel:
R. SCHMID, D.H. BERWICK, B. COMBES, R.B. D'AGOSTINO,
S.H. DANOVITCH, H.J. FALLON, O. JONASSON, C.E. MILLARD,
L. MILLER, F.G. MOODY, W.K. SCHUBERT, L. SHANDLER
and H.J. WINN

Introduction

Since performance of the first human orthotopic liver transplantation in 1963, over 540 such operations have been carried out in four medical centers in the United States and Western Europe. Additional liver transplantation procedures have been performed in other parts of the world, and more recently in several other American medical centers. Although extremely demanding and expensive, the operation has been shown to be technically feasible, and interpretable results have been reported from all four primary transplant centers. These clearly demonstrate that liver transplantation offers an alternative therapeutic approach which may prolong life in some patients suffering from severe liver disease that has progressed beyond the reach of currently available treatment and consequently carries a predictably poor prognosis. However, substantial questions remain regarding selection of patients who may benefit from liver transplantation; the stage of their liver disease at which transplantation should be performed; survival and clinical condition of patients beyond the initial year after transplantation; and overall long-range benefits and risks of transplantation in the management of specific liver diseases.

In order to resolve some of these questions, the National Institutes of Health on June 20–23, 1983, convened a Consensus Development Conference on Liver Transplantation. After 2 days of expert presentation of the available data, a Consensus Panel consisting of hepatologists, surgeons, internists, pediatricians, immunologists, biostatisticians, ethicists, and public representatives considered the offered evidence to arrive at answers to the following key questions:

1. Are there groups of patients for whom transplantation of the liver should be considered appropriate therapy?
2. What is the outcome (current survival rates, complications) in different groups?
3. In a potential candidate for transplantation, what are the principles guiding

selection of the appropriate time for surgery?
4. What are the skills, resources, and institutional support needed for liver transplantation?
5. What are the directions for future research?

1. Are there groups of patients for whom transplantation of the liver should be considered appropriate therapy?

Liver transplantation is a promising alternative to current therapy in the management of the late phase of several forms of serious liver disease. Candidates include children and adults suffering from irreversible liver injury who have exhausted alternative medical and surgical treatments and are approaching the terminal phase of their illness. In many forms of liver disease the precise indications and timing of liver transplantation remain uncertain or controversial.

Prolongation of life of good quality for patients who would otherwise have died has been reported in the following conditions:

- *Extrahepatic biliary atresia* is the most common cause of bile duct obstruction in the young infant. Patients who fail to respond to hepatoportoenterostomy (Kasai procedure) often benefit from liver transplantation. Recent data suggest that as many as two-thirds of these patients survive for 1 year or more after transplantation.
- *Chronic active hepatitis* is caused by viral infections or drug reactions, but many cases remain unexplained. Some patients with progressive liver failure are candidates for transplantation. Currently, exceptions seem to include drug-induced chronic active hepatitis, which usually responds to removal of the chemical agent, and hepatitis B-induced disease in which viremia persists. In the latter instance, rapid reappearance of infection with progressive liver failure has been reported following transplantation.
- *Primary biliary cirrhosis* is a slowly progressive cholestatic liver disease. Results of transplantation appear favorable for patients with end-stage liver injury. The procedure may improve the quality of life.
- *Inborn errors of metabolism* may cause end-stage liver damage or irreversible extrahepatic complications. Transplantation may be appropriate for such patients.
- *Hepatic vein thrombosis* (Budd-Chiari syndrome) often results in progressive liver failure, ascites, and death. Patients who have not responded to anticoagulation or appropriate surgery for portal decompression may be candidates for transplantation.
- *Sclerosing cholangitis*, a chronic non-suppurative inflammatory process of the bile ducts, may cause liver failure. Less favorable results following transplantation in this group may be due to prior multiple surgical procedures, a diseased extrahepatic bile duct, the presence of biliary infection, or other factors.

– *Primary hepatic malignancy* confined to the liver but no amenable to resection may be an indication for transplantation. Results to date indicate a strong likelihood of recurrence of the malignancy. Nonetheless, the procedure may achieve significant palliation.

– *Alcohol-related liver cirrhosis and alcoholic hepatitis* are the most common forms of fatal liver disease in America. Patients who are judged likely to abstain from alcohol and who have established clinical indicators of fatal outcome may be candidates for transplantation. Only a small proportion of alcoholic patients with liver disease would be expected to meet these rigorous criteria.

Although *fulminant hepatic failure* with massive hepatocellular necrosis induced by hepatitis viruses, hepatotoxins, or certain drugs may warrant liver transplantation, rapid progression of the disease and multi-organ system failure frequently preclude this option.

2. What is the outcome (current survival rates, complications) in different groups?

The survival and complication rates of patients who have undergone liver transplantation are the major criteria for judging efficacy. Data are available from four locations (Pittsburgh; Cambridge, England; Hanover, Germany; and Groningen, The Netherlands). The interpretation of the existing data on survival is extremely difficult because no control data are given for comparison, surgical techniques and drug therapies varied over time, and patient selection criteria and management differed across centers. While sufficient data for thorough assessment of liver transplantation are not available to date, today certain trends appear to emerge:

– Patients currently being accepted for transplantation have a high probability of imminent death and a low quality of life in the absence of transplantation.
– Patients undergoing transplantation have an operative mortality (within 1 month) of 20 to 40%.
– One-year survival among transplant recipients since 1980 is favorable when compared with their expected course in the absence of transplantation.
– Since 1980, 1-year survival appears improved over the earlier transplant experience.
– Individual patients have survived for many years with good quality of life after transplantation.
– Data are insufficient to evaluate survival rates beyond 1 year following transplantation with current technologies.
– Short-term quality of life is probably enhanced in many transplant survivors. We lack systematically gathered information on quality of life among long-term survivors.

Severe non-lethal complications of transplantation frequently occur and must be taken into account in judging efficacy of this procedure. Massive hemorrhage is the most serious intraoperative and early postoperative problem. Other postoperative complications include renal dysfunction, rejection, biliary tract complications, graft vascular obstruction, and infection. With accumulating expertise in medical and surgical management and with new developments in technology (e.g. intraoperative veno-venous bypass and cyclosporine), these complications can be expected to diminish.

3. In a potential candidate for transplantation, what are the principles guiding selection of the appropriate time for surgery?

Selecting an appropriate stage for a given illness for liver transplantation is a complex issue: transplantation just prior to death may significantly diminish the life-saving potential of the procedure since hepatic decompensation in its latest stages poses a formidable surgical risk. Transplantation early in the course of hepatic decompensation may deprive a patient of an additional period of useful life.

An ideally timed liver transplantation procedure would be in a late enough phase of disease to offer the patient all opportunity for spontaneous stabilization or recovery, but in an early enough phase to give the surgical procedure a fair chance of success. For most patients, these phases are difficult to define prospectively.

While no single best time for surgery can be specified, transplantation should be reserved for patients in any of the following phases of disease:
– When death is imminent.
– When irreversible damage to the central nervous system is inevitable.
– When quality of life has deteriorated to unacceptable levels.

The exact choice of the time for liver transplantation in an individual requires the judgment of a qualified medical team and a well-informed patient. The following are offered as guidelines for individual liver diseases.
– *Extrahepatic biliary atresia.* Biliary enteric anastomosis (hepatoportoenterostomy of Kasai) performed in the first 2 months of life provides significant improvement for at least 5 years in one-third of the patients, although cirrhosis and disappearance of the intrahepatic bile ducts occur with increasing age. While success of this procedure cannot be predicted for the individual patient, it should be used as initial therapy for extrahepatic biliary atresia. In the absence of severe hepatic decompensation in these children, liver transplantation should be delayed as long as possible to permit the child to achieve maximum growth. In children with successful hepatoportoenterostomy, liver transplantation should be deferred until progressive cholestasis, hepatocellular decompensation, or severe portal hypertension supervene. Multiple attempts at hepatoportoenterostomy or surgical porto-systemic shunting render even-

tual transplant surgery technically more difficult and operationally more dangerous and therefore should be avoided in favor of liver transplantation.

– *Chronic active hepatitis.* The potential for spontaneous remission and the complex course of chronic active hepatitis make valid predictions of the subsequent course difficult except in the latest stages of the disease. Using strict criteria, patients can be identified who have almost no chance of survival beyond 6 months. Such patients may be suitable candidates for transplantation.

– *Primary biliary cirrhosis.* The indolent course of primary biliary cirrhosis and the potential for spontaneous improvement even in patients with advanced disease make transplantation potentially suitable only in the final stages of liver failure or when the quality of life has deteriorated to an unacceptable level.

– *Alpha-1-antitrypsin deficiency.* Of the some 20 phenotypes in this genetic disorder, only Pi ZZ is associated with significant hepatic disease in children. Of infants with this phenotype, neonatal cholestasis occurs in 5.5%. Jaundice usually is transient, clearing before 6 months of age although biochemical evidence of activity may persist. Liver transplantation is indicated in children with Pi ZZ phenotype only when cirrhosis has developed and when evidence of hepatic failure is present.

Adults with alpha-1-antitrypsin deficiency may have liver disease associated with phenotype Pi ZZ, MZ, or SZ. If hepatic failure occurs, liver transplantation may be indicated.

– *Wilson's disease.* Patients with Wilson's disease usually are responsive to chelation therapy with penicillamine. However, some patients present with fulminant hepatic failure and/or progressive disease unresponsive to adequate chelation therapy. Liver transplantation may be indicated in these instances.

– *Crigler-Najjar syndrome.* Of the two types of this genetic disorder associated with severe unconjugated hyperbilirubinemia, patients with Type I invariably develop bilirubin encephalopathy usually before 15 months of age. Because of the inevitability of central nervous system damage and the limitations of phototherapy, liver transplantation is indicated in such patients at an early age.

– *Miscellaneous metabolic diseases.* A number of rare genetic diseases may involve the liver and cause cirrhosis and eventual hepatic failure.

Patients with tyrosinemia, Byler's disease, Wolman's disease, and glycogen storage diseases Types O and IV may be candidates for hepatic transplantation.

Liver transplantation may also be indicated for patients with certain genetic diseases associated with severe neurological complications, such as hereditary deficiency of urea cycle enzymes and disorders of lactate/pyruvate or amino acid metabolism.

– *Hepatic vein thrombosis.* The course of hepatic vein thrombosis is variable, and therefore transplantation should be reserved for patients with severe hepatic decompensation. The possibility of later transplant surgery should not dis-

courage the use of portal venous decompression when otherwise indicated.
- *Primary sclerosing cholangitis.* No clinical, biochemical, serologic, or histologic factors have proved to be of value in predicting outcome. When appropriate attempts at biliary tract diversion and dilatation have failed, and death from
liver failure is imminent, liver transplantation should be considered.
- *Alcoholic liver disease.* At least 50% of the cases of cirrhosis in the United
States are attributable to the abuse of alcohol, and alcohol abuse is the leading
cause of hepatic morbidity and mortality.

Alcoholic liver disease is most favorably affected by abstinence. The natural
history of untreated alcoholic hepatitis and/or cirrhosis is extremely variable,
and there are few precise prognostic indicators in any but the terminal phase of
the disease. Liver transplantation may be considered for the patients who
develop evidence of progressive liver failure despite medical treatment and
abstinence from alcohol.

4. What are the skills, resources, and institutional support needed for liver transplantation?

The requirements for conducting a liver transplantation program by a sponsoring
institution are formidable. Accordingly, any institution embarking on this program must make a major commitment to its support. In addition to the full array
of services required of a tertiary care facility and a program in graduate medical
education, an active organ transplantation program should exist. Few hospitals
are likely to meet these prerequisites.

Liver transplant recipients are seriously ill before surgery. The transplant effort
is prodigious, and the postoperative intensive care interval, averaging 2 weeks, is
punctuated by complications and frequent need for reoperation

In this context, experts in hepatology, pediatrics, infectious disease, nephrol-
ogy with dialysis capability, pulmonary medicine with respiratory therapy support, pathology, immunology, and anesthesiology are needed to complement a
qualified transplantation team. Extensive blood bank support to provide the
needed copious quantities of blood components is mandatory. Similarly, sophisticated microbiology, clinical chemistry, and radiology assistance are required.
Emotional support for patient and family warrants psychiatric participation.
Availability of effective social services to assist patients and families is indispens-
able.

The transplantation surgeon must be trained specifically for liver grafting and
must assemble and train a team to function whenever a donor organ is available.
Institutional commitment to the program mandates that operating room, recovery room, laboratory, and blood bank support exist at all times. Allocation of
intensive care and general surgical beds is important. Recruitment of a cohort of
specialized nurses and technicians to staff these areas is necessary. Access to

tissue typing capability; ongoing research programs in liver disease, organ preservation, and transplantation immunology; and available hemoperfusion and microsurgical techniques are desirable attributes of a transplantation effort.

Participation in a donor procurement program and network is essential, and an interdisciplinary deliberative body should exist to determine on an equitable basis the suitability of candidates for transplantation.

Institutions conducting liver transplantation are obligated to prospectively collect and share data in a coordinated, systematic, and comprehensive manner in all patients selected as transplantation candidates, so that the role of liver transplantation in the management of patients with liver disease can be assessed properly. Additional information permitting cost-benefit analysis should be secured.

Finally, the panel feels that adherence to these guidelines detailing the essentials to conduct a transplantation program offers the best assurance of high quality in performing this very difficult operation.

5. What are the directions for future research?

The Consensus Panel identified several broad areas related to liver transplantation in which critically important information is either unavailable or so incomplete as to defy meaningful interpretation. It is recommended that a registry or clearinghouse be established for collection and evaluation of all available data on liver transplantation. Such a center would develop unified criteria for selection of patients for transplantation and for reporting and evaluating all data related to the outcome of the operation and the patients' postoperative and long-term condition. As methods of immunosuppression improve and the logistic obstacles are resolved, the feasibility and desirability of randomized clinical trials of liver transplantation should be explored for suitable subgroups of patients with specific liver diseases.

High priority also should be given to research projects related to several aspects of the transplant procedure itself. Means should be developed to improve preservation of human liver *ex vivo* and criteria should be established to evaluate its viability. Improved control of organ rejection requires urgent attention; this includes thorough evaluation of the benefits and risks of cyclosporine as an immunosuppressive agent in liver transplantation. The design of the hemodynamic support system during transplantation needs evaluation and potential improvement. Research should be encouraged for developing better supportive measures for patients in liver failure, including maintenance of proper renal and cerebral function.

In the broad areas of the cause, pathogenesis, and natural course of chronic liver disease, present knowledge is fragmentary and incomplete, and research in these areas should be fostered and supported by all available means. Particular attempts should be made to determine the possible role of liver transplantation in the management of hepatocellular carcinoma at a stage when metastatic spread appears remote. Similarly, approaches should be sought to limit infection of the transplanted liver by hepatotropic viruses. Finally, liver transplantation should be explored as a modality of replacement therapy in genetically determined multi-organ enzyme deficiencies.

Conclusion

After extensive review and consideration of all available data, this panel concludes that liver transplantation is a therapeutic modality for end-stage liver disease that deserves broader application. However, in order for liver transplantation to gain its full therapeutic potential, the indications for and results of the procedure must be the object of comprehensive, coordinated, and ongoing evaluation in the years ahead. This can best be achieved by expansion of this technology to a limited number of centers where performance of liver transplantation can be carried out under optimal conditions.

Acknowledgments

The conference was sponsored by: National Institute of Arthritis, Diabetes, and Digestive and Kidney Diseases, Lester B. Salans, Director; Office of Medical Applications of Research, J. Richard Crout, Director.

Index